T0248849

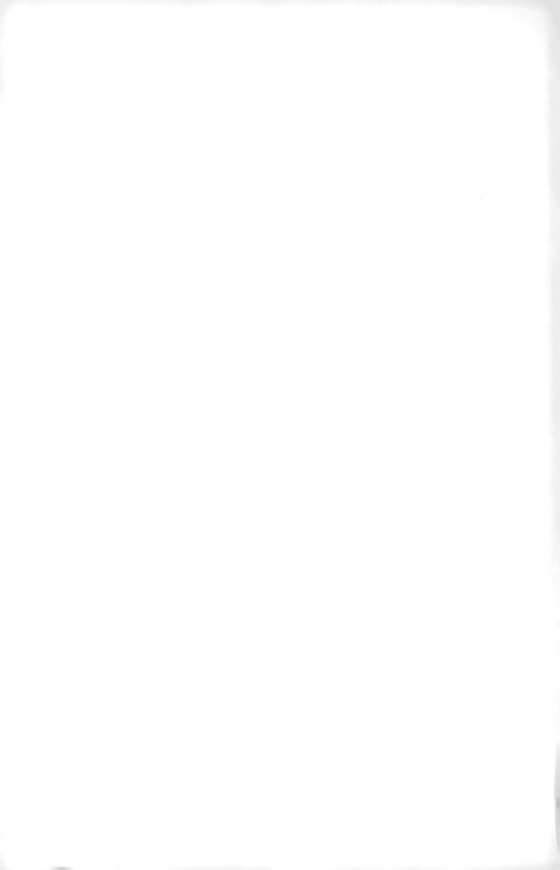

Tissue Regeneration: Biological Theory, Modeling and Applications

Volume II

Edited by **Shay Fisher**

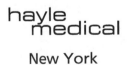

hayle
medical

New York

Published by Hayle Medical,
30 West, 37th Street, Suite 612,
New York, NY 10018, USA
www.haylemedical.com

Tissue Regeneration: Biological Theory, Modeling and Applications
Volume II
Edited by Shay Fisher

International Standard Book Number: 978-1-63241-373-4 (Hardback)

Contents

Preface

In a majority of incidents involving damage or injuries, the healing process involves formation of a scar, which is like a patch, reinstating structural integrity of the damaged tissue without reviving physiological functions. A far better option for a patient affected by tissue damage would be to replace the damaged tissue with something functionally similar. Increasing amount of study and research is being undertaken across the world in search for such a technology. This book provides a timely overview on crucial topics in tissue regeneration, in a well-researched manner, written by experts from around the globe. It facilitates better understanding of the application of stem cells, uses of scaffolds and modelling and evaluation of regeneration. This book will be a great source of reference for study and work undertaken by students, experts and medical professionals.

Various studies have approached the subject by analyzing it with a single perspective, but the present book provides diverse methodologies and techniques to address this field. This book contains theories and applications needed for understanding the subject from different perspectives. The aim is to keep the readers informed about the progress in the field; therefore, the contributions were carefully examined to compile novel researches by specialists from across the globe.

Indeed, the job of the editor is the most crucial and challenging in compiling all chapters into a single book. In the end, I would extend my sincere thanks to the chapter authors for their profound work. I am also thankful for the support provided by my family and colleagues during the compilation of this book.

Editor

Part 1

Application of Stem Cells

Towards Clinical Application of Mesenchymal Stromal Cells: Perspectives and Requirements for Orthopaedic Applications

Marianna Karagianni*, Torsten J. Schulze* and Karen Bieback
*Institute of Transfusion Medicine and Immunology;
Medical Faculty Mannheim, Heidelberg University;
German Red Cross Blood Donor Service Baden-Württemberg – Hessen
Germany*

1. Introduction

Mesenchymal stromal cells (MSC) possess a wide spectrum of interacting properties that contribute to their broad therapeutic potential: In pre- and clinical settings MSC have been demonstrated to reduce tissue damage, to activate the endogenous regenerative potential of tissues and to participate in tissue regeneration (Noort, Feye et al. 2010). Initially, MSC have been described to differentiate into derivates of the mesoderm: bone, adipose and cartilage tissue and were therefore applied to restore damaged tissue (Frohlich, Grayson et al. 2008). Subsequent analyses, however, indicated that the repair process does not only lay in the differentiation potential and plasticity of MSC. As demonstrated in later studies even if only few cells were detectable after MSC transplantation, the therapeutic effect was obvious (Fuchs, Baffour et al. 2001; Shake, Gruber et al. 2002). This could be attributed to paracrine properties with consecutive modification of the tissue microenvironment to decrease inflammatory and immune reactions. MSC are therefore beyond doubt promising candidates for cell therapy in various settings (Horwitz, Prockop et al. 2001; Le Blanc, Rasmusson et al. 2004; Prockop 2009; Pontikoglou, Deschaseaux et al. 2011).

The broad therapeutic efficacy of MSC renders them attractive candidates for cell therapy. However, translating basic research into clinical application is a complex multistep process (Bieback, Karagianni et al. 2011). It necessitates product regulation by the regulatory authorities and accurate management of the expected therapeutic benefits with the potential risks in order to balance the speed of clinical trials with a time-consuming, cautious risk assessment (Sensebe, Bourin et al. 2011). Despite their use in clinical studies, some questions remain open: What are the deviations among the MSC from different tissue sources? How shall MSC be adequately procured, isolated and cultivated? How should their therapeutic propensity, e.g. their homing properties, the secretion of bioactive factors, the differentiation pattern *in vivo* and their plasticity, be defined?

---

* Both authors contributed equally

It is obvious that MSC need to be further characterised in clinical studies with standardized protocols (Bieback, Karagianni et al. 2011; Sensebe, Bourin et al. 2011). Furthermore, despite immense work, still MSC cannot be identified as a distinct cell population by a set of marker proteins as CD34 defines hematopoietic stem cells. The field currently uses "minimal criteria" for MSC to describe them according to their *in vitro* behaviour (osteo-, adipo- and chondrogenic differentiation) and morphology (fibroblastoid, expressing a set of markers) (Dominici, Le Blanc et al. 2006). Nevertheless it has to be taken into account that *in vitro* data do not necessarily predict *in vivo* behaviour: MSC seem to alter their *in vitro* traits after *in vivo* transplantation and this might affect a future therapeutic outcome severely. For example MSC can express HLA-class II antigens and can therefore possibly trigger an immunreaction in the host after transplantation (Vassalli and Moccetti 2011) or may calcify spontaneously in uremic conditions and cause vessel occlusion in case of intravenous application (Kramann, Couson et al. 2011).

Using the example of bone defect regeneration, we will emphasize key parameters relevant for the translation of experimental data to clinical application. The focus on bone defect regeneration exemplifies the possibilities and challenges for MSC in combination with biomaterials in the light of regulatory frameworks in Europe, where MSC may be classified as "Advanced Therapy Medicinal Product - ATMP", or the US, where MSC fall under the term "Human Cells, Tissues, and Cellular and Tissue-Based Products -HCT/Ps". In this context, questions that need to be answered concern an adequate MSC tissue source with superior osteogenic potential compared to other tissues, the degree of cell differentiation prior to implantation and the adequate scaffold for tissue engineering (Seong, Kim et al. 2010).

1.1 MSC definition

Mesenchymal stromal cells (MSC) were initially isolated from bone marrow (BM) as described by Friedenstein and co-workers in 1968 (Friedenstein, Petrakova et al. 1968). They were identified as non hematopoietic, fibroblast-like cells adherent to plastic, with a colony-forming capacity (Friedenstein, Deriglasova et al. 1974), also as feeder cells for hematopoietic precursors (Eaves, Cashman et al. 1991; Wagner, Saffrich et al. 2008). Subsequent characterisation revealed their mesodermal differentiation and immune modulatory capacity, raising the interest in these cells (Le Blanc, Rasmusson et al. 2004; Bieback, Hecker et al. 2009; Mosna, Sensebe et al. 2010). Consequently, numerous terms for these cells were established: mesenchymal stem cells, mesenchymal stromal cells, adult stromal cells, multipotent and non hematopoietic adult precursor cells (Horwitz, Le Blanc et al. 2005; Dominici, Le Blanc et al. 2006). These conflicting nomenclature suggestions in the literature lead to a complex information exchange upon MSC (Prockop 2009). In an attempt to clarify and define the nomenclature, the ISCT (International Society for Cell Therapy) set "minimal criteria" for MSC, such as:

- adherence to plastic when maintained in standard culture conditions,
- expression of CD105, CD73 and CD90, and lack of expression of CD45, CD34, CD14 or CD11b, CD79 alpha or CD19 and HLA-DR surface molecules,
- as well as differentiation ability into osteoblasts, adipocytes and chondroblasts *in vitro* (Dominici, Le Blanc et al. 2006).

In the last decade there has been rapid movement from bench to bedside. Based on their stromal origin, MSC were initially applied in co-transplantation studies with hematopoietic precursor cells (Koc, Day et al. 2002). Later, due to their mesodermal differentiation potential, Horwitz et al. were able to perform seminal studies applying MSC to children with osteogenesis imperfecta (Horwitz, Prockop et al. 2001). MSC were then applied as immunosuppressants in patients with graft versus host disease (Le Blanc, Rasmusson et al. 2004). Further studies introduced them as promising candidates for tissue regeneration in bone and cartilage repair (Frohlich, Grayson et al. 2008), epithelial regeneration (Long, Zuk et al. 2010), cardiovascular regeneration (Noort, Feye et al. 2010; Rangappa, Makkar et al. 2010), immunomodulation in graft versus host disease (GvHD) (Ringden, Uzunel et al. 2006), and inflammatory neurological diseases (Momin, Mohyeldin et al. 2010). MSC are expected to reduce tissue damage, to activate the endogenous regenerative potential of tissues and to participate in the regeneration (Noort, Feye et al. 2010). However, in all these studies it became apparent that MSC function mainly through paracrine effects rather than differentiating into cells or tissues (Caplan and Correa 2011).

1.2 MSC from different tissue sources

Bone marrow (BM) was the first source of MSC identified by Friedenstein and co-workers (Friedenstein, Gorskaja et al. 1976). BM-MSC are already being tested worldwide in clinical studies with currently over 1500 found in the Clinical Trials registry of the NIH (www.clinicaltrials.gov). Due to the long lasting research on BM-MSC they became the gold standard for any MSC research and therapeutic application. Nevertheless, a limitation for BM MSC clinical application is the low cell frequency in source tissue. Thus large volume bone marrow aspiration is necessary even in autologous settings, feasible only in general anaesthesia which is associated with an additional patient morbidity. In consequence, investigators have developed protocols for isolating MSC from a variety of different tissues and sources other than bone marrow. Latest studies led to the conclusion that MSC are not limited to a certain tissue source: the MSC niche is rather localized in the perivascular area of virtually all tissues (Crisan, Yap et al. 2008; da Silva Meirelles, Caplan et al. 2008). Thus numerous tissues containing MSC have been identified, for example adipose tissue (AT), cord blood (CB), fetal membranes and amniotic fluid, pancreatic islet, lung parenchyma, intestinal lamina propria, oral and nasal mucosa, eye limbus, dental tissues and synovial fluid (Jakob, Hemeda et al. ; Karaoz, Ayhan et al. ; Marynka-Kalmani, Treves et al. ; Pinchuk, Mifflin et al. ; Powell, Pinchuk et al. ; Zuk, Zhu et al. 2002; Kern, Eichler et al. 2006; Phinney and Prockop 2007; Jones, Crawford et al. 2008; Polisetty, Fatima et al. 2008; Huang, Gronthos et al. 2009; Ilancheran, Moodley et al. 2009; Karoubi, Cortes-Dericks et al. 2009).

Among all tissue sources, AT shows several important clinical advantages compared to BM: AT procurement can be achieved via tumescent-lipoaspiration in local anaesthesia, a lower risk operating procedure. Adipose tissue is abundant even in older individuals. AT-MSC are shown to have similar functional properties to BM-MSC while their frequency is definitely higher than in BM (Zuk, Zhu et al. 2002; Kern, Eichler et al. 2006). AT-MSC are currently being applied in clinical trials, at least 33 trials can be found in the NIH registry. The high frequency of MSC in AT renders it possible to isolate the mononuclear cell fraction directly at the patients bedside without the need for expansion in a GMP facility (Duckers, Pinkernell et al. 2006). There are divergent outcomes in those studies directly comparing freshly isolated with expanded cells (Garcia-Olmo, Herreros et al. 2009). Despite the advantages of processing at the patient's bedside, direct application of the freshly isolated mononuclear cells in one session procedure gives no opportunity to control the clinical outcome, for an amount of diverse undefined cell populations are effective in these settings. However, this is still being exercised as autologous treatment.

Studies are being performed in order to compare BM-MSC, AT-MSC and MSC of other tissue sources. They show that MSC are not one distinct cell population. Among their tissue sources MSC differ concerning their isolating rate, their expansion potential, their differentiating capacities (Kern, Eichler et al. 2006), their immunosuppressive and migratory properties (Najar, Raicevic et al. ; Constantin, Marconi et al. 2009). These differences have probably an impact on their quality and therapeutic ability, which only can be definitely clarified in "*in vivo*" studies. Summarizing, there is a complex algorithm, which should be followed in order to find the adequate tissue source for MSC cell therapy. Very important are:

- the patient's risk associated with the tissue procurement,
- the MSC frequency in the origin tissue stroma,
- the potential of MSC to be enrolled in its therapeutic function *in vivo*.

All this can rather be answered gradually applying standardized protocols. After procurement and expansion MSC have to be analysed regarding their functional properties through well defined *in vitro* potency assays. Finally functional properties have to be compared *in vivo* through animal studies and phase I clinical trials.

2. MSC protocols for clinical applications

Translating MSC into cell therapy settings requires a manufacturing process and manufacturing authorisation congruent to the local regulatory framework. Regulatory standards in the EU and USA comply with the good manufacturing practice (GMP) regulations and are set in order to control the therapeutics' safety process, e.g. tissue procurement, cell isolation, selection and expansion and have to be validated according to the quality criteria as defined by the manufacturer. Furthermore it is essential to control the quality, purity and potency of the cell product prior to their administration by well defined and validated quality control and potency assays to ensure safety.

2.1 Isolation and expansion of MSC for clinical applications

For clinical applications, MSC shall be isolated under aseptic conditions in GMP facilities. MSC are a subpopulation among the mononuclear cell fraction. They can be isolated after density gradient centrifugation or if MSC are embedded in extracellular matrix after enzymatic digestion. In general, the low frequency of human MSC within their origin tissues necessitates their expansion prior to clinical use. This raises the risk for contaminations (Bieback, Karagianni et al. 2011; Sensebe, Bourin et al. 2011). Furthermore, in long term cell culture the proliferation rate decays, the cell size increases, differentiation potential becomes affected and chromosomal instabilities and neoplastic transformation may arise (Prockop, Brenner et al.; Lepperdinger, Brunauer et al. 2008; Wagner, Horn et al. 2008) raising the risk for adverse reactions.

Similarly, the cultivation media potentially affect MSC, exposing them to pathogens and immunogens (Heiskanen, Satomaa et al. 2007; Sundin, Ringden et al. 2007; Bieback, Hecker et al. 2009). In order to achieve controlled conditions and a safe cell product for clinical use it is necessary to define quality criteria to monitor the cell product (Bieback, Schallmoser et al. 2008; Bieback, Karagianni et al. 2011; Sensebe, Bourin et al. 2011). For expansion aiming at clinical application it is obligatory to use GMP-grade supplements and sera if available. However, these reagents are just under development. Accordingly we, amongst others, tested human blood-derived components, like human serum or platelet derivatives to replace fetal bovine serum commonly used to expand MSC (Kocaoemer, Kern et al. 2007; Mannello and Tonti 2007; Bieback, Schallmoser et al. 2008; Bieback, Hecker et al. 2009). Human blood components offer the advantage that they are both well controlled and already in clinical use for decades. Still, human serum as well as platelet lysate is a very crude protein cocktail. Essential growth factors for optimal MSC culture have not yet been defined. Platelet derived growth factor (PDGF), epidermal growth factor (EGF), transforming growth factor (TGF-ß), and insulin growth factor (IGF) have been subjected to investigation. Basic fibroblast growth factor (bFGF) has demonstrated most promising effects in expanding MSC whilst maintaining stem cell properties and reducing replicative senescence (Tsutsumi, Shimazu et al. 2001). Recently, Pytlik et al described a human serum and growth factor supplemented clinical-grade medium, which allowed high cell expansion mediated by loss of contact inhibition (Pytlik, Stehlik et al. 2009). Anyhow, the ideal solution is a chemically defined clinical-grade medium permitting both adhesion and expansion of MSC and numerous attempts are ongoing to develop this (Mannello and Tonti 2007).

2.2 Quality control

In order to obtain a manufacturing authorization for cell therapeutics the quality criteria ought to meet the regulatory standards. Quality controls are instrumented within the manufacturing process to prove according to the set quality criteria. Essential quality criteria are the traceability of the cell product through donor identification and product labelling, the prevention of introduction and spreading of infection and communicable diseases through donor screening and aseptic cell processing and proof of the therapeutic safety, lot consistency, potency and purity of the cell product (European Parliament 2007; FDA 2010).

2.2.1 Therapeutic safety, purity and potency

Safety is a key issue in cell therapy. In addition to the above mentioned aspects regarding reagents (fetal bovine serum has been elaborated on) and sterility testing (bacterial, fungal, viral, mycoplasma), cellular aspects have to be considered as well. In long term cell culture current testing methods of chromosomal aberrations and neoplastic transformation are fluoerescence in situ hybridization (FISH), karyotype analysis or detection of proto-oncogenes or activators of tumorigenesis like myc-assosiated proteins (Agrawal, Yu et al. 2010). Further lately developed testing methods are BAC-based (Bacterial Artificial Chromosome) Array to detect DNA copy number or oligonucleotide-based Array CGH (Chromosomal Comparative Genomic Hybridization) to detect small genomic regions with amplification or deletion (Wicker, Carles et al. 2007). Additionally, detection of telomerase activation is often performed, as telomerase plays a role in malignant transformation *in vitro* (Yamaoka, Hiyama et al. 2011). All these assays indicate that there is a low risk of transformation of MSC in *in vitro* expansion. However, more safety studies – especially long term follow up *in vivo* - are required to exclude risks and to enable to value risks against therapeutic value.

Further aspects that are critical for the therapeutic safety and need to be analysed are the spontaneous or the induced *in vivo* differentiation potential of MSC. It has to be proven that MSC after *in vivo* application serve their therapeutic function and do not develop into unwanted cell types for example BM-MSC into adipocytes or osteocytes when intended for epithelial or myogenic regeneration. The latter could possibly lead to threatening thrombembolic incidents after intravascular application. In general, intravascular injection is associated with a higher risk than direct application into the site of injury or into the neighbouring parenchyma (Furlani, Ugurlucan et al. 2009).

MSC are not a distinct cell fraction in fresh tissue isolates. Accordingly purity is a key issue to be taken into account. To isolate MSC, mononuclear cells of fresh tissue isolates are seeded on plastic culture dishes, MSC adhere, proliferate and form colonies. Those expanded MSC should have a distinct immune phenotype, defined by the ISCT, they do not express haematopoietic markers and have a characteristic fibroblastoid morphology (Dominici, Le Blanc et al. 2006). Based on these criteria, contaminations of MSC with hematopoietic or endothelial cells can be assessed and consequently purity of the MSC cell product can be proven via flow cytometry. This is further amended by description of expanded MSC morphology and colony assays (CFU-F-assay) to quantify the precursor frequency. Quality controls of MSC expanded in scaffolds or in bioreactors vs. 2D cell culture regarding population purity is probably more complex.

MSC are applied in various clinical settings, as they possess a variety of functional properties. MSC can work as progenitor cells in tissue modelling, due to their adipo-, osteo-, chondrogenic potential, or as immunomodulatory agents in GvHD, autoimmune disease or as anti-inflammatory agents through their paracrine abilities. Due to this extremely broad range it is difficult to establish potency assays. These standardized *in vitro* functional assays have to be performed to predict the consistency of the manufacturing process and the functionality of the cell product. Quality control assays, including potency assays, have to be well established and validated to be capable of addressing the consistent quality of the cellular product. It is certainly difficult to reproduce the *in vivo* setting within *in vitro* conditions,. This is probably why *in vitro* potency assays often fail to predict the *in vivo* outcome (Sensebe, Bourin et al. 2011). Anyhow, it is a demand for the manufacturing facility to implement potency assays capable of predicting therapeutic capacity. These assays have to be quantitative and directly related to the mechanism of action. Where possible surrogate assays can replace time-consuming functional assays (e.g. cell surface marker expression, growth factor release, gene or protein expression analysis). Finally, the manufacturing process in order to conduct clinical trials in Europe and the US has to be validated and approved by the authorities in accordance to the pharmaceutical regulations.

2.3 Pharmaceutical guidelines

2.3.1 Advanced therapy medicinal products as described in the Regulation (EC) No 1394/2007 of the European Parliament

In cases where MSC are to be used in a medicinal product the donation, procurement and testing of the cells are covered in Europe by the Tissues and Cells Directive (2004/23/EC). To make innovative treatments available to patients, and to ensure that these novel treatments are safe, the EU institutions agreed on a "regulation on advanced therapies"

(EC1394/2007). Furthermore, a number of products also combine biological materials, cells and tissues with scaffolds. This regulation defines those products as "advanced therapy medicinal products (ATMP)" that are:

- "a gene therapy medicinal product" (Part IV of Annex I to Directive 2001/83/EC),
- "a somatic cell therapy medicinal product" (Part IV of Annex I to Directive 2001/83/EC) and
- "a tissue engineered product".

Cells or tissues shall be considered 'engineered' if they fulfil at least one of the following conditions:

- "the cells or tissues have been subject to substantial manipulation, in order to unfold their biological characteristics, physiological functions or structural properties" or
- "the cells or tissues are not intended to be used for the same essential function or functions in the recipient as in the donor" (Official Journal of the European Union 10.12.2007).

The scope of this regulation is to set standards for advanced therapy medicinal products which are intended to be placed on the market in European member states. It indicates the setting of manufacturing guidelines specific for ATMP as to properly reflect the particular nature of their manufacturing process. The directive 2004/23/EC amends to this regulation setting standards of quality and safety in tissue procurement and donor testing. Regarding clinical trials on ATMP, they should be conducted in accordance with the Directive 2001/20/EC. Additionally Directive 2005/28/EC laid down principles and detailed guidelines for good clinical practice as well as the requirements for authorisation of the manufacturing and importation of ATMP. Considering tissue engineered cell products, medicinal devices incorporated in the ATMP (combined medicinal products) are regulated by the directive 93/42/and the directive 90/385/ EEC.

2.3.2 Human cells, tissues, and cellular and tissue-based products (HCT/P's) as described by the US Food and Drug Administration (FDA)

The quality system for Food and Drug Administration (FDA) regulated products is known as current good manufacturing practices (cGMP). For globally operating pharmaceutical facilities it is mandatory to fulfil the requirements of both FDA and EU. The Code of Federal Regulation (CFR) Title 21, part 1271 has the purpose to create a unified registration and listing system for human cells, tissues, and cellular and tissue-based products (HCT/P's) and to establish donor-eligibility, current good tissue practice, and other procedures to "prevent the introduction, transmission, and spread of communicable diseases by HCT/P's" (www.FDA.gov).

Whereas cell products, only minimally manipulated or subjected to homologous use without systemic effect, are regulated solely by the Public Health Service (PHS) Act Section 361 and do not require to undergo premarket review (GEN Mar. 15, vol 25, no 6), they still must comply with Good Tissue practice (GTP) (Burger 2003). Clinical trials of higher-risk involving "more-than-minimally manipulated" HCT/P's require the Investigational New Drug (IND) mechanism.

3. Example for MSC in regenerative medicine: Attempts for orthopaedic applications in bone defect healing

Orthopaedic surgery provides a fascinating field for the application of MSC (Horwitz, Prockop et al. 2001; Le Blanc, Gotherstrom et al. 2005; Bernhardt, Lode et al. 2009; Chanda, Kumar et al. 2010; Diederichs, Bohm et al. 2010; Mosna, Sensebe et al. 2010; Parekkadan and Milwid 2010; Levi and Longaker 2011). Bone defects appear in increasing numbers in orthopaedic clinics due to aseptic loosening of hip endoprosthesis after 10 to 20 years. These defects are then covered primarily with either bone cement or acellular bone from a bone bank prior to insertion of a new endoprosthesis in order to provide primary stability - that is immediate mechanical support of a new implant (Gruner and Heller 2009).

An ideal scaffold must offer osteoinduction – induction of bone growth – and osteoconduction – providing the guiding structure that paves the way for future bone growth - and eventually osteointegration, becoming part of the bone architecture of a body (Frohlich, Grayson et al. 2008; Ferretti, Ripamonti et al. 2010). The advantages and disadvantages of bone cement have been controversially discussed regarding different rates of implant failure in follow up examinations (Kavanagh, Ilstrup et al. 1985; Izquierdo and Northmore-Ball 1994; Stromberg and Herberts 1996). Recent works suggest to proceed without use of bone cement if possible, and recommend other surgical techniques to implant a total hip endoprosthesis. Bone cement is stiff and strong with a gradual increasing resorption area at its limits. Where bone cement is placed, immediate primary stability is provided, however, at the expense of bone regeneration that does not take place anymore (Izquierdo and Northmore-Ball 1994; Gruner and Heller 2009). Depending on the localization of the bone cement and the mechanical stress, this can gradually lead to a decreased stability. In case another revision operation is needed but great bone defects and osteolysis can impede or even inhibit surgical possibilities (Kavanagh, Ilstrup et al. 1985; Izquierdo and Northmore-Ball 1994; Stromberg and Herberts 1996; Gruner and Heller 2009). Fresh autologous bone or allogenous acellular bone from a bone bank can support bone growth. These preparations are osteoconductive and are, if preserved as a cancellous bone even osteoinductive but fail to provide immediate stability alone. These scaffolds have osteoconductive potential, however regular radiological controls often demonstrate gradually increasing resorption at sites of the implanted acellular bone. In the consequence, stability may be compromised (Gruner and Heller 2009).

Given the potential of MSC to differentiate into bone, MSC became attractive candidates. For hard tissue replacement, cells alone are not adequate. Thus surgical procedures treating bone defects in which a combination of MSC and scaffolds are applied, may provide both immediate stability and permanent integration into the recipient's bone. Different techniques are described for the implantation of MSC. Still it remains unclear if implants shall carry completely osteogenically differentiated MSC, or more likely optimize adaptive possibilities within the host organism. The more differentiated the MSC the more initial stability they provide for implants in areas with high mechanical force exposure (Bernhardt, Lode et al. 2008). Less differentiated MSC on the other prove more plasticity (Niemeyer, Krause et al. 2004; Bieback, Kern et al. 2008). In the worst case, undesired differentiation or even dedifferentiation might occur. Medication, integrated drugs or even genetically engineered cells may prove a possible control *in vivo*.

3.1 *In vitro* 3D culture, choice of scaffold

Tissue engineering aims at regenerating or replacing tissues or even organs. Therefore a complex architecture is needed, which cannot be generated by simple two-dimensional (2D) cultures. Investigation on MSC concentrates on characterization *in vitro* in a 2D culture, as mentioned above, to assess both the differentiation potential and the influence of the biomaterial surface on growth and development. MSC can be driven towards osteogenic differentiation by use of dexamethasone, β-glycerophosphate and ascorbate in addition to osteogenic basal medium (Jaiswal, Haynesworth et al. 1997; Pittenger, Mackay et al. 1999; Augello and De Bari 2010). Cells can be used as undifferentiated, pre- or terminally differentiated cells in combinations with scaffolds to achieve tissue-like conditions. Compared to 2D, 3D cultures better mimic physiological conditions. Static 3D cultures are mainly used to investigate the suitability of a certain biomaterial (Bernhardt, Lode et al. 2009). Increasing attention is recently been paid to dynamic 3D culture, assuring a more homogenous cell distribution within a scaffold, a higher number of cells and all in all less manipulation (Diederichs, Roker et al. 2009; Stiehler, Bunger et al. 2009). Flow perfusion cultures itself, even in absence of dexamethasone, may lead to differentiation into bone tissue (Holtorf, Jansen et al. 2005). Nevertheless, cell expansion of MSC in order to achieve a high cell dose prior to use in animal or humans may not always be advantageous, since uncontrolled growth can also lead to benign or malign tumours.

There is a broad choice of biomaterials for scaffolds for clinical applications. However, only bone cement and bone of bone banks are regularly favoured for bone defect surgeries, when available. Bone itself has become the biomaterial per se as a natural scaffold supply. Bone cement on the other hand can be stored as powder, provides immediate stability and is easily prepared and applied during an operation. Within a few minutes, the cement becomes firm (Gruner and Heller 2009). Although acellular scaffolds prove stability immediately following implantation, a better option would be to seed them with cells. For MSC application a great variety of materials, ranging from sterilised original bone to nanostructures and bioglass-collagen composites are being utilised (Karageorgiou and Kaplan 2005; Tanner 2010). Eventually, in order to approach the therapeutic effect of scaffold-MSC composites, studies are currently being performed on several stages: cell culture either in a dish or in a bioreactor, animal models and individual attempts in human (Bernstein, Bornhauser et al. 2009; Diederichs, Roker et al. 2009; Diederichs, Bohm et al. 2010). Further key parameters for the choice of the suitable biomaterial is the ability to support cell growth, cellular ingrowth, osteogenic differentiation and antimicrobial functions (Costantino, Hiltzik et al. 2002; Bernstein, Bornhauser et al. 2009). For that reason, additional osteogenic cytokines such as bone morphogenetic proteins (BMP) or bioactive peptides that become integrated into scaffolds are of interest (Keibl, Fugl et al. 2011).

An optimum scaffold must allow bone cells to grow into it. Pores of 300 to 500µm are requested (De Long, Einhorn et al. 2007; Stiehler, Bunger et al. 2009). Apart from this an optimum scaffold has to be adapted to bone structures. Defects in facial areas, in the skull, femur or hip require different stabilities and shapes. Only hip re-implantation seems to provide some standardised features (Gruner and Heller 2009).

Building suitable biomaterials to be combined with MSC has led to very different approaches: Collagen as a basis of any bone tissue was modified and calcified at all pore sizes. Integration of MSC is easily achieved but primary stability is comparably low (Bernhardt, Lode et al. 2009; Nienhuijs, Walboomers et al. 2011). Hydroxyapatite is a ubiquitous part of the vertebrate bone. Hydroxyapatite ceramics become easily integrated and also prove enough primary stability (John, Varma et al. 2009; Nair, Bernhardt et al. 2009; Nair, Varma et al. 2009). Beta-tricalciumposphate is a completely resorbable scaffold with high purity. It is available at all sizes, all porous degrees, it can be supplied as granules or as plates and therefore serves as comparison to newly developed biomaterials (Wiedmann-Al-Ahmad, Gutwald et al. 2007). Due to its low tissue reactivity and good stability titanium based structures not only serve well as implants but also as scaffolds. Titanium or TiO_2 does not become degraded or resorbed, instead as a whole it becomes very firmly integrated into any tissue (Gotman 1997; Olmedo, Tasat et al. 2009). Due to the fact that titanium is not resorbable it holds the risks of infection, be it acute or slowly increasing, so that an explantation must be performed. Since titanium becomes very well integrated into the host's body, an explantation is often associated with a great tissue loss. Application of titanium has to be carefully considered. In sum, since tissue reactions to titanium are quite well characterised as an implant it serves well as an example of future challenges and possibilities of other biomaterials. Silver nanoparticles are matter of current discussion due to their antimicrobial and toxic effects that can also be used within polymeric nanocomposites. Titanium nanostructures alone have been proven to act antimicrobially (Dallas, Sharma et al. 2011; Ercan, Taylor et al. 2011).

3.2 Analysis of 3D cultures and biomaterials

Once a 3D scaffold has been seeded, the efficiency of the seeding procedure, cell growth and differentiation must be determined, e.g. by quantifying the DNA content and mineralisation by histochemical stains or RT-PCR (Stiehler, Bunger et al. 2009; Peister, Woodruff et al. 2011). Homogeneic seeding and / or cell growth can be determined by fluorescence microscopy or μCT (Zou, Hunter et al. 2011). Mechanical tests are not standardized. For *in vitro* generated bone tissue from MSC crush tests, i.e. the use of a defined force until a scaffold breaks, are the most simple. For *in vivo* generated bone tissue shear and bending tests give additional data concerning the stability of the MSC composite within the animal's original bone. However, *in vitro* and *in vivo* experiments are only conclusive when scaffolds used are comparable in size and porosity (De Long, Einhorn et al. 2007; Stiehler, Bunger et al. 2009). The same applies to standardisation of surgical procedures and animal models used (Reichert, Saifzadeh et al. 2009).

3.3 Tissue source

As already mentioned, tissue engineering requires a scaffold next to the cells to seed it. Since MSC can be isolated from different tissue sources, the question remains: which cells are best suited? MSC derived from different tissues show different osteogenic differentiation properties: human embryonic stem cells (hESC), CB-MSC, AT-MSC, BM-MSC and even amniotic membrane-derived MSC can undergo osteogenic differentiation. Historically, most work had been performed on BM-MSC, so at least BM-MSC are the source to compare with, when MSC behaviour in a scaffold is analysed (Lindenmair, Wolbank et al. 2010; Guven, Mehrkens et al. 2011; Stockmann, Park et al. 2011; Weinand, Nabili et al. 2011). In recent studies, aspects of differentiation in 2D tissue culture and in 3D tissue culture have been examined. Comparisons between BM-MSC and amniotic fluid derived stem cells (AFS) showed different properties in differentiation in 2D and 3D. In 2D tissue culture, AFS produce more mineralized matrix but delayed peaks in osteogenic markers. Differentiation towards bone tissue occurred faster in BM-MSC, however, after weeks mineralization slowed down. AFS differentiated more slowly but mineralized until the end of the observation period 15 weeks, producing 5 fold higher amounts of mineral matrix. Human term placenta derived MSC seem to be less prone to osteogenic differentiation than BM-MSC (Pilz, Ulrich et al. 2011). These characteristics might be of interest, when fast ingrowth is needed (Peister, Woodruff et al. 2011). As initially mentioned, for some groups AT-MSC are the most promising candidates in bone tissue engineering (Levi and Longaker 2011). Osteogenic capacity does not decrease with age in contrast to BM-MSC (Khan, Adesida et al. 2009). Also due to a relatively high and still increasing rate of obesity in the western hemisphere it can be considered that adipose tissue has a great potential as main source for MSC. So, metabolic disease can be of benefit when it comes to autologous MSC implantation (Diederichs, Bohm et al. 2010). All in all an ideal cell source has yet not been identified. Further research is important to compare the advantages of all tissue sources. Moreover, for each biomaterial the MSC differentiation properties have to be determined. The adequate MSC will depend both on availability and differentiating / functional properties.

3.4 Clinical trials

There is no on-going clinical trial that deals with the use of MSC and a suitable biomaterial in healing of bone defects in humans. Osteogenesis imperfecta has been successfully treated with MSC alone, even with allogenic MSC (Horwitz, Prockop et al. 2001; Le Blanc, Gotherstrom et al. 2005). The Iranian Royan Institute, Teheran, announced a clinical trial in 2008 (http://www.clinicaltrials.gov). The study aimed to establish the influence of MSC in non-union fracture healing. However, in 2011 the state of the study is still unknown and cannot be verified. One case report from 2009 refers to a clinical trial in preparation. The benefit of the use of decellularized bone and MSC was demonstrated in a case of large hip transplant loosening. Follow-up radiological exams could confirm the stable position of a new hip implant (Bernstein, Bornhauser et al. 2009). So far, no clinical trial on the use of MSC for bone fracture healing has been published. Various preclinical studies predict benefits in bone tissue healing and stability by use of MSC (Bernhardt, Lode et al. 2008; Bernhardt, Lode et al. 2009; John, Varma et al. 2009; Nair, Bernhardt et al. 2009; Nienhuijs, Walboomers et al. 2011). However the methods and more importantly the animal models to prove beneficial effects of MSC are not yet standardized. This is of great importance since the forces exerted on a fracture cannot be compared between animal species, nor can it be to humans. Comparisons between different procedures, cells and scaffolds are thus not reliable. A recent article proposes rules for comparable preclinical bone defects model that amongst others affect standardized surgical procedures and measurements. In this work tibia fracture and segmental defect models are preferred (Reichert, Saifzadeh et al. 2009).

3.5 Animal model and interpretation

Unfortunately, the criteria to evaluate the outcome of studies - be it *in vitro* or *in vivo* - differ considerably. Regarding the major requirement of mechanical stability, a variety of mechanical tests exist that determine stability. However, till date none of them has been defined as standard (Hak, Makino et al. 2006; Jones, Atwood et al. 2009; Reichert, Saifzadeh et al. 2009). In animal models success criteria of implanted MSC and scaffold are restricted mainly to analysis of regenerated bone e.g. by histologiacal findings, CT-scan technology, x-ray or simply by measuring the weight of the created bone as well as by mechanical torsion tests (Zou, Hunter et al. 2011). The fate of implanted scaffold and MSC, in terms of material resorption and MSC engraftment into the host body, is rarely studied (Bernstein, Bornhauser et al. 2009). Since there is no standard in animal models, experiments are being carried out on various models. The rat model is broadly used because of availability. Bio-mechanical properties similar to humans are found in sheep, especially in hip arthroplasty (Korda, Blunn et al. 2008). Usually a fracture is induced as described by Matsumoto et al or Mifune et al (Matsumoto, Kawamoto et al. 2006; Mifune, Matsumoto et al. 2008). In a first step a tibia is fractured. Then a collagen scaffold is inserted containing saline and either BM-MSC or hESC. Then Undale et al compared the bone tissue healing properties of BM-MSC and hESC in rats after an induced fracture. BM-MSC resulted to be more efficient than hESC to bridge and heal a critical bone fracture. Moreover, in this setting hESC tended to produce benign bony tumours compromising the use of these cells in clinical settings (Undale, Fraser et al. 2011).

Bone fracture healing or integration into the animal's bone tissue can be demonstrated by follow-up conventional radiology in two weeks intervals. The limbs are both fully extended so that the broken and fractured limb can be compared. In recent studies μCT, a specialized CT for small animal structure, is used. Precise 3D models can be built from the data, allowing a comparison between the original and the newly built bone. Eight weeks after fracturing the animals can be euthanized and the limbs can be analysed histologically or biomechanically. Biomechanical stability of the fracture healing can be assessed by torsional load to evaluate normal and abnormal fracture healing (Undale, Fraser et al. 2011).

In summary, MSC from different sources appear as complementation to biomaterial implants. Depending on the tissue source and culture, different patterns of differentiation into bone, cartilage or fibre can be obtained. Depending on the precise situation different sorts of MSC-biocomposites may facilitate wound healing and functional regeneration of bone defects with high long term stability. However, the handling of biomaterial MSC composites is far more complex than conventional methods and oblige to adhere to regulatory standards: Since living cells are worked with, purity, a lack of bacterial contamination and absence of cell transformation has to be proven before clinical application. Conventional methods, that are acellular implants, may be limited because of rigidity and even lack of stability on the long run, but actually, in contrast to MSC biocomposites, they can be well compared regarding their advantages and disadvantages. MSC may differ much more as a matter of treatment, culture conditions and the cells itself need further investigation, experimental and clinical studies to evaluate their true potential at best in comparative studies. But the prospect of individual medicine with the patients' easily extractable and expandable own cells may support future research and applications in regenerative medicine.

3.6 Future prospects

Future orthopaedic research that may one day provide suitable personalized scaffolds to cover bone defects must integrate vascularisation as well. A balanced attempt to support both bone growth and blood supply must be established to create a stable long lasting graft that becomes completely integrated into bone. Osteoinduction is difficult to obtain. Local application of osteoinductive factors such as FGF, the bone morphogenic proteins BMP-2, BMP-4, BMP-7 and vascular endothelial growth factor VEGF does either not lead to results due to degradation or does lead to too strong responses since it cannot be well regulated. Recent work shows promising results in this regard. However no standard can be proposed in terms of choice of growth factor, dose and modification (Keibl, Fugl et al. 2011). Recent work demonstrated the feasibility of plasmid DNA-integration into a scaffold that lead to a higher bone differentiation ratio (Hosseinkhani, Hosseinkhani et al. 2008). Future research must also deal with possibly breaking the border between autologous and allogenic MSC in treatment, in case patients cannot donate autologous MSC of any source. Allogeneic MSC in treatment of patients with osteogenesis imperfecta defects could be recently demonstrated (Le Blanc, Gotherstrom et al. 2005).

The optimal degree of differentiation in culture prior to implantation in an animal model or a human remains unclear: Should implants carry completely osteogenically differentiated MSC, or more likely quite the opposite to provide an optimum of adaptive possibilities within the host organism? The more differentiated the MSC the more initial stability they provide for implants in areas in which great forces act. Less differentiated MSC on the other hand prove more plasticity. In the worst case undesired differentiation or even dedifferentiation might occur. Medication, integrated drugs or even genetically engineered cells may provide a possible control *in vivo*.

The specifications defined by the regulatory framework focussing on the clinical use of MSC are becoming increasingly detailed (Burger 2003). These are more complex when it comes to MSC and biomaterial composites as there are no standards for quality controls. *In vitro* and *in vivo* interactions between scaffolds and in-growing cells, as well as between scaffolds and host tissues, need to be investigated further.

4. Conclusion

In vitro studies indicate that MSC possess a wide spectrum of properties in tissue regeneration as adult progenitor cells or by secreting immunomodulatory and antiinflammatory factors. Still various manufacturing protocols, cultivating media and methods hinder to correlate and interpret scientific findings. Nevertheless MSC are very promising candidates for cell therapy and have moved extremely quickly in the last ten years from the bench to the bedside. For controlled clinical trials there are several obstacles to overcome in order to define a safe and efficacious therapeutic. There is a need to determine factors that may influence the cell quality and consequently the clinical outcome in terms of the tissue source, the isolating, expansion and cultivating conditions. Above that, protocols and *in vitro* and safety animal studies need to be performed in compliance with GMP requirements. To be able to conduct clinical trials on MSC, the manufacturing process has to fulfil several regulatory standards. Advances in clinical application of MSC can be exemplified in the field of orthopaedic bone regeneration. The osteogenic potential of MSC is seen to be of great benefit in bone defect healing. However, only in rare conditions are MSC alone beneficial. The choice of a suitable biomaterial to both carry MSC and provide good primary stability is crucial for clinical applications in hard tissue regeneration. Different sources of MSC that have different differentiation properties can be used. To assess compatibility of both MSC and biomaterial *in vitro*, MSC can be cultured on 2D or in 3D structures. Stability testing of seeded scaffolds helps determine the biomechanical properties of the biocomposite. Different animal models are being used, but no standard has yet been proposed that allows comparison of biomaterials and biomaterial/MSC. No biomaterial/MSC composite is in regular use in human for bone regeneration at present. Future efforts to establish treatments with these biocomposites must therefore concentrate on standardised procedures both in evaluation of tissue culture experiments and, more importantly, in animal models. The choice of the animal and the precise comparable procedures need to be defined. The prospect is individual autologous healing.

5. References

Agrawal, P., K. Yu, et al. (2010). "Proteomic profiling of Myc-associated proteins." Cell Cycle 9(24): 4908-4921.
Augello, A. and C. De Bari (2010). "The regulation of differentiation in mesenchymal stem cells." Hum Gene Ther 21(10): 1226-1238.
Bernhardt, A., A. Lode, et al. (2008). "Mineralised collagen--an artificial, extracellular bone matrix--improves osteogenic differentiation of bone marrow stromal cells." J Mater Sci Mater Med 19(1): 269-275.
Bernhardt, A., A. Lode, et al. (2009). "In vitro osteogenic potential of human bone marrow stromal cells cultivated in porous scaffolds from mineralized collagen." J Biomed Mater Res A 90(3): 852-862.
Bernstein, P., M. Bornhauser, et al. (2009). "[Bone tissue engineering in clinical application : assessment of the current situation]." Orthopade 38(11): 1029-1037.
Bieback, K., A. Hecker, et al. (2009). "Human alternatives to fetal bovine serum for the expansion of mesenchymal stromal cells from bone marrow." Stem Cells 27(9): 2331-2341.
Bieback, K., M. Karagianni, et al. (2011). "Translating research into clinical scale manufacturing of mesenchymal stromal cells." Stem Cells Int 2010: 193519.
Bieback, K., S. Kern, et al. (2008). "Comparing mesenchymal stromal cells from different human tissues: bone marrow, adipose tissue and umbilical cord blood." Biomed Mater Eng 18(1 Suppl): S71-76.
Bieback, K., K. Schallmoser, et al. (2008). "Clinical Protocols for the Isolation and Expansion of Mesenchymal Stromal Cells." Transfus Med Hemother 35(4): 286-294.
Burger, S. R. (2003). "Current regulatory issues in cell and tissue therapy." Cytotherapy 5(4): 289-298.
Caplan, A. I. and D. Correa (2011). "The MSC: An Injury Drugstore." Cell Stem Cell 9(1): 11-15.
Chanda, D., S. Kumar, et al. (2010). "Therapeutic potential of adult bone marrow-derived mesenchymal stem cells in diseases of the skeleton." J Cell Biochem 111(2): 249-257.
Constantin, G., S. Marconi, et al. (2009). "Adipose-derived mesenchymal stem cells ameliorate chronic experimental autoimmune encephalomyelitis." Stem Cells 27(10): 2624-2635.
Costantino, P. D., D. Hiltzik, et al. (2002). "Bone healing and bone substitutes." Facial Plast Surg 18(1): 13-26.

Crisan, M., S. Yap, et al. (2008). "A perivascular origin for mesenchymal stem cells in multiple human organs." Cell Stem Cell 3(3): 301-313.

da Silva Meirelles, L., A. I. Caplan, et al. (2008). "In search of the in vivo identity of mesenchymal stem cells." Stem Cells 26(9): 2287-2299.

Dallas, P., V. K. Sharma, et al. (2011). "Silver polymeric nanocomposites as advanced antimicrobial agents: Classification, synthetic paths, applications, and perspectives." Adv Colloid Interface Sci.

De Long, W. G., Jr., T. A. Einhorn, et al. (2007). "Bone grafts and bone graft substitutes in orthopaedic trauma surgery. A critical analysis." J Bone Joint Surg Am 89(3): 649-658.

Diederichs, S., S. Bohm, et al. (2010). "Application of different strain regimes in two-dimensional and three-dimensional adipose tissue-derived stem cell cultures induces osteogenesis: implications for bone tissue engineering." J Biomed Mater Res A 94(3): 927-936.

Diederichs, S., S. Roker, et al. (2009). "Dynamic cultivation of human mesenchymal stem cells in a rotating bed bioreactor system based on the Z RP platform." Biotechnol Prog 25(6): 1762-1771.

Dominici, M., K. Le Blanc, et al. (2006). "Minimal criteria for defining multipotent mesenchymal stromal cells. The International Society for Cellular Therapy position statement." Cytotherapy 8(4): 315-317.

Duckers, H. J., K. Pinkernell, et al. (2006). "The Bedside Celution system for isolation of adipose derived regenerative cells." EuroIntervention 2(3): 395-398.

Eaves, C. J., J. D. Cashman, et al. (1991). "Molecular analysis of primitive hematopoietic cell proliferation control mechanisms." Ann N Y Acad Sci 628: 298-306.

Ercan, B., E. Taylor, et al. (2011). "Diameter of titanium nanotubes influences anti-bacterial efficacy." Nanotechnology 22(29): 295102.

European Parliament, E. C. (2007). "REGULATION (EC) No 1394/2007 OF THE EUROPEAN PARLIAMENT AND OF THE COUNCIL." Available from: http://ec.europa.eu/health/files/eudralex/vol-1/reg_2007_1394/reg_2007_1394_en.pdf.

FDA (2010). "FDA : Code of Federal Regulations Title 21." Available from: http://www.accessdata.fda.gov/scripts/cdrh/cfdocs/cfcfr/CFRSearch.cfm?CFRPart=1271&showFR=1

Ferretti, C., U. Ripamonti, et al. (2010). "Osteoinduction: translating preclinical promise into clinical reality." Br J Oral Maxillofac Surg 48(7): 536-539.

Friedenstein, A. J., U. F. Deriglasova, et al. (1974). "Precursors for fibroblasts in different populations of hematopoietic cells as detected by the in vitro colony assay method." Exp Hematol 2(2): 83-92.

Friedenstein, A. J., J. F. Gorskaja, et al. (1976). "Fibroblast precursors in normal and irradiated mouse hematopoietic organs." Exp Hematol 4(5): 267-274.

Friedenstein, A. J., K. V. Petrakova, et al. (1968). "Heterotopic of bone marrow. Analysis of precursor cells for osteogenic and hematopoietic tissues." Transplantation 6(2): 230-247.

Frohlich, M., W. L. Grayson, et al. (2008). "Tissue engineered bone grafts: biological requirements, tissue culture and clinical relevance." Curr Stem Cell Res Ther 3(4): 254-264.

Fuchs, S., R. Baffour, et al. (2001). "Transendocardial delivery of autologous bone marrow enhances collateral perfusion and regional function in pigs with chronic experimental myocardial ischemia." J Am Coll Cardiol 37(6): 1726-1732.

Furlani, D., M. Ugurlucan, et al. (2009). "Is the intravascular administration of mesenchymal stem cells safe? Mesenchymal stem cells and intravital microscopy." Microvasc Res 77(3): 370-376.

Garcia-Olmo, D., D. Herreros, et al. (2009). "Expanded adipose-derived stem cells for the treatment of complex perianal fistula: a phase II clinical trial." Dis Colon Rectum 52(1): 79-86.

Gotman, I. (1997). "Characteristics of metals used in implants." J Endourol 11(6): 383-389.

Gruner, A. and K. D. Heller (2009). "[Revision hip arthroplastiy of the hip joint. Revision of the femur: which implant is indicated when?]." Orthopade 38(8): 667-680.

Guven, S., A. Mehrkens, et al. (2011). "Engineering of large osteogenic grafts with rapid engraftment capacity using mesenchymal and endothelial progenitors from human adipose tissue." Biomaterials 32(25): 5801-5809.

Hak, D. J., T. Makino, et al. (2006). "Recombinant human BMP-7 effectively prevents non-union in both young and old rats." J Orthop Res 24(1): 11-20.

Heiskanen, A., T. Satomaa, et al. (2007). "N-glycolylneuraminic acid xenoantigen contamination of human embryonic and mesenchymal stem cells is substantially reversible." Stem Cells 25(1): 197-202.

Holtorf, H. L., J. A. Jansen, et al. (2005). "Flow perfusion culture induces the osteoblastic differentiation of marrow stroma cell-scaffold constructs in the absence of dexamethasone." J Biomed Mater Res A 72(3): 326-334.

Horwitz, E. M., K. Le Blanc, et al. (2005). "Clarification of the nomenclature for MSC: The International Society for Cellular Therapy position statement." Cytotherapy 7(5): 393-395.

Horwitz, E. M., D. J. Prockop, et al. (2001). "Clinical responses to bone marrow transplantation in children with severe osteogenesis imperfecta." Blood 97(5): 1227-1231.

Hosseinkhani, H., M. Hosseinkhani, et al. (2008). "DNA nanoparticles encapsulated in 3D tissue-engineered scaffolds enhance osteogenic differentiation of mesenchymal stem cells." J Biomed Mater Res A 85(1): 47-60.

Huang, G. T., S. Gronthos, et al. (2009). "Mesenchymal stem cells derived from dental tissues vs. those from other sources: their biology and role in regenerative medicine." J Dent Res 88(9): 792-806.

Ilancheran, S., Y. Moodley, et al. (2009). "Human fetal membranes: a source of stem cells for tissue regeneration and repair?" Placenta 30(1): 2-10.

Izquierdo, R. J. and M. D. Northmore-Ball (1994). "Long-term results of revision hip arthroplasty. Survival analysis with special reference to the femoral component." J Bone Joint Surg Br 76(1): 34-39.

Jaiswal, N., S. E. Haynesworth, et al. (1997). "Osteogenic differentiation of purified, culture-expanded human mesenchymal stem cells in vitro." J Cell Biochem 64(2): 295-312.

Jakob, M., H. Hemeda, et al. "Human nasal mucosa contains tissue-resident immunologically responsive mesenchymal stromal cells." Stem Cells Dev 19(5): 635-644.

John, A., H. K. Varma, et al. (2009). "In vitro investigations of bone remodeling on a transparent hydroxyapatite ceramic." Biomed Mater 4(1): 015007.

Jones, E. A., A. Crawford, et al. (2008). "Synovial fluid mesenchymal stem cells in health and early osteoarthritis: detection and functional evaluation at the single-cell level." Arthritis Rheum 58(6): 1731-1740.

Jones, J. R., R. C. Atwood, et al. (2009). "Quantifying the 3D macrostructure of tissue scaffolds." J Mater Sci Mater Med 20(2): 463-471.

Karageorgiou, V. and D. Kaplan (2005). "Porosity of 3D biomaterial scaffolds and osteogenesis." Biomaterials 26(27): 5474-5491.

Karaoz, E., S. Ayhan, et al. "Isolation and characterization of stem cells from pancreatic islet: pluripotency, differentiation potential and ultrastructural characteristics." Cytotherapy 12(3): 288-302.

Karoubi, G., L. Cortes-Dericks, et al. (2009). "Identification of mesenchymal stromal cells in human lung parenchyma capable of differentiating into aquaporin 5-expressing cells." Lab Invest 89(10): 1100-1114.

Kavanagh, B. F., D. M. Ilstrup, et al. (1985). "Revision total hip arthroplasty." J Bone Joint Surg Am 67(4): 517-526.

Keibl, C., A. Fugl, et al. (2011). "Human adipose derived stem cells reduce callus volume upon BMP-2 administration in bone regeneration." Injury.

Kern, S., H. Eichler, et al. (2006). "Comparative analysis of mesenchymal stem cells from bone marrow, umbilical cord blood, or adipose tissue." Stem Cells 24(5): 1294-1301.

Khan, W. S., A. B. Adesida, et al. (2009). "The epitope characterisation and the osteogenic differentiation potential of human fat pad-derived stem cells is maintained with ageing in later life." Injury 40(2): 150-157.

Koc, O. N., J. Day, et al. (2002). "Allogeneic mesenchymal stem cell infusion for treatment of metachromatic leukodystrophy (MLD) and Hurler syndrome (MPS-IH)." Bone Marrow Transplant 30(4): 215-222.

Kocaoemer, A., S. Kern, et al. (2007). "Human AB serum and thrombin-activated platelet-rich plasma are suitable alternatives to fetal calf serum for the expansion of mesenchymal stem cells from adipose tissue." Stem Cells 25(5): 1270-1278.

Korda, M., G. Blunn, et al. (2008). "Use of mesenchymal stem cells to enhance bone formation around revision hip replacements." J Orthop Res 26(6): 880-885.

Kramann, R., S. K. Couson, et al. (2011). "Exposure to Uremic Serum Induces a Procalcific Phenotype in Human Mesenchymal Stem Cells." Arterioscler Thromb Vasc Biol.

Le Blanc, K., C. Gotherstrom, et al. (2005). "Fetal mesenchymal stem-cell engraftment in bone after in utero transplantation in a patient with severe osteogenesis imperfecta." Transplantation 79(11): 1607-1614.

Le Blanc, K., I. Rasmusson, et al. (2004). "Treatment of severe acute graft-versus-host disease with third party haploidentical mesenchymal stem cells." Lancet 363(9419): 1439-1441.

Lepperdinger, G., R. Brunauer, et al. (2008). "Controversial issue: is it safe to employ mesenchymal stem cells in cell-based therapies?" Exp Gerontol 43(11): 1018-1023.

Levi, B. and M. T. Longaker (2011). "Concise review: adipose-derived stromal cells for skeletal regenerative medicine." Stem Cells 29(4): 576-582.

Lindenmair, A., S. Wolbank, et al. (2010). "Osteogenic differentiation of intact human amniotic membrane." Biomaterials 31(33): 8659-8665.

Long, J. L., P. Zuk, et al. (2010). "Epithelial differentiation of adipose-derived stem cells for laryngeal tissue engineering." Laryngoscope 120(1): 125-131.

Mannello, F. and G. A. Tonti (2007). "Concise review: no breakthroughs for human mesenchymal and embryonic stem cell culture: conditioned medium, feeder layer, or feeder-free; medium with fetal calf serum, human serum, or enriched plasma; serum-free, serum replacement nonconditioned medium, or ad hoc formula? All that glitters is not gold!" Stem Cells 25(7): 1603-1609.

Marynka-Kalmani, K., S. Treves, et al. "The lamina propria of adult human oral mucosa harbors a novel stem cell population." Stem Cells 28(5): 984-995.

Matsumoto, T., A. Kawamoto, et al. (2006). "Therapeutic potential of vasculogenesis and osteogenesis promoted by peripheral blood CD34-positive cells for functional bone healing." Am J Pathol 169(4): 1440-1457.

Mifune, Y., T. Matsumoto, et al. (2008). "Local delivery of granulocyte colony stimulating factor-mobilized CD34-positive progenitor cells using bioscaffold for modality of unhealing bone fracture." Stem Cells 26(6): 1395-1405.

Momin, E. N., A. Mohyeldin, et al. (2010). "Mesenchymal stem cells: new approaches for the treatment of neurological diseases." Curr Stem Cell Res Ther 5(4): 326-344.

Mosna, F., L. Sensebe, et al. (2010). "Human bone marrow and adipose tissue mesenchymal stem cells: a user's guide." Stem Cells Dev 19(10): 1449-1470.

Nair, M. B., A. Bernhardt, et al. (2009). "A bioactive triphasic ceramic-coated hydroxyapatite promotes proliferation and osteogenic differentiation of human bone marrow stromal cells." J Biomed Mater Res A 90(2): 533-542.

Nair, M. B., H. K. Varma, et al. (2009). "Triphasic ceramic coated hydroxyapatite as a niche for goat stem cell-derived osteoblasts for bone regeneration and repair." J Mater Sci Mater Med 20 Suppl 1: S251-258.

Najar, M., G. Raicevic, et al. "Mesenchymal stromal cells use PGE2 to modulate activation and proliferation of lymphocyte subsets: Combined comparison of adipose tissue, Wharton's Jelly and bone marrow sources." Cell Immunol 264(2): 171-179.

Niemeyer, P., U. Krause, et al. (2004). "Evaluation of mineralized collagen and alpha-tricalcium phosphate as scaffolds for tissue engineering of bone using human mesenchymal stem cells." Cells Tissues Organs 177(2): 68-78.

Nienhuijs, M. E., X. F. Walboomers, et al. (2011). "The Evaluation of Mineralized Collagen as a Carrier for the Osteoinductive Material COLLOSS((R))E, In Vivo." Tissue Eng Part A 17(13-14): 1683-1690.

Noort, W. A., D. Feye, et al. (2010). "Mesenchymal stromal cells to treat cardiovascular disease: strategies to improve survival and therapeutic results." Panminerva Med 52(1): 27-40.

Olmedo, D. G., D. R. Tasat, et al. (2009). "The issue of corrosion in dental implants: a review." Acta Odontol Latinoam 22(1): 3-9.

Parekkadan, B. and J. M. Milwid (2010). "Mesenchymal stem cells as therapeutics." Annu Rev Biomed Eng 12: 87-117.

Peister, A., M. A. Woodruff, et al. (2011). "Cell sourcing for bone tissue engineering: Amniotic fluid stem cells have a delayed, robust differentiation compared to mesenchymal stem cells." Stem Cell Res 7(1): 17-27.

Phinney, D. G. and D. J. Prockop (2007). "Concise review: mesenchymal stem/multipotent stromal cells: the state of transdifferentiation and modes of tissue repair--current views." Stem Cells 25(11): 2896-2902.

Pilz, G. A., C. Ulrich, et al. (2011). "Human term placenta-derived mesenchymal stromal cells are less prone to osteogenic differentiation than bone marrow-derived mesenchymal stromal cells." Stem Cells Dev 20(4): 635-646.

Pinchuk, I. V., R. C. Mifflin, et al. "Intestinal mesenchymal cells." Curr Gastroenterol Rep 12(5): 310-318.

Pittenger, M. F., A. M. Mackay, et al. (1999). "Multilineage potential of adult human mesenchymal stem cells." Science 284(5411): 143-147.

Polisetty, N., A. Fatima, et al. (2008). "Mesenchymal cells from limbal stroma of human eye." Mol Vis 14: 431-442.

Pontikoglou, C., F. Deschaseaux, et al. (2011). "Bone Marrow Mesenchymal Stem Cells: Biological Properties and Their Role in Hematopoiesis and Hematopoietic Stem Cell Transplantation." Stem Cell Rev.

Powell, D. W., I. V. Pinchuk, et al. "Mesenchymal Cells of the Intestinal Lamina Propria." Annu Rev Physiol.

Prockop, D. J. (2009). "Repair of tissues by adult stem/progenitor cells (MSCs): controversies, myths, and changing paradigms." Mol Ther 17(6): 939-946.

Prockop, D. J., M. Brenner, et al. "Defining the risks of mesenchymal stromal cell therapy." Cytotherapy 12(5): 576-578.

Pytlik, R., D. Stehlik, et al. (2009). "The cultivation of human multipotent mesenchymal stromal cells in clinical grade medium for bone tissue engineering." Biomaterials 30(20): 3415-3427.

Rangappa, S., R. Makkar, et al. (2010). "Review article: current status of myocardial regeneration: new cell sources and new strategies." J Cardiovasc Pharmacol Ther 15(4): 338-343.

Reichert, J. C., S. Saifzadeh, et al. (2009). "The challenge of establishing preclinical models for segmental bone defect research." Biomaterials 30(12): 2149-2163.

Ringden, O., M. Uzunel, et al. (2006). "Mesenchymal stem cells for treatment of therapy-resistant graft-versus-host disease." Transplantation 81(10): 1390-1397.

Sensebe, L., P. Bourin, et al. (2011). "Good manufacturing practices production of mesenchymal stem/stromal cells." Hum Gene Ther 22(1): 19-26.

Seong, J. M., B. C. Kim, et al. (2010). "Stem cells in bone tissue engineering." Biomed Mater 5(6): 062001.

Shake, J. G., P. J. Gruber, et al. (2002). "Mesenchymal stem cell implantation in a swine myocardial infarct model: engraftment and functional effects." Ann Thorac Surg 73(6): 1919-1925; discussion 1926.

Stiehler, M., C. Bunger, et al. (2009). "Effect of dynamic 3-D culture on proliferation, distribution, and osteogenic differentiation of human mesenchymal stem cells." J Biomed Mater Res A 89(1): 96-107.

Stockmann, P., J. Park, et al. (2011). "Guided bone regeneration in pig calvarial bone defects using autologous mesenchymal stem/progenitor cells - A comparison of different tissue sources." J Craniomaxillofac Surg.

Stromberg, C. N. and P. Herberts (1996). "Cemented revision total hip arthroplasties in patients younger than 55 years old. A multicenter evaluation of second-generation cementing technique." J Arthroplasty 11(5): 489-499.

Sundin, M., O. Ringden, et al. (2007). "No alloantibodies against mesenchymal stromal cells, but presence of anti-fetal calf serum antibodies, after transplantation in allogeneic hematopoietic stem cell recipients." Haematologica 92(9): 1208-1215.

Tanner, K. E. (2010). "Bioactive composites for bone tissue engineering." Proc Inst Mech Eng H 224(12): 1359-1372.

Tsutsumi, S., A. Shimazu, et al. (2001). "Retention of multilineage differentiation potential of mesenchymal cells during proliferation in response to FGF." Biochem Biophys Res Commun 288(2): 413-419.

Undale, A., D. Fraser, et al. (2011). "Induction of fracture repair by mesenchymal cells derived from human embryonic stem cells or bone marrow." J Orthop Res.

Vassalli, G. and T. Moccetti (2011). "Cardiac repair with allogeneic mesenchymal stem cells after myocardial infarction." Swiss Med Wkly 141: w13209.

Wagner, W., P. Horn, et al. (2008). "Replicative senescence of mesenchymal stem cells: a continuous and organized process." PLoS One 3(5): e2213.

Wagner, W., R. Saffrich, et al. (2008). "The Stromal Activity of Mesenchymal Stromal Cells." Transfus Med Hemother 35(3): 185-193.

Weinand, C., A. Nabili, et al. (2011). "Factors of Osteogenesis Influencing Various Human Stem Cells on Third-Generation Gelatin/beta-Tricalcium Phosphate Scaffold Material." Rejuvenation Res 14(2): 185-194.

Wicker, N., A. Carles, et al. (2007). "A new look towards BAC-based array CGH through a comprehensive comparison with oligo-based array CGH." BMC Genomics 8: 84.

Wiedmann-Al-Ahmad, M., R. Gutwald, et al. (2007). "Growth of human osteoblast-like cells on beta-tricalciumphosphate (TCP) membranes with different structures." J Mater Sci Mater Med 18(4): 551-563.

Yamaoka, E., E. Hiyama, et al. (2011). "Neoplastic transformation by TERT in FGF-2-expanded human mesenchymal stem cells." Int J Oncol 39(1): 5-11.

Zou, W., N. Hunter, et al. (2011). "Application of polychromatic microCT for mineral density determination." J Dent Res 90(1): 18-30.

Zuk, P. A., M. Zhu, et al. (2002). "Human adipose tissue is a source of multipotent stem cells." Mol Biol Cell 13(12): 4279-4295.

Technologies Applied to Stimulate Bone Regeneration

Arnaldo Rodrigues Santos Jr.[1], Christiane Bertachini Lombello[2]
and Selma Candelária Genari[3]
*[1]Centro de Ciências Naturais e Humanas (CCNH),
Universidade Federal do ABC, Santo André, SP;
[2]Centro de Engenharia e Ciências Sociais Aplicadas (CECS),
Universidade Federal do ABC, Santo André, SP;
[3]Centro Estadual de Educação Tecnológica Paula Souza,
Faculdade de Tecnologia de Bauru (FATEC), Bauru, SP;
Brazil*

1. Introduction

Regenerative medicine constantly encounters situations where specific tissues do not have sufficient regenerative capacity to cope with lesions. Routine techniques involve varied surgical procedures, and often involve mechanical, functional and/or aesthetic discomfort. The need to develop alternative techniques for reducing these inconveniences is therefore necessary.

Techniques that stimulate normal tissue repair represent a major advance in biology and regenerative medicine. Frequently applied to the repair of bone lesions and reconstructive surgery, these new biomedical technologies and procedures have afforded technical simplification, elimination of some surgical processes, ease in handling, availability, good levels of predictability and effectiveness, and cost reduction. All this results in an improvement in the quality of life of the patients involved.

All the components of the skeletal system, bones and cartilage as well as the connective tissue present in tendons and ligaments, are capable of repair after an injury. During morphogenesis, bone is formed in a particular sequence of events. First, mesenchymal cells proliferate and differentiate into chondroblasts. This process leads to the production of cartilaginous skeleton. In the following stages, cartilage hypertrophy is observed with mineralization of the cartilaginous matrix. The cartilage cells then replaced by osteoblasts. Vascular invasion is necessary for this stage. The bone is then remodeled. Such events are seen during bone morphogenesis and, in the adult, during fracture consolidation (Reddi, 2001; Tsonis, 2002).

A bone fracture results in the loss of mechanical stability, discontinuity of the bone tissue and partial destruction of its blood supply. Repair is a complex process of tissue regeneration, resulting in stabilization of the fragments, consolidation through bone union, reconstruction of the tips of the avascular and partially necrotic fragments and, finally, internal and external remodeling of the newly formed tissue.

Hemorrhage caused by the blood vessel lesion, destruction of matrix and death of bone cells occurs at the site of a bone fracture. For the repair to begin, the blood clot and the cellular remnants from the matrix must be removed by the macrophages. The *periosteum* and the *endosteum* that are close to the fractured area respond with intense proliferation, forming tissue that is very rich in osteoprogenitor cells which constitute a collar around the fracture that will penetrate between the ruptured bone extremities, making a ring or collar that is located between the fractured bone extremities. This leads to the appearance of immature bone tissue, both through endochondral ossification of small pieces of cartilage that form there and through intramembranous ossification (Kierszenbaum, 2004; Junqueira & Carneiro, 2008). Areas of cartilage, areas of intramembranous ossification and areas of endochondral ossification can be found at the repair site. This process evolves with the appearance after a while of a bone callus covering the extremity of the fractured bones. The callus is formed of immature bone tissue that will temporarily join together the extremities of the fractured bone (Kierszenbaum, 2004; Junqueira & Carneiro, 2008).

Bone repair is also mediated by Mesenchymal stem cells (MSCs) (Bruder et al., 1994). These cells can be stimulated to differentiate into osteoblasts, cultivating them in the presence of serum, dexamethasone, beta-glycerophosphate and ascorbic acid. Moreover, MSCs can differentiate into osteoblasts due to the influence of vitamin D and BMP-2 (Pittenger et al, 1999). Human adipose tissue also contains stroma cells that are able to differentiate into chondrocytes and osteoblasts (Halvorsen et al, 2001).

The traction and pressure applied to the bone during fracture repair, and soon after the patient resumes normal activities, cause the remodeling of the bone callus and its complete substitution with lamellar bone tissue. When these tractions and pressures are identical to those applied to the bone before the fracture, the bone structure returns to its previous state; unlike other connective tissues, bone tissue, despite its rigidity, heals without scar formation (Kessel, 2001; Junqueira & Carneiro, 2008). Bone formation depends on the existence of an extensive vascular network and on the stability of the fracture focus that facilitates local vascularization, giving rise to the differentiation of the osteoprogenitor cells into osteoblasts; moreover, it is well established that the osteoblasts only synthesize the bone matrix in the presence of high oxygen tension.

The mechanical instability of the fracture hinders local vascularization and under these conditions the osteoprogenitor cells differentiate preferentially into chondroblasts. Accordingly, the fracture focus will initially be filled with cartilage (avascular tissue), which will provide a certain degree of stability to this focus, subsequently favoring vascularization of the site (Kierszenbaum, 2004). The quantity of cartilage formed during embryogenesis and at the site of a fracture (bone granulation tissue) is inversely proportional to the quantity of osteoprogenitor cells and of blood capillaries present at the site. If the bone callus tissue and the capillaries develop at the same time, the osteoprogenitor cells will differentiate into a vascularized environment and will consequently form bone. If there are proportionally few vessels or movement of the fracture segments, there will be cartilage formation followed by its substitution with bone tissue (endochondral ossification). If, however, the movement is excessive and the vascular supply limited, the establishment of local fibrous connective tissue (fibrosis) is probable (Kierszenbaum, 2004).

In the *regeneration of a fracture without loss of bone mass*, the repair process occurs in a biologically determined order. The first priority is stabilization and consolidation through callus formation on the edges and between the fragments, followed by its remodeling, besides revascularization and substitution of the necrotic areas. External factors can deeply affect the regeneration process, but the tissues act according to biological rules that control proliferation and cell differentiation as well as the production of matrix, which may occur regardless of, yet influenced by, external interferences.

However, *fractures with loss of bone mass* call for the use of grafts or implants. The latter serve as a support to bone regeneration, interacting with the interface of the receptor fragments and stimulating the tissue restoration process. These devices developed to be implanted are currently known as biomaterials (Hench, 1998), and will be addressed subsequently over the course of this text, constituting the basis of procedures such as guided tissue regeneration and tissue engineering. We will also address other technologies applied to bone regeneration, seeking optimization and acceleration of the process.

2. Regeneration biology without loss of bone mass

The bone repair process can be characterized by 6 physiological stages: impact, induction, inflammation, formation of cartilaginous callus, formation of bone callus and remodeling (Heppenstall, 1980).

Impact consists of the period of energy absorption until the fracture. The quantity of energy absorbed depends on the bone volume and is related to the loading rate. The impact stage of the fracture occurs until energy dissipation.

The *induction* stage involves modulation and differentiation of cellular elements required during the regeneration process. In fractures there is always local hemorrhage caused by injury to the blood vessels of the bone and of the periosteum, besides destruction of the matrix and death of the bone cells adjacent to the fractured site (Fawcett, 1986). This process triggers the inflammatory stage that will persist until the remodeling stage, with phagocytic activity of macrophages that will remove tissue and clot remnants. Cells from the periosteum and from the endosteum, close to the fractured area, will be activated (induction stage) and will respond with intense proliferation of their fibroblasts. Mesenchymal tissues, undifferentiated osteogenic and chondrogenic cells will differentiate into functional osteoblasts and chondrocytes, respectively. The stimulus for this induction can be electrical, low oxygen tension, low pH, release of lysosomal enzymes, release of cytosine and the presence of a series of inductor proteins, including bone morphogenetic proteins (BMP) and cartilage growth factors (Reddi, 1981; Canalis, 1983; Zellin *et al.*, 1996; Lieberman *et al.*, 2002; Oringer, 2002). The induction stage actually occurs through a series of sub-stages in which the inducing phenomena for each subsequent repair stage can be quite distinct, with unique characteristics toward specific target cells (for example: chondrocytes in the cartilaginous callus and osteoblasts in the bone callus).

During the *cartilaginous callus formation* stage, there is a considerable increase of vascularity and cellularity, and of the production of collagen, proteoglycans and lipids.

The callus is electronegative and the osteoclasts continue to remove the necrotic bone. The cartilage formed undergoes modifications, with hypertrophy of the chondrocytes that generate compression on the preexisting cartilaginous matrix, and consequent enlargement of its gaps, being gradually reduced to fenestrated thin septa and spicules of irregular shapes (Probst & Spiegel, 1997). The hyaline matrix from this hypertrophic region becomes calcified, and small granular aggregates and crystals of calcium phosphate are deposited on it.

The *bone callus formation* stage is marked by the substitution of calcified cartilage in primary bone tissue (Heppenstall, 1980; Probst & Spiegel, 1997; Mandracchia *et al.*, 2001). Cells with osteogenic potential, originating from the endosteum and particularly from the periosteum, are activated and a thin layer of bone (a periosteal ring or collar) is deposited around the central portion of the calcified cartilage. At the same time, periosteal blood vessels grow, invading the irregular cavities of the cartilaginous matrix created by the enlargement of the chondrocytes and by the confluence of its gaps. Vessels with thin walls branch out and grow into the cavities of the cartilaginous matrix with blind bottoms. Pluripotent cells are carried to the perivascular tissue of these blood vessels and, some differentiate into hematopoietic elements of the bone marrow. Other cells differentiate into osteoblasts, which deposit an aligned layer similar to an epithelium on the irregular walls of the spicules of the calcified cartilaginous matrix, and start the production of bone matrix. The osteoblasts covered by matrix become osteocytes and start to maintain contact with one another through cytoplasmic processes in a system of canaliculi. The callus remains electronegative, while the osteoclasts finish removing the necrotic bone. The cartilaginous matrix is gradually replaced by primary bone tissue.

During *remodeling*, the conversion of the primary bone tissue into secondary or lamellar bone tissue is completed. The collagen fibers are thicker and present preferential orientation alternating between layers or lamellae. These lamellae can be compacted if deposited on a flattened or concentric surface covering a blood vessel. The collagen fibers extend between the lamellae, thus increasing the bone strength. The blood vessels are contained in central canals (the Haversian canals), which intercommunicate through Volkmann's canals. Moreover, there are several canaliculi that extend to nourish the osteocytes. This assembly is known as the *osteon* or classically as *Haversian system*. Secondary osteons are formed when part of the concentric lamellar bone is converted into Haversian systems (Fawcett, 1986). The medullary canal is reestablished and the diameter and electronegativity of the callus decrease until they disappear.

3. Regeneration biology with loss of bone mass

As mentioned previously, the natural phenomenon of bone regeneration is insufficient, on its own, to reestablish the integrity of fractures with substantial loss of bone mass. For bone regeneration process to take place, it is necessary to have four components: a) a morphogenetic signal, b) host cells that respond to the signal, c) an appropriate carrier of this signal that can deliver it to the specific sites and thus serve as support to the growth of responsive cells of the host and d) a viable and well-vascularized bed (Burg *et al.*, 2000). Consequently, the need to use materials that would serve as support for the regeneration process is present and currently appears as an alternative to the use of grafts, where there are difficulties involved in obtaining bone tissue and in molding for the fracture in question.

These devices produced to serve as implants are known as biomaterials (Hench, 1998) and should exhibit characteristics that stimulate (osteoinduction) and/or guide (osteoconduction) the bone regeneration process.

Osteoinduction consists of a set of chemical, humoral or physical signals that initiate and sustain the various stages of the bone regeneration process and several factors may be involved (Nakagawa & Tagawa, 2000). The concept of osteoinduction was explored in 1965 by Urist, who showed ectopic bone formation when the demineralized bone matrix was implanted in muscles of rabbits, rats, mice and guinea pigs (Urist, 1965). Afterwards, it was concluded that a protein, called *bone morphogenetic protein* (BMP), was involved in the sequence of events involving chemotaxis, mitosis, bone differentiation and formation (Urist *et al.*, 1979). BMP is a glycoprotein of 17,500 daltons, and one of the factors currently identified in bone formation (Adriano *et al.*, 2000; Nakagawa & Tagawa, 2000; Reddi, 2000). Nowadays, several groups have shown that BMPs have the capacity to induce new formation of bone tissue by the endochondral route when implanted in ectopic sites in animals used for experimentation (Habibovic & de Groot, 2007). Besides BMP, other factors such as electromagnetic fields and direct currents also manifest inductive properties. The common result of osteoinduction is the modulation and differentiation of cells for bone production.

Osteoconduction, in turn, is related to the establishment of an appropriate environment model on which osteoprogenitor cells, when adequately stimulated, can produce bone (Heppenstall, 1980). Osteoconduction also facilitates production and bone deposition in the appropriate three-dimensional arrangement and increases the ability of the regeneration process in large segmental defects. Collagen, a natural organic component of bone and of bone surfaces, is the prototype of an osteoconductive substance (Kimura *et al.*, 2000; Lee *et al.*, 2001). A large number of natural and manufactured substances can also stimulate a favorable environment for bone formation (Mandracchia *et al.*, 2001; Pineda *et al.*, 1996), as discussed below. Osteoconduction is the phenomenon in which a single vehicle physically conducts the proliferation of osteogenic cells.

Many studies have investigated the inductive signals for bone morphogenesis, but the greatest emphasis has been placed on BMPs (Reddi, 2000). These proteins were found to have highly specialized patterns of expression during bone repair (Bostrom, 1998; Groeneveld & Burger, 2000). During the initial phases of consolidation, some primordial cells express BMPs in the bone callus. Expression is greater in MSCs and chondrocytes when endochondral ossification occurs. Expression decreases as the cartilaginous component of the callus matures. BMPs are expressed by osteoblasts, but decrease as the primary bone is replaced by lamellar bone. BMP-2, -3, -4, -5, -7, and -8 are responsible for the induction of bone and cartilage formation. BMP-12, -13 and -14, are cartilage derived. BMPs have also been used in clinical trials for the treatment fractures and pseudarthrosis, for example (Reddi, 2001).

A large number of natural substances can be extracted and/or manufactured to stimulate a favorable environment for bone formation (Mandracchi *et al.*, 2001; Pineda *et al.*, 1996). Among all the biomaterials of natural origin that aim to assist in bone regeneration, special emphasis is placed on those of bovine origin, where different protocols of chemical treatment of the bovine bone are evaluated with the purpose of preserving the organic components and inorganic components, such as collagen and hydroxyapatite repectively, which results in a mixed bovine bone (MBB) with an increase of the material's mechanical resistance. The MBB scaffold used in tissue regeneration has the appearance of a porous sponge that will occupy the space of the bone defect, preventing the migration of epithelial and connective cells, so that the osteoblastic cells have access to the regenerating tissue and start to populate the scaffold. Another role of the scaffold is its use as a vehicle for drugs that induce tissue regeneration and inhibit the progression of the disease.

Autogenous bone grafts are considered very advantageous, since they avoid complications of immunological rejection and supply cells that can immediately start the regenerative process (Cunha et al., 2005, 2006). The use of bone grafts is becoming frequent in orthopedics, as a method for resolution of comminuted fractures, (fractures in which the bone is splintered or crushed) thus significantly reducing the need to amputate an affected limb (Cavassini *et al.*, 2001).

One option in the treatment of partial bone defects is to perform the transportation of small bone fragments - called parietal transportation. In this technique (seldom reported in medical literature), the viable bone segment contiguous to the bone cavity is preserved. A bone fragment is created in the healthy region adjacent to the cavity and transported, according to the Llizarov method, filling a cavity of approximately 50% of the bone diameter (Rodrigues & Mercadante, 2005). The option of performing resection of viable bone occupying the complete cortical, transforming the partial defect into segmental for application of the conventional bone transportation technique, appears to us to be absolute nonsense: removing healthy bone when this is what is missing. The main advantage of parietal transportation is bone formation, even during infection.

The exact mechanism of osteoinduction by biomaterials is still largely unknown. Neither is it known whether the mechanisms of osteoinduction by BMPs and biomaterials are the same. In a recent review (Habibovic & de Groot, 2007) striking differences were shown in osteoinduction by BMPs and biomaterials, namely: (1) bone induced by biomaterials is always intramembranous, while bone induced by BMP is formed mainly by the endochondral route; (2) in small animals, just as in rodents, the bone is very rarely induced by biomaterials, but easily by BMPs; (3) bone is never observed on the edge of biomaterials but instead is always formed inside their pores, while bone formation by BMPs is regularly seen on the outside of the carrier and the soft tissue distant from the surface of this carrier.

4. Bone regeneration scaffolds

4.1 Autogenous grafts and allografts

The advantages cited for autogenous grafts in the bone regeneration process allow us to classify it as "gold standard". The presence of osteoprogenitor cells and osteoblasts confer the property of *osteogenesis*; the proteins that are contained in the bone matrix (for example, transforming growth factor β (TGF–β) , and the BMPs) confer the aspect of *osteoinduction;* and the actual mineralized bone matrix provides a structural base for the growth of newly formed tissue, favoring the lodging of cells, the growth of blood vessels, and the deposition of bone matrix, characterizing *osteoconduction* (Bauer & Muschler, 2000).

The autogenous graft of *spongy* or *cortical* origin, whether vascularized or not, presents good integration with the adjacent tissue (Khan et al., 2005). In general autogenous grafts are obtained from the iliac crest, due to ease of access and as the obtainment of spongy bone of good quality, which is considered more osteoconductive, osteogenic and osteoinductive than the cortical bone graft, once it favors the diffusion of nutrients and revascularization of the treated area, and presents in its structure osteoprogenitor cells and osteoinductor proteins. Cortical bone graft acts mainly as a support for bone regeneration, changing the direction of the tissue regeneration process (Cypher & Grossman, 1996).

As regards *mechanical resistance*, the spongy graft does not offer immediate resistance at the grafting site. But the osseointegration process favors the acquisition of resistance during bone neoformation, and in an interval of 6 to 12 months it acquires resistance similar to that offered by the cortical graft (Dell et al., 1985; Stevenson, 1999). The opposite occurs with the cortical bone graft, which initially presents good mechanical resistance; however, over the first 6 months of grafting, this resistance is decreased by the presence of a mixture of newly formed bone and necrotic bone at the grafting site (Goldberg & Stevenson, 1992).

The different properties of spongy and cortical autogenous grafts establish the direction of their clinical use. The spongy autogenous graft can be used in cases involving difficulty in the consolidation of long bone fractures, and in the reconstruction of depressed lateral tibial plateau fractures (Marsh, 2006; Marino & Ziran, 2010; Nandi et al., 2010). A case report on autograft use in osteotomy for ulnar lengthening demonstrates the use of the trabecular autograft in functional recovery of the humeroulnar joint, resulting from difficulty in bone union. The patient presented recovery of movements in the two years of follow-up, achieving 105°of humeroulnar movement (Doornberg & Marti, 2010).

The cortical bone graft can be used in cases that require greater initial mechanical resistance at the graft site, even with the need for stabilization of the fracture with implants. Bone defects larger than 5 or 6cm are indications for the use of cortical grafts, as they require immediate mechanical support and a longer period of graft use (Nandi et al., 2010).

In spite of clinical results demonstrating the efficacy and safety of use of autogenous grafts in bone regeneration, some *disadvantages* of their clinical application limit their use (Arrington et al., 1996). We can mention high morbidity of the graft obtainment procedure, the aesthetic discomfort of this route, complications related to the surgical technique that mainly include infection and hemorrhage, and the actual limitations of indication, such as young or elderly patients and cases of recurring surgeries (Seiler & Johnson, 2000; Giannoudis et al., 2005).

As possible alternatives to autograft surgeons have allografts, demineralized bone matrix and natural or synthetic bone graft substitutes at their disposal.

Allografts have a growing clinical use, favored by the upgrading of techniques for obtaining, preparing and storing these materials. Fresh, frozen or freeze-dried grafts can be obtained, but fresh materials are used less often due to their technical difficulty and associated risks (Boyce et al., 1999; Keating & McQueen, 2001). Frozen and freeze-dried allografts are kept in specific tissue banks, properly processed and sterilized prior to storage. Their processing ends up eliminating cells naturally present in the graft, so there is no osteogenic activity here. It is considered that the allograft retains osteoinductive activity, and in spite of its processing some proteins are maintained. But its main activity is conduction of bone formation. However, even the osteoconductive activity can be affected by the material processing. The freezing, drying and sterilization stages, normally using Gamma rays, end up weakening the graft structure, reducing its mechanical properties (Pelker & Friedlaender, 1987; Henman & Finlayson, 2000).

The advantages of allograft use include immediate availability in a sufficient quantity for any treatment and in varied forms, facilitating clinical handling of this graft (Nandi et al., 2010). Li and collaborators described allograft use in the treatment of malignant humeral resection in patient treated between 2005 and 2008, with bone regeneration occurring at 26.3 weeks on average (Li et al., 2011). In another study, Virolainen and collaborators performed a survey of 10 years of allograft use for the treatment of periprosthetic fractures. This type of fracture can entail some surgical complication, and in this case the fractures occur soon after the prosthesis implant surgery, while fractures occurring at a later stage usually result from osteolytic lesions or osteoporosis. In both cases there is bone impairment at the implant site, hindering corrective surgical treatment. There were 71 patients treated between 1999 and 2008 with the use of cortical allograft and stabilization of the site with metal implants, and the patients presented a bone union rate of 91%. Allograft use was considered adequate, allowing biomechanical stability of the site (Virolainen et al., 2010).

4.2 Demineralized bone matrix

An alternative to bone tissue regeneration induction is the use of demineralized bone matrix (DBM) (Pietrzak et al., 2005). This type of biomaterial, obtained by acid hydrolysis of the bone matrix, through the action of hydrochloric acid, basically presents osteoinductive properties (Tuli & Singh, 1978; Katz et al., 2009). Its principle of action is based on preservation of the trabeculated collagen structure of the matrix and of bone formation inductor proteins, even with the processing of the tissue, obtained preferentially from human or bovine bones. The use of DBM to replace grafts should be observed with restrictions, as it does not present osteoconductive properties, due to the absence of the calcified bone matrix, and osteogenic properties, since processing for demineralization ends up killing the cells initially present in the tissue.

Nowadays there is a wide variety of available forms of DBM, either rigid or malleable. One of their main applications is the treatment of unconsolidated fractures (Pietrzak et al., 2005), in addition to the filling of bone cysts and cavities (Docquier & Delloye, 2005) and long bone fractures (Tiedeman et al., 1995; Keating & McQueen, 2001). Pieske and collaborators presented data on 20 patients with unconsolidated diaphyseal long bone fractures, treated between the years 2000 and 2006. The patients received autogenous grafts (n=10) or demineralized bone matrix (n=10), with bone formation having been observed in all the patients treated with DBM, while 20% of the patients treated with autogenous graft did not obtain the expected result (Pieske et al., 2009). The use of demineralized bone matrix has also been indicated for treatments of arthrodesis of the spinal column on account of its bone formation inducing action, and there may be an association with osteoconductive graft substitutes (Morone and Boden, 1998; Park et al., 2009). However, one of the disadvantages of demineralized bone matrix is related to the significant variability of donor sources, and corresponding variability of results obtained (Pietrzak et al., 2005).

Therefore in spite of the *availability* of natural materials as autogenous grafts, allografts and demineralized bone matrix, some limitations of use or clinical disadvantages of these materials drive the development of new technologies for bone tissue regeneration. *Natural and synthetic bone graft substitutes* are available to perform this role. The synthetic bone graft substitutes include ceramic and polymeric biomaterials, while biopolymers represent natural bone graft substitutes, including collagen and chitosan.

4.3 Bioceramics

Bioceramics are biocompatible biomaterials with a long history of clinical applications for bone regeneration. Among the advantages of these biomaterials we can cite their synthetic origin, eliminating the risk of autograft morbidity, or the risk of immunorejection and transmission of diseases of allografts or even biomaterials of human and animal origin. The structural similarity between some bioceramics, such as hydroxyapatite and beta-tricalcium phosphate, and spongy bone, allows us to classify them as biomimetic in relation to physical structure and chemical composition (Giannoudis et al., 2005). This mimicry favors the differentiation of osteoprogenitor cells and the deposition of bone matrix, characterizing bioceramics as essentially *osteoconductive*. The porous structure of bioceramics, or even the crystalline structure of calcium sulfate, also allows neoangiogenesis, which is essential in the osteoconduction process. Bioceramics of interest in the bone tissue regeneration process are those classified as temporary, since they are gradually replaced by newly formed bone (Tormala et al., 1998). Calcium sulfate and beta-tricalcium phosphate do this. Resorption time varies depending on the bioceramic in question, but is generally consistent with the bone callus formation time, sustaining tissue regeneration as osteoconductive agents. Hydroxyapatite is not considered resorbable by many authors, since the resorption process of this bioceramic averages 5 years, which corresponds to the period of natural bone remodeling of the body. Therefore it is considered that this bioceramic is integrated to the newly formed bone tissue and its resorption occurs during the intrinsic remodeling of the tissue.

Calcium Sulfate is one of the synthetic biomaterials with a long history of clinical use as a graft substitute for bone regeneration (Peltier et al., 1957; Tay et al., 1999). The dihydrated form of calcium sulfate, also called "gypsum", presents a crystalline structure that is not very uniform, and is currently used as a raw material in a calcination process that results in hemi-hydrated calcium sulfate ($CaSO_4.\frac{1}{2}H_2O$), also called "Plaster of Paris" (Peltier et al., 1957). Calcium sulfate presents optimal biocompatibility, with reports of sporadic cases of inflammatory reaction after its use, with good evolution and spontaneous resolution in most cases. The length of stay in the organism is 8 weeks on average, a relatively short time, yet sufficient for bone callus formation to begin (Coetzee , 1980; Kelly et al., 2001). Calcium sulfate has ample clinical application potential, including bone defects resulting from trauma or created surgically, such as osteotomies and resection of tumors (Finkemeier, 2002; Kelly et al., 2001), as well as spinal surgery, for filling or bone fusion (Hadjipavlou et al., 2001).

More recently there was a proposal for the expansion of the clinical use of calcium sulfate as an *antibiotic release* agent, since it ensures high local concentration of the drug, avoiding its systemic circulation (Gogia et al., 2009). Reports demonstrate the control of osteomyelitis through the application of calcium sulfate pellets with antibiotics such as tobramycin, vancomycin and gentamicin (Bibbo & Patel, 2006; Chang et al., 2007). A randomized, prospective clinical study, published in 2010, presents data on local control of chronic osteomyelitis of long bones and cases of infection at non-bone consolidation sites. Thirty patients were treated, with half receiving calcium sulfate associated with tobramycin and the other half bone cement (polymethyl methacrylate) impregnated with antibiotic. The results demonstrated the mean follow-up of the patients for 38 months (ranging between 24 and 38 months) with the resolution of 86% of the cases in both experimental groups, concluding on the efficacy of calcium sulfate application in the local control of osteomyelitis (McKee et al., 2010).

In turn, *calcium phosphates* constitute bioceramics with a nanoparticulated physical structure, porous with pores of 100µm to favor the osteoconductive aspect of the biomaterial. The pore density can range between 40% and 60%, with Ca:P stequiometric ratio similar to spongy bone, imitating it (Gautier et al., 1998; Tanaka et al., 2008; Porter et al., 2009). Osteoconduction with calcium phosphate, often used in beta conformation, as *beta-tricalcium phosphate* (β-TCP, CA3(PO4)2), results in resorption of the biomaterial and osseointegration of the treated region in approximately 12 weeks. The bioresorption process occurs through a combination of dissolution and osteoclastic resorption at the implant site (Dong et al., 2002).

The persistence of the biomaterial favors the treatment of cavities resulting from bone resection, filling of osteotomy regions, defects of critical size of the bone (Gaasbeek et al., 2005; Tanaka et al., 2008) or even spinal fusion. Le Huec and collaborators reported the use of β-TCP for spinal fusion in 30 patients in association with bone graft, in comparison to another 24 patients treated with cortical allograft. The authors did not report pseudarthrosis and demonstrated the formation of bone callus 6 months after the β-TCP implant, with full resorption in 2 years (Le Huec et al., 1997).

The physical properties of β-TCP favor its association with liquids such as blood and bone marrow aspirate. In an experimental study with dogs, Bruder and collaborators demonstrated bone formation and the refinement of the bioceramic in association with mesenchymal cells obtained from bone marrow aspirate (Bruder et al., 1998). In 2007 the same author published, together with collaborators, the result of an experimental application of β-TCP grafts in sheep for posterolateral fusion (Gupta et al., 2007). In this experiment the authors compared the results of the fusion process with the use of autograft, biomaterial enriched with mesenchymal cells, biomaterial associated with total bone marrow aspirate and pure biomaterial. The radiological findings, in line with histological data, demonstrated a high rate of bone formation after 6 months in the presence of autograft (25%) and in the presence of the biomaterial enriched with cells (33%), whereas the biomaterial associated with the total bone marrow aspirate presented a low rate of bone formation (8%) and no bone formation was observed with the use of pure biomaterial, reinforcing the need for association of characteristics such as osteogenesis for guided tissue regeneration.

Unlike beta-tricalcium phosphate, *hydroxyapatite* ($Ca_{10}(PO_4)_6(OH)2$) a bioceramic with a low resorption rate and greater mechanical resistance, is commonly used in association with beta-tricalcium phosphate, in the proportion of 60/40 to improve osseointegration of the graft substitute (Balcik et al., 2007). The porosity of the biomaterial is essential for its action, requiring pores of 100-200µm, at a density of 60 to 65% for cellular lodging and vascularization of the treated area, confirming the osteoconductive action of hydroxyapatite (Giannoudis et al., 2005). The regeneration of defects of critical size and defects in long bones, created surgically or resulting from trauma, are general indications for its use, either pure or in association with β-TCP. Hydroxyapatite can also be used in spinal fusion procedures. The report on the use of hydroxyapatite in orthopedic lesions, including the resection of bone tumors, and the treatment of cystic lesions in rheumatoid arthritis, without the occurrence of adverse reactions and with good clinical evolution of the patients, was published by the group of Yoshikawa and collaborators (2009).

Bioactive glass, or *bioglass*, is a biocompatible bioceramic that allows good integration with newly formed tissue (Hench et al., 1971). It is basically composed of silica, sodium oxide, calcium oxide and phosphates. Some factors influence the integration of bioglass with the surrounding environment, such as composition of the biomaterial, pH of the environment, temperature, and porosity, directing its osteoconductive function (Nandi et al., 2010). Bioglass is indicated for filling bone cavities in general, in reconstructive surgery, including craniofacial defects, besides spinal column fusion procedures (Asano et al., 1994; Suominen &, Kinnunen, 1996).

4.4 Polymeric biomaterials

Among the polymeric, biocompatible and bioresorbable biomaterials used for bone tissue regeneration, the poly (L-lactic acid) (PLLA), poly (glycolic acid) (PGA), polycaprolactone (PCL) polyesters, and their copolymers, such as poli (D,L-lactic-co-glycolic acid) (PLGA) (Santos & Wada, 2007; Santos, 2010) deserve special emphasis. These polymers are often associated with bone formation induction proteins, such as BMPs or even with osteoconductive bioceramics, such as hydroxyapatite. One of the advantages of the use of polymers for tissue regeneration resides in the wide variety of possible applications, not just as graft substitutes, but also as fastening elements, including screws and plates. Bone tissue regeneration is guided by the polymer structure used, whereas proliferation induction and cellular differentiation are observed in these specific scaffolds (Ishaug-Riley et al., 1998; Santos et al., 2001; Santos et al., 2004). The PLGA copolymers implanted in bones induce bone tissue neoformation at the implant site, over a variable period of time, depending on the ratio of polyesters present in the copolymers (Reed & Gilding, 1981).

Polymer/bioceramic composites have the advantage of conferring on polymers the intrinsic biomechanical property of calcium phosphates, such as hydroxyapatite, favoring osteoconductive characteristic of the biomaterial (Hutmacher et al., 2007). Osteoblast cell cultures in porous PLLA/hydroxyapatite composites (PLLA-HA) enable cell proliferation, the lodging of cells throughout the scaffold of the biomaterial and the differentiation of these cells with synthesis of mineralized matrix (Ma et al., 2001). These results are corroborated by the study of Rizzi and collaborators with the biomaterial of PLA-HA and PCL-HA (Rizzi et al. 2001). HA induces the activity of the bone cells preferentially adhered to these particles, exposed on the surface of the composite.

The application of HA-PLLA to two cases of mandibular reconstruction after tumor resection was published recently (Matsuo et al., 2010). The plates were designed with the use of computed tomography. In one of the cases there was association of the composite biomaterial with growth factors obtained from platelets harvested from the patient and in the second case there was a dental graft. Both cases presented good clinical evolution, without the observation of bone resorption in two years of follow-up, and with the formation of good quality bone.

4.5 Other biomaterials

Besides the synthetic bioceramics and polymeric biomaterials, some biomaterials obtained in nature present considerable potential for application in bone regeneration: coralline hydroxyapatites and chitosan.

Similar to hydroxyapatite, *coralline hydroxyapatites* have been explored recently for their osteoconductive potential. They derive from marine corals, with a calcium carbonate base, a porous structure, and pore size ranging between 100 and 500μm, suitable for the proposed function. They can be obtained directly in nature (and processed mainly for sterilization), or obtained from hydroxyapatite (Keating & McQueen, 2001). Indications for use include long bone fractures and tibial plateau fractures, presenting a behavior similar to the autogenous graft (Bucholz et al., 1989).

Chitosan is another biocompatible biomaterial with potential for clinical application under analysis, and is considered very promising for the area of tissue regeneration. It is a natural biopolymer, obtained from the polysaccharide chitin, common in the exoskeleton of crustaceans (such as shrimps and lobsters). It presents encouraging results demonstrating its performance as an osteoconductive biomaterial guiding osseointegration. A study published in 2003 uses chitosan glutamate associated with hydroxyapatite for the treatment of defects of critical size in rat calvaria. The results were obtained after 9 and 18 weeks. The association with osteoprogenitor cells obtained from bone marrow proved ideal for tissue regeneration according to the protocol under investigation, including with mineralization of the treated areas (Mukherjee et al., 2003).

A recently published study (Jayasuriya & Kibbe, 2010) demonstrates the preparation of chitosan microparticles on a wide scale, and the incubation of these particles in concentrated physiological fluid for the stimulation of in vitro biomineralization and subsequent incorporation of insulin-like growth factor (IGF-1). The study evidenced the release of IGF-1 over a 30-day period, characterizing the possibility of the biomaterial's use as a drug release agent.

Collagen, in turn, exhibits a series of possible clinical applications, such as a scaffold for the regeneration of various tissues, including skin, cartilage and bone. It is a natural biopolymer, obtained from animal tissue, generally bovine, with low toxicity and immunogenicity. It can be made available in the form of gels, films and sponges, favoring cell adhesion and resorption, driving the regenerative process. In the case of bone regeneration, collagen is often associated with osteoconductive materials such as beta-tricalcium phosphate or hydroxyapatite (Wahl & Czernuszka, 2006). These composites aim to reproduce the natural conditions of bone and thus to drive cell behavior, with the differentiation of osteoblasts and the synthesis of mineralized bone matrix (Zhang et al., 2010). A randomized, prospective clinical study brings data on the clinical application of collagen biomaterial associated with calcium phosphate bioceramic in the treatment of long bone fractures, having the use of autogenous grafts as a form of control. The fractures were stabilized with metal implants suitable for each case. There was a follow-up on 213 patients, and a total of 249 fractures. According to the authors the collagen-based composite had the same performance observed for the autograft as regards fracture union rate and functional measurements, and is a possible treatment alternative (Chapman et al., 1997).

Associations of biomaterials, initially used as *scaffolds* for the conduction of bone formation, with tissue regeneration *inductor proteins*, are not just a promise for regenerative medicine, but are already taking shape as potential and usual clinical applications. At the same time associations with *osteoprogenitor cells* or bone marrow aspirate are also consolidating for the refinement of the functions of these scaffolds.

5. Stem cells and bone regeneration

Cells are the essential elements during repair and regeneration, with *stem cells* playing an important role in this process, as already mentioned previously. Nowadays there are a growing number of studies seeking therapeutic strategies and applications using stem cells to minimize clinical problems caused by injury or diseases in the bone tissue (Meyer, et al., 2006; Charbord, 2010), which present increasing demand, considering the demographic growth of the population and the rise in the number of elderly citizens, where the frequency of diseases in the musculoskeletal system is higher (De Peppo et al., 2010).

6. Stem cells and their application to regeneration and to bioengineering of bone tissue

Stem cells correspond to a group of *undifferentiated cells* with the capacity for unlimited self-renewal, as they are capable of successive divisions throughout the entire lifetime of the organism. Moreover, these cells, once stimulated by specific signals and under ideal conditions, will be able to differentiate into cell types with specialized forms and functions and that will maintain the homeostasis of the body. Therefore the proliferative capacity associated with the potential to differentiate into different specific cell types, confer immense potential for application to different areas of biomedicine including gene therapy and tissue engineering on stem cells (Kirschstein & Skirboll, 2001).

Thus, the success of tissue engineering depends on the use of the appropriate cells, on the ability to predict the cell response and on culture techniques for proliferation and differentiation into specific cell types. Nowadays tissue engineering applications are allowing, among others, the use of cells from the actual patient (autologous cells), from donors (allogenic), from different species (xenogeneic), from immortalized lineages (both allogeneic and xenogeneic) and fetal and adult stem cells (Parenteau, 2002); which can be cultivated on molds of biocompatible materials, and subsequently implanted to the injured tissue or inoculated directly or onto the biomaterials at the implant sites. This methodology opens vast perspectives for application in the medical area, allowing the performance of graft implants in injured tissues leading to a greater benefit to the patient, with the initial use of a small number of cells, which will be expanded *in vitro* by means of culture techniques, and also due to the fact that it will be possible to either minimize or avoid immunological problems such as rejection of non-autogenous transplants (Calvert et al.,

2000; Temenoff & Mikos, 2000a,b). To this effect, several strategies are being applied to improve the efficiency of tissue engineering such as growth factors and recombinant differentiation factors, use of autologous cells, gene therapy through the incorporation of vectors and genetic engineering of cells (Satija et al., 2007).

7. Embryonic stem cells

The self-renewal capacity of *human embryonic stem cells (ESCs)* over prolonged periods and their ability to differentiate into different tissues from the three embryonic layers, were characterized by Thomson and collaborators (Thomson et al., 1998). These oocyte-derived cells fertilized in the morule phase or derived from the inner cell mass of embryos in the blastula phase, are able to divide in an unlimited manner, keeping their original characteristics and genetic information, besides being pluripotent, that is, they can differentiate into practically all cell types, derived from the three embryonic germ layers, mesoderm, ectoderm and endoderm (Figure 1) (Doetschman et al., 1985; Smith, 2001).

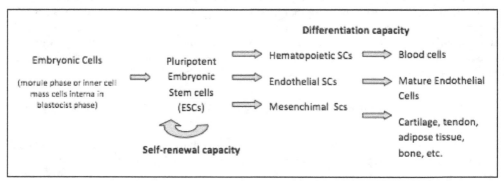

Fig. 1. Diagram showing pluripotent property of embryonic stem cells and their capacity to originate cell types from the three embryonic germ layers.

Although there is immense potential for the use of embryonic stem cells, due to their pluripotency, in practical terms their use is still very limited due to problems including cell regulation, immunological incompatibility, and possible development of neoplasias upon their administration (Passier & Mummery, 2003). These complications are also accentuated by ethical and religious issues and government regulations vis-à-vis the use of human embryonic cells in research (Zuk et al., 2001; Lee et al., 2003, Undale et al. 2009). Such factors led scientists to seek options with greater application potential, such as adult stem cells.

8. Adult stem cells

Although they decrease with age, *adult stem cells* are present in a wide variety of tissues throughout the lifetime of an individual. These cells, like the ESCs, also have the capacity for unlimited self-renewal and the potential to differentiate into cell types with specific morphologic and functional characteristics. This differentiation process generally involves intermediate cell types called precursor or progenitor cells that, although with a reduced self-renewal capacity, can split up to produce specific cell types (Robey, 2000; Gamradt & Lieberman, 2004). Accordingly, adult stem cells are being identified by different methods and there is a growing number of tissues and organs identified as carriers of the so-called mesenchymal stem cells (MSCs), including the bone marrow, peripheral blood, brain, spinal cord, dental pulp, blood vessels, skeletal muscle, epithelium of the skin and of the digestive system, cornea, retina, liver, pancreas and others, whereas the umbilical cord and the placenta are also carriers of cells similar to the mesenchymal stem cells. In spite of the fact that they have similar characteristics, MSCs of different origins present varied differentiation and gene expression potentials. Bone marrow is known to present considerable potential for obtaining stem cells and they have been studied with clinical and therapeutic objectives for fractures with substantial loss of bone mass and metabolic diseases involving the bone tissue.

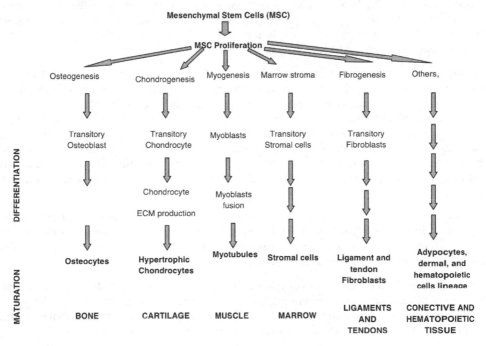

Fig. 2. Summary diagram showing the capacity of mesenchymal stem cells (MSCs) to differentiate into bone, cartilage, muscle, tendons/ligaments and other tissues. Each stage of this differentiation and maturation process involves the control and the interaction of growth factors and cytokines (Caplan, 2010).

9. Bone marrow stem cells

The pioneer studies that evidenced the separation of a population of cells with the capacity to differentiate into a variety of cell types including osteoblasts, chondrocytes, adipocytes and hematopoietic cells, were carried out by Friedenstein *et al*, in the sixties (Friedenstein et. al., 1968). Their studies demonstrated the existence of precursor *mesenchymal cells*, with the potential to differentiate into osteoblasts and fibrous tissue (Figure 2) (Charbord, 2010; Hidalgo-Bastida et al., 2010).

These stem cells in the muridae are frequently obtained from femoral or tibial flushing, obtaining the bone marrow mononuclear cells (BMMNCs) that are isolated by density gradient centrifugation then cultivated *in vitro*. On the other hand, human cells are aspirated from the iliac crest and cultivated directly, since gradient centrifugation techniques have not been seen to increase the separation efficiency and frequently present contamination with hematopoietic cells. This methodology is used to obtain populations that undergo a cloning process, and are characterized by the presence of both positive markers (Stro-1, CD29, CD73, CD90, CD105, CD166 and CD44) and negative markers (CD43, CD45, CD14, CD11b, CD19, CD79a and HLA-DR). The positive expression for Stro-1, identifies cells with osteogenic potential and expression of the three markers for osteoblast differentiation: alkaline phosphatase, 1,25-dihydroxy-vitamin D that has induction dependent on the specific bone protein: osteocalcin and hydroxyapatite production (mineralized matrix). Recent studies have pointed to other markers present in mesenchymal stem cells of the bone marrow that present osteogenic potential (Undale et al., 2009).

The molecular regulatory mechanism involved in the MSC differentiation control process has been extensively studied *in vitro*, whereas *in vivo* control is little known due to the difficulties inherent in the study process. However, the properties of the MSCs *in vivo* and *in vitro* vary according to the method of removal of these cells from their natural environment and the use of chemical and physical factors to keep them in culture, which can lead to alterations in their characteristics. Heterogeneity and diversity of types of MSCs and their ability to undergo phenotypic rearrangements in culture, modifies the expression of markers and hinders the comparison of data or renders it unfeasible in some situations (Augello & De Bari, 2010).

In vitro, the classical methodology to induce osteogenic differentiation in human MSCs consists of incubation with bovine fetal serum, in a medium supplemented with ascorbic acid, β-glycerophosphate and dexamethasone, which leads to the increase of alkaline phosphatase and calcium deposition (Jaiswal et al, 1997; Pittenger et al. 1999).

On the other hand, *in vivo*, the information obtained from studies of embryonic development indicates that different signaling routes and transcription factors may play a critical role in the differentiation of MSCs. Different molecules have been described in the regulation of MSC differentiation, including Wnt and the TGF-β superfamily.

Wnt proteins, coded by a family of 19 genes in humans and in mice, are involved in cell proliferation, differentiation and apoptosis. They act directly on MSCs, and are crucial for embryonic development and regeneration of different tissues in adults, including bone. Etheridge and collaborators (2004) demonstrated that MSCs express a series of ligands including Wnt2, Wnt4, Wnt5a, Wnt11, and Wnt16, and different Wnt receptors, FZD2, 3, 4, 5, and 6, as well as several co-receptors and inhibitors.

Several studies have shown that osteogenic differentiation *in vitro* is upregulated by some molecules related to the Wnt family and downregulated by others. For example, the administration of exogenous Wnt3 leads to osteogenesis repression. The TGF–β superfamily represents a set of growth factors and morphogens that play a role in skeletogenesis and in postnatal skeletal homeostasis. The TGF–β superfamily of ligands includes BMPs, growth and differentiation factors (GDFs), anti-mullerian hormone (AMH), activin, nodal, and TGF–β (Piek et al., 1999; Derynck & Miyazono, 2008).

The expression of growth factors from the TGF–β family is crucial for bone repair in adults and has been described during the embryonic phase as essential for the development of cartilage and bones. TGF–β1 promotes the specific gene expression, initializing chain events with the participation of the SMAD proteins, which lead to the process of chondrogenesis and differentiation of the MSCs (Tuli et al., 2003).

BMPs are important morphogens involved in the regulation of chondrogenesis and osteogenesis during normal embryonic development (Hogan, 1996). The effects of BMPs on MSCs has been investigated, demonstrating that the culture of MSCs in the presence of BMP2 increases alkaline phosphatase activity and osteocalcin expression, both indicators of osteoblast differentiation, whereas this effect is intensified in the presence of dexamethasone. Other factors are also known to influence the differentiation of MSCs, interacting at different levels with the metabolism of the Wnts and/or TGF–β/BMP. One of these factors is FGF-2 (fibroblast growth factor - 2), which promotes cell proliferation and maintains the populations of MSCs undifferentiated for prolonged periods of time (Martin et al., 1997).

10. Applications and clinical potential

Different characteristics of MSCs, including their availability, potential for autologous use and absence of immunological rejection, make them very promising for clinical and therapeutic applications, especially in fractures with significant bone loss and metabolic diseases (Caplan, 2010). In spite of the major advances that have occurred in orthopedic surgery, fractures that involve considerable bone loss and non-union still represent a very important clinical problem. During the normal regeneration of a fracture, as seen previously, undifferentiated MSCs, with the assistance of BMPs and regulatory cytokines, proliferate and differentiate into chondrocytes and osteoblasts, which will form bone tissue reconstituting the lesion. Although related to the site where they occur, around 5 to 20% or more of fractures present failure in regeneration and consolidation (Kimelman et al., 2007; Undale, et al, 2009). Experiments on animal models using autologous MSCs and different scaffolds have resulted in bone regeneration (Arinzeh et al, 2003; Bruder et al. 1998a, b; Kon et al, 2000; Petite et al, 2000). Clinical studies on humans with the use of MSCs aspirated from the iliac crest and subsequently expanded in cultures on different biomaterials (Quarto et al., 2001; Marcacci et al, 2007), or percutaneously injected (Hernigou et al., 2005), have also been conducted, indicating clinical success positively correlated with greater capacity for *in vitro* formation of colonies and concentration of injected MSCs. Clinical applications in humans have also been described in patients with metabolic diseases of the bone tissue such as osteogenesis imperfecta and hypophosphatasia. Cultures of allogeneic MSCs and intravenous administration have mainly been used in these diseases, demonstrating the ability of these stem cells to stimulate bone mineralization and regeneration (Undale et al., 2009)

11. Mesenchymal stem cells of the adipose tissue

Stem cells play a crucial role for the body's homeostasis, as they maintain the functional state of the tissues and also replace cells killed by injury or disease. These cells are very rare in the adult (Kirschstein & Skirboll, 2001). For example, it is estimated that in the bone marrow only one among ten to fifteen thousand cells is a hematopoietic source cell (Weissman, 2000).

Although the bone marrow is the place where the presence and the differentiation process of MSCs is currently best known and characterized, they are also found in other places (Gamradt & Lieberman, 2004).

Studies have indicated that MSCs are also found in animal (Lee et al., 2002) and human (Zuk et al., 2002) *adipose tissue*, and can be obtained by the lipoaspiration process. They are frequently referred to in literature as PLA (processed lipoaspirative) or ADAS (adipose-derived adult stem cells). Different studies have evidenced that mesenchymal stem cells obtained from the adipose tissue, when stimulated by different factors, can also differentiate into adipose cells (Halbleib et al., 2003), osteoblasts (Hicok et al., 2004), chondroblasts, myocytes and neural cells, which means that they draw great interest for applications in regenerative medicine and in tissue engineering (Barry & Murphy, 2004; Ogawa et al., 2004a,b). Since they are easily and abundantly obtained by lipoaspirative process, which is therefore less invasive, using local anesthesia, mesenchymal cells from the adipose tissue offer advantages over the bone marrow (Mizuno & Hyakusoku, 2003; Macleod et al, 2010). In the latter, the obtainment of mesenchymal cells is generally performed using aspiration and flushing of the upper part of the iliac crest, involving a process that is extremely painful for the patient, with the risk of a general or spinal anesthesia, usually implying morbidity of the donor site, resulting in a small number of functional cells. Now the obtainment of mesenchymal cells from the adipose tissue has presented more homogeneous populations with normal karyotype, and can be kept *in vitro* for long periods, with constancy in the cell doubling time and low levels of senescence (Zuk et al., 2002; Aust et al., 2004). Comparative studies between the mesenchymal cells of the bone marrow and of adipose tissue have shown that they both exhibit similarity in their ability to differentiate into adipose cells, from the bone, cartilaginous and muscle tissues; share similarities in the kinetics of growth and senescence, with the capacity for gene transduction and also among the cell surface markers (Mizuno & Hyakusoku, 2003; De Urgate et al., 2003a,b; Mosna et al., 2010)

Thus the autologous mesenchymal stem cells of the adipose tissue are also being used in the construction of three-dimensional scaffolds and applied to patients with severe problems of bone mass loss (Gamradt & Lieberman, 2004).

12. Stem cells and gene therapy: prospects of future applications

Genetic engineering of adult stem cells with genes presenting osteogenic potential has gained considerable emphasis in the repair of fractures and bone tissue formation. Studies have indicated that these genetically modified cells can produce autocrine and paracrine effects on the stem cells present in the actual patient, leading to a greater response in the osteogenic effect. These strategies involve both the use of viral and non-viral vectors, presenting genes that code different BMPs, as well as genetically modified cells containing these implanted transgenes. The advance of these studies may be essential for the future prospects of clinical use of stem cells for bone regeneration (Kimelman et al, 2007), bringing more efficient solutions in the field of orthopedics.

The proliferation capacity of MCSs is a measure of the number of cell divisions that can occur *in vitro* after the culture has been started. Many studies suggest that MCSs have doubling capacity of up to 50 times; after this period the culture is characterized by alteration of a series of cellular characteristics and properties, followed by senescence or even cell transformation. The senescence process is characterized by modifications to morphology and increase of cell volume, reduction in surface marker expression and decrease in differentiation potential. Several molecular mechanisms have already been identified in the senescence process, including DNA injury, accumulation of the cyclin-dependent kinase inhibitor, oxidative stress, telomeric modifications, action of epigenetic factors, and others (Wagner et al, 2010).

Accordingly, the safe and efficient clinical application of stem cells to bone tissue regeneration depends on the elucidation of mechanisms associated with senescence. Moreover, it is essential to understand the mechanisms of action and interaction with other cell types, with different biomaterials, soluble factors, extracellular matrix components (Hidalgo-Bastida et al, 2010) and biochemical and mechanical agents present in the micro-environment *in vitro* and *in vivo*, as well as to keep the proliferation of stem cells restricted to the implanted site and to know the gene control mechanism for safe induction of the desired functions (Gronthos et al., 2000; Discher et al., 2009). The identification of growth factors and the signaling mechanisms involved in the actual control of stem cell renewal and differentiation will allow the design of strategies to block senescence and to safely drive cellular differentiation (Satija et al, 2007).

13. References

Andriano, K.P.; Chandrashekar, B.; McEnery, K.; Dunn, R.L.; Moyer, K.; Balliu, C.M.; Holland, K.M.; Garrett, S.; Huffer, W.E. (2000) Preliminary in vivo studies on the osteogenic potential of bone morphogenetic proteins delivered from an absorbable puttylike polymer matrix. J. Biomed. Mater. Res., Vol. 53, No.1, pp.36-43.

Arinzeh, T.L.; Peter, S.J.; Archambault, M.P.; van den Bos, C.; Gordon, S.; Kraus, K.; Smith, A.; Kadiyala, S. (2003) Allogeneic mesenchymal stem cells regenerate bone in a critical-sized canine segmental defect. J. Bone Joint Surg. Am. Vol., Vol. 85-A, No. 10, pp.1927-1935.

Arrington, E.D.; Smith, W.J.; Chambers, H.G.; Bucknell, A.L.; Davino, N.A. (1996) Complications of iliac crest bone graft harvesting. Clin. Orthop. Rel. Res., Vol. 329, pp.300-309.

Asano, S.; Kaneda, K.; Satoh, S.; Abumi, K.; Hashimoto, T.; Fujiya, M. (1994) Reconstruction of an iliac crest defect with a bioactive ceramic prosthesis. Eur. Spine J., Vol.3, No. 1, pp.39-44.

Augello, A.; De Bari, C. (2010) The regulation of differentiation in mesenchymal stem cells. Human Gene Therapy, Vol. 21, No. 10, pp.1226–1238.

Aust, L.; Devlin, B.; Foster, S.J.; Halvorsen, Y.D.; Hicok, K.; Du Laney, T.; Sen, A.; Willingmyre, G.D.; Gimble, J.M. (2004) Yield of human adipose-derived adult stem cells from liposuction aspirates. Cytotherapy, Vol.6, No. 1, pp.7-14.

Balcik, C.; Tokdemir, T.; Senköylü, A.; Koç, N.; Timuçin, M.; Akin, S, Korkusuz P.; Korkusuz, F. (2007) Early weight bearing of porous HA/TCP (60/40) ceramics in vivo: a longitudinal study in a segmental bone defect model of rabbit. Acta Biomater., Vol. 3, No. 6, pp.985-996.

Barry, F.P.; Murphy, J.M. (2004) Mesenchymal stem cells: clinical applications and biological characterization. Int. J. Biochem. Cell Biol., Vol. 36, No. 4, pp.568-584.

Bauer, T.W.; Muschler, G.F. (2000) Bone graft materials. An overview of the basic science. Clin. Orthop. Relat. Res., Vol. 371, pp.10-27.

Bibbo, C.; Patel, D.V. (2006) The effect of demineralized bone matrix-calcium sulfate with vancomycin on calcaneal fracture healing and infection rates: A prospective study. Foot Ankle Int., Vol. 27, No. 7, pp.487–493.

Bostrom, M.P. (1998) Expression of bone morphogenetic proteins in fracture healing. Clin. Orthop., Vol. 355, pp. S116–S123.

Boyce, T.; Edwards, J.; Scarborough, N. (1999) Allograft bone: the influence of processing on safety and performance. Orthop. Clin. North Am., Vol. 30, No. 4, pp.571-81.

Bruder, S.P.; Kraus, K.H.; Goldberg, V.M.; Kadiyala, S. (1998) The effect of implants loaded with autologous mesenchymal stem cells on the healing of canine segmental bone defects. J. Bone Joint. Surg. Am., Vol. 80, No. 7, pp.985-996.

Bruder, S.P.; Kraus, K.H.; Goldberg, V.M.; Kadiyala, S. (1998) The effect of implants loaded with autologous mesenchymal stem cells on the healing of canine segmental bone defects. J. Bone Joint Surg. Am., Vol. 80, No. 7, pp.985-996.

Bruder, S.P.; Fink, D.J.; Caplan, A.I. (1994) Mesenchymal stem cells in bone development, bone repair, and skeletal regeneration therapy. J. Cell Biol., Vol. 56, No. 3, pp.283–294.

Bucholz, R.W.; Carlton, A.; Holmes, R. (1989) Interporous hydroxyapatite as a bone graft substitute in tibial plateau fractures. Clin. Orthop. Relat. Res., Vol. 240, pp.53-62.

Burg, K.J.L.; Porter, S.; Kellam, J.L. (2000) Biomaterial developments for bone tissue engineering. Biomaterials, Vol. 21, No. 23, pp.2347-2359.

Canalis, E. (1983) The hormonal and local regulation of bone formation. Endocr. Rev., Vol. 4, No. 1, pp.62-77.

Caplan, A. I. (2010) Mesenchymal stem cells: cell-based reconstructive therapy in orthopedics. In: Advances in tissue engineering: stem cells. Vol 2: Stem Cells. Peter C. Johnson & Antonios G. Mikos, eds., pp. 32-45. Mary Ann Liebert, Inc., New Rochelle, NY.

Cavassini, M.M.; Moraes, J.R.E.; Padilha, F.J.G. (2001) Função osteoindutora de fragmentos ósseos conseervados em glicerina a 98%: estudo experimental em ratos. Cienc. Rural, Vol. 31, No. 3, p.445-448.

Chang, W.; Colangeli, M.; Colangeli, S.; Di Bella, C.; Gozzi, E.; Donati, D. (2007) Adult osteomyelitis: Debridement versus debridement plus Osteoset T pellets. Acta Orthop .Belg., Vol. 73, No. 2, pp.238-243.

Chapman, M.W.; Bucholz, R.; Cornell, C. (1997) Treatment of acute fractures with a collagen-calcium phosphate graft material. A randomized clinical trial. J Bone Joint Surg. Am., Vol. 79, No. 4, pp.495-502.

Charbord, P. (2010) Bone marrow mesenchymal stem cells: historical overview and concepts. Human Gene Therapy, Vol.21, No. 9, pp.1045–1056.

Coetzee, A.S. (1980) Regeneration of bone in the presence of calcium sulfate. Arch. Otolaryngol., Vol.106, No. 7, pp.405–409.

Cunha, M.R. Implantes tridimensionais de colágeno polianiônico em falhas ósseas produzidas no fêmur de ratas ovariectomizadas. Tese de doutorado, IB-Unicamp, Campinas, 2006.

Cunha, M.R.; Santos Jr., A.R.; Genari, S.C. (2005) Cultura de osteoblastos sobre membranas de colágeno polianiônico: avaliação preliminar do potencial de indução da formação de tecido ósseo visando reparação tecidual. Bol. Med. Vet., Vol. 1, No. 1, pp.73-85.

Cypher, T.G.; Grossman, J.P. (1996) Biological principles of bone graft healing. J. Foot Ankle Surg., Vol. 35, No. 5, pp.413-417.

De Peppo, G.M.; Sjovall, P.; Lennera, M.; Strehl, R.; Hyllner, J.; Thomsen, P.; Karlsson, C. (2010) Osteogenic potential of human mesenchymal stem cells and human embryonic stem cell-derived mesodermal progenitors: a tissue engineering perspective. Tissue Eng. Part A, Vol. 16, No 11, pp.3413-3423.

De Urgate, D.A.; Alfonso, Z.; Zuk, P.A.; Elbarbary, A.; Zhu, M.; Ashijan, P.; Benhaim, P.; Hedrick, M.H., Fraser, J.K. (2003a) Differential expression of stem cells mobilization-associated molecules on multilineage cells from adipose tissue and bone marrow. Immunol. Lett., Vol. 89, No. 2-3, pp.267-270.

De Urgate, D.A.; Morizono, K.; Elbarbary, A.; Alfonso, Z.; Zuk, P.A.; Zhu, M.; Dragoo, J.L.; Ashijan, P.; Thomas, B.; Benhaim, P.; Chen, I., Hedrick, M.H. (2003b) Comparison of multi-lineage cells from human adipose tissue and bone marrow. Cells tissue organs, Vol. 174, No. 3, pp.101-109.

Dell, P.C.; Burchardt, H.; Glowczewskie Jr, F.P. (1985) A roentgenographic, biomechanical, and histological evaluation of vascularized and non-vascularized segmental fibular canine autografts. J. Bone Joint Surg. Am., Vol. 67, No. 1, pp.105-112.

Derynck, R.; Miyazono, K. (2008) TGF-b and the TGF-b family. In: The TGF-β family, R. Derynck and K. Miyazono, eds., pp. 29-44, Cold Spring, NY.

Discher, D.E.; Mooney, D.J.; Zandstra, P.W. (2009) Growth factors, matrices, and forces combine and control stem cells. Science, Vol. 324, No. 5935, pp.1673-1677.

Docquier, P.L.; Delloye, C. (2005) Treatment of aneurysmal bone cysts by introduction of demineralized bone and autogenous bone marrow. J. Bone Joint Surg. Am., Vol. 87, No. 10, pp.2253-2258.

Doetschman, T.; Eistetter, H.; Katz, M.; Schmit, W.; Kemier, R. (1985) The in vitro development of blastocyst-derived embryonic stem cell lines: formation of visceral yolk sac, blood islands and myocardium. J. Embriol. Exp. Morph., Vol. 87, pp.27-45.

Dong, J.; Uemura, T.; Shirasaki, Y.; Tateishi, T. (2002) Promotion of bone formation using highly pure porous beta-TCP combined with bone marrow-derived osteoprogenitor cells. Biomaterials., Vol. 23, No. 23, pp.4493-4502.

Doornberg, J.N.; Marti, R.K. (2009) Osteotomy and autograft lengthening for intra-articular malunion of the proximal ulna: a case report. Case Report Med., Article: 647126, pp.1-3.

Etheridge, S.L.; Spencer, G.J.; Heath, D.J.; Genever, P.G. (2004). Expression profiling and functional analysis of Wnt signaling mechanisms in mesenchymal stem cells. Stem Cells, Vol. 22, No. 5, pp.849–860.

Fawcett, D.W. (1986) Bone. In: A Textbook of Histology, D.W. Fawcett, ed., pp. 199-238, W.B. Saunders, Igaku-Shoin.

Finkemeier, C.G. (2002) Bone-grafting and bone-graft substitutes. J. Bone Joint Surg. Am., Vol. 84A, No. 3, pp.454-464.

Gaasbeek, R.D.; Toonen, H.G.; van Heerwaarden, R.J.; Buma, P. (2005) Mechanism of bone incorporation of beta-TCP bone substitute in open wedge tibial osteotomy in patients. Biomaterials, Vol. 26, No. 33, pp.6713-6719.

Gamradt, S.C.; Lieberman, J.R. (2004) Genetic modification of stem cells to enhance bone repair. Annals Biom. Engineering, Vol. 32, No. 1, pp.136-147.

Gauthier, O.; Bouler, J.M.; Aguado, E.; Pilet, P.; Daculsi, G. (1998) Macroporous biphasic calcium phosphate ceramics: influence of macropore diameter and macroporosity percentage on bone ingrowth. Biomaterials, Vol. 19, No. 1-3, pp.133-139.

Giannoudis, P.V.; Dinopoulos, H.; Tsiridis, E. (2005) Bone substitutes: an update. Injury. Int. J. Care Injured; Vol. 36, Suppl. 3, pp.S20-S27.

Gogia, J.S.; Meehan, J.P.; Di Cesare, P.E.; Jamali, A.A. (2009) Local antibiotic therapy in osteomyelitis. Semin., Plast. Surg., Vol.23, No. 2, pp.100-107.

Goldberg, V. M.; Stevenson, S. (1992) Biology of autografts and allografts, In: Allografts in orthopaedic practice, A. A. Czitrom and A. E. Gorss, eds, pp. 1-13, Williams & Wilkins, Baltimore.

Groeneveld, E.H.; Burger, E.H. (2000) Bone morphogenetic proteins in human bone regeneration. Eur. J. Endocrinol., Vol. 142, No.1, pp.9-21.

Gronthos, G.; Akitoye, S.O.; Wang, C.Y.; Shi, S. (2006) Bone marrow stromal stem cells for tissue engineering. Periodontology, Vol. 41, No. 41, pp.188-195.

Gupta, M.C.; Theerajunyaporn, T.; Maitra, S.; Schmidt, M.B.; Holy, C.E.; Kadiyala, S.; Bruder, S.P. (2007) Efficacy of mesenchymal stem cell enriched grafts in an ovine posterolateral lumbar spine model. Spine, Vol. 32, No.7, pp.720-726.

Habibovic, P.; de Groot, K. (2007) Osteoinductive biomaterials – properties and relevance in bone repair. J. Tissue Eng. Regen. Med., Vol. 1, No. 1, pp.25-32.

Hadjipavlou, A.G.; Simmons, J.W.; Tzermiadianos, M.N.; Katonis, P.G.; Simmons, D.J. (2001) Plaster of Paris as bone substitute in spinal surgery. Eur. Spine J., Vol. 10, Suppl. 2, pp.S189-S196.

Halbleib, M.; Skurk, T.; De Luca, C.; Von Heimburg, D.; Hauner, H. (2003) Tissue engineering of white adipose tissue using hyaluronic acid-based scaffolds. I: in vitro differentiation of human adipocyte precursor cells on scaffolds. Biomaterials, Vol. 24, No. 18, pp.3125-3132.

Halvorsen, Y-D.C.; Franklin, D.; Bond, A.L.; Hitt, D.; Auchter, C.; Boskey, A.L.; Paschalis, E.P.; Wilkison, W.O.; Gimble, J.M. (2001) Extracellular matrix mineralization and osteoblast gene expression by human adipose tissue-derived stromal cells. Tissue Eng., Vol. 7, No. 6, pp.729-741.

Hench, L.L.; Splinter, R.J.; Allen, W.C.; Greenlee, T.K. Jr. (1971) Bonding mechanisms at the interface of ceramic prosthetic materials. J. Biomed. Mater. Res. Symp., Vol. 2, pp.117-141.

Hench, L.L. (1998) Biomaterials: a forecast for the future. Biomaterials, Vol. 19, No. 16, pp.1419-1423.

Henman, P.; Finlayson, D. (2000) Ordering allograft by weight: suggestions for the efficient use of frozen bone-graft for impaction grafting. J. Arthroplasty, Vol. 15, No. 3, pp.368-371.

Heppenstall, R.B. (1980) Fracture Healing. In: Fracture Treatment and Healing, R.B. Heppenstall, ed., pp. 35-64, WB Saunders, Philadelphia.

Hernigou, P.; Poignard, A.; Beaujean, F.; Rouard, H. (2005) Percutaneous autologous bone-marrow grafting for nonunions: influence of the number and concentration of progenitor cells. J. Bone Joint Surg. Am., Vol. 87, No. 7, pp.1430-1437.

Hicok, K.C.; Du Laney, T.V.; Zhou, Y.S.; Halvorsen, Y.D.; Hitt, D.C.; Cooper, L.F. Gimble, J.M. (2004) Human adipose-derived adult stem cells produce osteoid in vivo. Tissue Eng., Vol. 10, No. 3-4, pp.371-380.

Hidalgo-Bastida, L.A.; Cartmell, S.H. (2010) Mesenchymal stem cells, osteoblasts and extracellular matrix proteins: enhancing cell adhesion and differentiation for bone tissue engineering. Tissue Eng., Part B, Vol. 16, No. 4, pp.405-412.

Hogan, B.L. (1996). Bone morphogenetic proteins: Multifunctional regulators of vertebrate development. Genes Dev., Vol. 10, No. 13, pp.1580–1594.

Hutmacher, D.W.; Schantz, J.T.; Lam, C.X.; Tan, K.C.; Lim, T.C. (2007) State of the art and future directions of scaffold-based bone engineering from a biomaterials perspective. J. Tissue Eng. Reg. Med., Vol. 1, No. 4, pp.245–260.

Ishaug-Riley, S.L.; Crane-Kruger, G.M.; Yaszemski, M.J.; Mikos, A.G. (1998) Three-dimensional culture of rat calvarial osteoblasts in porous biodegradable polymers. Biomaterials, Vol. 19, No. 15, pp.1405-1412.

Jaiswal, N.; Haynesworth, S.E.; Caplan, A.I.; Bruder, S.P. (1997). Osteogenic differentiation of purified, ultureexpanded human mesenchymal stem cells in vitro. J. Cel. Biochem., Vol. 64, No. 2, pp.295–312.

Jayasuriya, A.C.; Kibbe, S. (2010) Rapid biomineralization of chitosan microparticles to apply in bone regeneration. J. Mater. Sci. Mater. Med., Vol. 21, No. 2, pp.393-398.

Junqueira, L.C.; Carneiro, J. (2008) Histologia Básica. 11ª ed., Guanabara Koogan, Rio de Janeiro.

Katz, J.M.; Nataraj, C.; Jaw, R.; Deigl, E.; Bursac, P. (2009) Demineralized bone matrix as an osteoinductive biomaterial and in vitro predictors of its biological potential. J. Biomed. Mater. Res. B Appl. Biomater., Vol. 89, No. 1, pp.127-134.

Keating, J.F.; McQueen, M.M. (2001) Substitutes for autologous bone graft in orthopaedic trauma. J. Bone Jt. Surg. Br., Vol. .83, pp.3-8.

Kelly, C.M.; Wilkins, R.M.; Gitelis, S.; Hartjen, C.; Watson, J.T.; Kim, P.T. (2001) The use of a surgical grade calcium sulfate as a bone graft substitute: Results of a multicenter trial. Clin. Orthop. Relat. Res., Vol. 382, pp.42-50.

Kessel, R.G. (2001) Histologia Médica Básica - A Biologia das Células, Tecidos e Órgãos, Guanabara Koogan, Rio de Janeiro.

Khan, S.N.; Cammisa Jr, F.P.; Sandhu, H.S.; Diwan, A.D.; Girardi, F.P.; Lane, J.M. (2005) The biology of bone grafting. J. Am. Acad. Orthop. Surg., Vol. 13, No. 1, pp.77-86.

Kierszenbaum, A.L. (2004) Histologia e Biologia Celular - Uma Introdução à Patologia, Elsevier, Rio de Janeiro.

Kimelman, N.; Pelled, G, Helm, G.A.; Huard, J.; Schwarz, E.M.; Gazit, D. (2007) Review: Gene and stem cell–based therapeutics for bone regeneration and repair. Tissue Eng., Vol. 13, No. 6, pp.1135-1150.

Kimura, M.; Zhao, M.; Zellin, G.; Linde, A. (2000) Bone-inductive efficacy of recombinant human bone morphogenetic protein- 2 expressed in Escherichia coli: an experimental study in rat mandibular defects. Scand. J. Plast. Reconstr. Surg. Hand Surg., Vol. 34, No. 4, pp.289-299.

Kirschstein, R.; Skirboll, L.R. (2001) The Stem Cell. In: Stem Cells: Scientific Progress and Future Research Directions. Report Prepared by the National Institute of Health, pp. 1-4, Terese Winslow ed. , Virginia.

Kon, E.; Muraglia, A.; Corsi, A.; Bianco P.; Marcacci, M.; Martin, I.; Boyde A.; Ruspantini I.; Chistolini, P.; Rocca M.; Giardino, R.; Cancedda, R.; Quarto, R. (2000) Autologous bone marrow stromal cells loaded onto porous hydroxyapatite ceramic accelerate bone repair in criticalsize defects of sheep long bones. J. Biomed. Mater. Res., Vol. 49, No. 3, pp.328-337.

Le Huec, J.C.; Lesprit, E.; Delavigne, C.; Clement, D.; Chauveaux, D.; Le Rebeller, A. (1997) Tri-calcium phosphate ceramics and allografts as bone substitutes for spinal fusion in idiopathic scoliosis as bone substitutes for spinal fusion in idiopathic scoliosis: comparative clinical results at four years. Acta Orthop. Belg., Vol. 63, No. 3, pp.202-211.

Lee, G.H.; Khoury, J.G.; Bell, J.E.; Buckwalter, J.A. (2002) Adverse reactions to OsteoSet bone graft substitute, the incidence in a consecutive series. Iowa Orthop. J., Vol. 22, pp.35-38.

Lee, C.H.; Singla, A.; Lee, Y. (2001) Biomedical applications of collagen. Int. J. Pharm., Vol. 221, No. 1-2, pp.1-22.

Lee, J.A.; Parret, B.M.; Conejero, J.A.; Laser, J.; Chen, J.; Kogon, A.J.; Nanda, D.; Grant, R., Breitbart, A.S. (2003) Biological Alchemy: Enginnering bone and fat from fat-derived stem cells. Ann. Pastic Surgery, Vol. 50, No. 6, pp.610-617.

Li, J.; Wang, Z.; Pei, G.X.; Guo, Z. (2011) Biological reconstruction using massive bone allograft with intramedullary vascularized fibular flap after intercalary resection of humeral malignancy. J. Surgical Oncol. Vol 104, No.3, pp. 244-249

Lieberman, J.R.; Daluiski, A.; Einhorn, T.A. (2002) The role of growth factors in the repair of bone. Biology and clinical applications. J. Bone Joint Surg. Am., Vol. 84-A, pp.1032-1044.

Macload, L.C.; James, A.W.; Carre, A.L.; Longaker, M.T.; Lorenz, H.P. (2010) A Review of the Therapeutic Potential of Adipose-Derived Stem Cells. Advances In Wound Care, Mary Ann Liebert, Inc., New Rochelle, NY.

Mandracchia, V.J.; Nelson, S.C.; Barp, E.A. (2001) Current concepts of bone healing. Clin. Podiatr. Med. Surg., Vol. 18, pp.55-77.

Marcacci, M.; Kon, E.; Moukhachev, V.; Lavroukov A.; Kutepov, S.; Quarto, R.; Mastrogiacomo, M.; Cancedda, R. (2007) Stem cells associated with macroporous bioceramics for long bone repair: 6- to 7-year outcome of a pilot clinical study. Tissue Eng., Vol. 13, No. 6, pp.947-955.

Marino, J.T.; Ziran, B.H. (2010) Use of solid and cancellous autologous bone graft for fractures and nonunions. Orthop Clin North Am., Vol. 41, No. 1, pp.15-26.

Marsh, J.L. (2006) Principles of bone grafting: non-union, delayed union. Surgery, Vol. 24, No. 6, pp.207-210.

Martin, I.; Muraglia, A.; Campanile, G.; Cancedda, R.; Quarto, R. (1997). Fibroblast growth factor-2 supports ex vivo expansion and maintenance of osteogenic precursors from human bone marrow. Endocrinology, Vol. 138, pp.4456–4462.

Matsuo, A.; Chiba, H.; Takahashi, H.; Toyoda, J.; Abukawa, H. (2010) Clinical application of a custom-made bioresorbable raw particulate hydroxyapatite/poly-L-lactide mesh tray for mandibular reconstruction. Odontology, Vol. 98, No. 1, pp.85-88.

McKee, M.D.; Li-Bland, E.A.; Wild, L.M.; Schemitsch, E.H. (2010) A prospective, randomized clinical trial comparing an antibiotic-impregnated bioabsorbable bone substitute with standard antibiotic-impregnated cement beads in the treatment of chronic osteomyelitis and infected nonunion. J. Orthop. Trauma, Vol. 24, No. 8, pp.483-490.

Meyer, U.; Wiesman, H.; Berr, K.; Kübler, N.; Handschel, J. (2006) Cell-based bone reconstruction therapies - principles of clinical approaches. Inter. J. Oral & Maxillofacial Implant, Vol. 21, No. 6, pp.899-906.

Mizuno, H.; Hyakusoku, H. (2003) Mesengenic potential and future clinical perspective of human processed lipoaspirate cells. J Nippon Med Sch., Vol. 70, No. 4, pp.300-306.

Morone, M.A.; Boden, S.D. (1998) Experimental posterolateral lumbar spinal fusion with a demineralized bone matrix gel. Spine, Vol. 23, No. 2, pp.159-167.

Mosna, F.; Sensebe, L.; Krampera, M. (2010) Human bone marrow and adipose tissue mesenchymal stem cells: a user's guide. Stem Cells Dev., Vol. 19, No. 10, pp.1449-1470.

Mukherjee, D.P.; Tunkle, A.S.; Roberts, R.A.; Clavenna, A.; Rogers, S.; Smith, D. (2003) An animal evaluation of a paste of chitosan glutamate and hydroxyapatite as a synthetic bone graft material. J. Biomed. Mater. Res. B Appl. Biomater., Vol. 67, No. 1, pp.603-609.

Nakagawa, T.; Tagawa, T. (2000) Ultrastructural study of direct bone formation induced by BMPs-collagen complex implanted into an ectopic site. Oral Dis., Vol. 6, No. 3, pp.172-179.

Nandi, S.K.; Roy, S.; Mukherjee, P.; Kundu, B.; De, D.K.; Basu, D. (2010) Orthopaedic applications of bone graft & graft substitutes: a review. Indian J. Med. Res., Vol. 132, No. 1, pp.15-30.

Ogawa, R.; Mizuno, H.; Hyakusoku, H.; Watanabe, A.; Migita, M.; Shimada, T. (2004b) Chondrogenic and osteogenic differentiation of adipose-derived stem cells isolated from GFP transgenic mice. J. Nippon Med. Sch., Vol. 71, No. 4, pp.240-241.

Ogawa, R.; Mizuno, H.; Watanabe, A.; Migita, M.; Shimada, T.; Hyakusoku, H. (2004a). Osteogenic and chondrogenic differentiation by adipose-derived stem cells harvested from GFP transgenic mice. Biopchem. Biophys. Res. Comm., Vol. 313, No. 4, pp.871-877.

Oringer, R.J. (2002) Biological mediators for periodontal and bone regeneration. Compend. Contin. Educ. Dent., Vol. 23, No. 6, pp.501-510.

Parenteau, N.L. (2002). Cells. In: Tissue Engineering Research, pp 19-32. International Technology Research Institute, Baltimore, Maryland.

Park, H.W.; Lee, J.K.; Moon, S.J.; Seo, S.K.; Lee, J.H.; Kim, S.H. (2009) The efficacy of the synthetic interbody cage and Grafton for anterior cervical fusion. Spine, Vol. 34, No. 17, pp. E591-E595.

Passier, R.; Mummery, C. (2003) Origin and use of embryonic and adult stem cells in differentiation and tissue repair. Cardiovascular Res., Vol. 58, No. 2, pp.324-335.

Pelker, R.R.; Friedlaender, G.E. (1987) Biomechanical aspects of bone autografts and allografts. Orthop. Clin. North Am., Vol. 18, No. 2, pp.235-239.

Peltier, L.F.; Bickel, E.Y.; Lillo, R.; Thein, M.S. (1957) The use of plaster of Paris to fill defects in bone. Ann Surg., Vol. 146, No. 1, pp.61-69.

Petite, H.; Viateau, V.; Bensaïd, W.; Meunier, A.; de Pollak, C.; Bourguignon, M.; Oudina, K.; Sedel L.; Guillemin, G. (2000) Tissue-engineered bone regeneration. Nat. Biotechnol., Vol. 18, No. 9, pp.959-963.

Piek, E.; Heldin, C.H.; Ten Dijke, P. (1999). Specificity, diversity, and regulation in TGF-b superfamily signaling. FASEB J., Vol. 13, No. 15, pp.2105-2124.

Pieske, O.; Wittmann, A.; Zaspel, J.; Löffler, T.; Rubenbauer, B.; Trentzsch, H.; Piltz, S. (2009) Autologous bone graft versus demineralized bone matrix in internal fixation of ununited long bones. J. Trauma Management Outcomes., Vol. 3, pp. 11.

Pietrzak, W.S.; Perns, S.V.; Keyes, J.; Woodell-May, J.; McDonald. (2005) Demineralized bone matrix graft: a scientific and clinical case study assessment. J. Foot Ankle Surg., Vol. 44, No. 5, pp.345-353.

Pineda, L.M.; Busing, M.; Meinig, R.P.; Gogolewski, S. (1996) Bone regeneration with resorbable polymeric membranes. III. Effect of poly (L-lactide) membrane pore size on the bone healing process in larger defects. J. Biomed. Mater. Res., Vol. 31, No. 3, p.385-394.

Pittenger, M.F.; Mackay, A.M.; Beck., S.C. Jaiswal, R.K.; Douglas, R.; Mosca, J.D.; Moorman, M.A.; Simonetti, D.W. Craig, S.; Marshak, D.R. (1999) Multilineage potential of adult human mesenchymal stem cells. Science, Vol. 284, No. 5411, pp.143-147.

Porter, J.R.; Ruckh, T.T.; Popat, K.C. (2009) Bone tissue engineering: a review in bone biomimetics and drug delivery strategies. Biotechnol. Prog., Vol. 25, No. 6, pp.1539-1560.

Probst, A.; Spiegel, H.U. (1997) Cellular mechanisms of bone repair. J. Invest. Surg., Vol. 10, No. 3, pp.77-86.

Quarto, R.; Mastrogiacomo, M.; Cancedda, R.; Kutepov, S.M.; Mukhachev, V.; Lavroukov, A.; Kon, E.; Marcacci, M. (2001) Repair of large bone defects with the use of autologous bone marrow stromal cells. N. Engl. J. Med., Vol. 344, No. 5, pp.385-386.

Reddi, A.H. (2001) Bone morphogenetic proteins: From basic science to clinical applications. J. Bone Joint Surg., Vol. 83A, Suppl. A, Part 1, pp.S63-S69.

Reddi, A.H. (1981) Cell Biology and biochemistry of endochondral bone development. Coll. Relat. Res., Vol. 1, No. 2, pp.209-226.

Reddi, A.H. (2000) Morphogenesis and tissue engineering of bone and cartilage: inductive signals, stem cells, and biomimetic biomaterials. Tissue Eng, Vol. 6, No. 4, pp.351-359.

Reed, A.M.; Gilding, D.K. (1981) Biodegradable polymers for use in surgery — poly(glycolic)/poly(lactic acid) homo and copolymers: In vitro degradation. Polymer, Vol. 22, No. 4, pp.494-498.

Rizzi, S.C.; Heath, D.J.; Coombes, A.G.; Bock, N.; Textor, M.; Downes, S. (2001) Biodegradable polymer/hydroxyapatite composites: surface analysis and initial attachment of human osteoblasts. J. Biomed. Mater. Res., Vol. 55, No. 4, pp.475-486.

Robey, P.G. (2000) Stem cells near the century mark. J. Clin. Invest., Vol. 105, No. 11, pp.1489-1491.

Rodrigues, F.L.; Mercadante, M.T. (2005) Tratamento da falha óssea parcial pelo transporte ósseo parietal. Acta Ortop. Bras., Vol. 13, No. 1, pp.9-12.

Rubin, E.; Farber, J.L. (2002) Patologia. 6.ed., Guanabara Koogan, Rio de Janeiro.

Santos, A.R. Jr. Barbanti, S.H.; Duek, E.A.R.; Dolder, H.; Wada, R.S.; Wada, M.L.F. (2001) Growth and differentiation of Vero cells on poly(L-lactic acid) membranes of different pore diameters. Artif. Organs, Vol. 25, No. 1, pp.7-13.

Santos, A.R. Jr. Ferreira, B.M.P.; Duek, E.A.R.; Dolder, H.; Wada, R.S.; Wada, M.L.F. (2004) Differentiation pattern of Vero Cells cultured on poly(l-lactic acid)/poly(hydroxybutyrate-co-hydroxyvalerate) blends. Artif. Organs, Vol. 28, No. 4, pp.381-89.

Santos, A.R. Jr. Wada, M.L.F. (2007) Polímeros biorreabsorvíveis como arcabouços para cultura de células e engenharia tecidual. Polímeros Cienc Tecnol, Vol. 17, No. 4, pp.308-317.

Santos, A.R. Jr. (2010) Bioresorbable polymers for tissue engineering. In: Tissue engineering, pp. 235-246, Daniel Eberlin, ed., In-Teh, Olajnica.

Satija, N.K.; Gurudutta, G.U.; Sharma, S.; Farhat Afrin, F.; Guptta, P.; Kumar, R.Y.; Singh, V.K.; Tripathi, R.P. (2007) Mesenchymal stem cells: molecular targets for tissue engineering. Stem Cells Dev., Vol. 16, No. 1, pp.7-23.

Seiler, J.G.; Johnson, J. (2000) Iliac crest autogenous bone grafting: donor site complications. J. South Orthop. Assoc., Vol. 9, No. 2, pp.91-97.

Stevenson, S. (1999) Biology of bone grafts. Orthop. Clin. North Am., Vol. 30, No. 4, pp.543-552.

Suominen, E.; Kinnunen, J. (1996) Bioactive glass granules and plates in the reconstruction of defects of the facial bones. Scand. J. Plast. Reconstr. Surg. Hand Surg., Vol. 30, No. 4, pp.281-289.

Tanaka, T.; Kumagae, Y.; Saito, M.; Chazono, M.; Komaki, H.; Kikuchi, T.; Kitasato, S.; Marumo, K. (2008) Bone formation and resorption in patients after implantation of beta-tricalcium phosphate blocks with 60% and 75% porosity in opening-wedge high tibial osteotomy. J. Biomed. Mater. Res. B Appl. Biomater., Vol. 86B, No. 2, pp.453-459.

Tay B.K.; Patel V.V.; Bradford D.S. (1999) Calcium sulfate- and calcium phosphate-based bone substitutes. Mimicry of the mineral phase of bone. Orthop Clin North Am., Vol. 30, No. 4, pp.615-623.

Temenoff, J.S.; Mikos, A.G. (2000a) Review: tissue engineering for regeneration of articular cartilage. Biomaterials, Vol. 21, No. 5, pp. 431-440.

Temenoff, J.S.; Mikos, A.G. (2000b) Injectable biodegradable materials for orthopedic tissue engineering. Biomaterials, Vol. 21, No. 23, pp. 2405-2415.

Thomson J.A.; Itskovitz-Eldor J.; Shapiro S.S.; Waknitz M.A.; Swiergiel J.J.; Marshall V.S.; Jones J.M. (1998) Embryonic stem cell lines derived from human blastocysts. Science, Vol. 282, No. 5391, pp.1145-1147.

Tiedeman, J.J.; Garvin, K.L.; Kile, T.A.; Connolly, J.F. (1995) The role of a composite, demineralized bone matrix and bone marrow in the treatment of osseous defects. Orthopedics, Vol. 18, No. 12, pp.1153-1158.

Törmälä, P.; Pohjonen, T.; Rokkanen, P. (1998) Bioabsorbable polymers: materials technology and surgical applications. Proc. Instn. Mech. Eng. Part H - J. Eng. Med., Vol. 212, No. 2, pp.101-111.

Tsonis, P.A. (2002) Regenerative biology: the emerging field of tissue repair and restoration. Diferentiation, Vol. 70, No. 8, pp.397-409.

Tuli, S.M.; Singh, A.D. (1978) The osteoinductive property of decalcified bone matrix. An experimental study. J. Bone Joint Surg. Br., Vol. 60, No. 1, pp.116-123.

Tuli, R.; Tuli, S.; Nandi, S.; Huang, X.; Manner, P.A.; Hozack, W.J.; Danielson, K.G.; Hall, D.J.; Tuan, R.S. (2003). Transforming growth factor-b-mediated chondrogenesis of human mesenchymal progenitor cells involves N-cadherin and mitogen-activated protein kinase and Wnt signaling cross-talk. J. Biol. Chem., Vol. 278, No. 42, pp.41227–41236.

Undale, A.H.; Westendorf, J.J.; Yaszemski, M.J., Khosla, S. (2009) Mesenchymal stem cells for bone repair and metabolic bone desease. Mayo Clin. Proc., Vol. 84, No. 10, pp.893-902.

Urist, M.R. (1965) Bone: formation by autoinduction. Science, Vol. 150, No. 698, pp.893-899.

Urist, M.R.; Grant, T.T.; Lindholm, T.S.; Mirra, J.M.; Hirano, H.; Finerman, G.A. (1979) Induction of new-bone formation in the host bed by human bone-tumour transplants in athymic nude mice. J. Bone Joint Surg. Am., Vol. 61, No. 8, pp.1207-1216.

Virolainen, P.; Mokka, J.; Seppänen, M.; Mäkelä, K. (2010) Up to 10 years follow up of the use of 71 cortical allografts (strut-grafts) for the treatment of periprosthetic fractures. Scand. J. Surg., Vol. 99, No. 4, pp.240-243.

Wagner, W; Ho, A.D.; Zenke, M. (2010) Different facets of aging in human mesenchymal stem cells. Tissue Eng. Part B., Vol. 16, No. 4, pp.445-453.

Wahl, D.A.; Czernuszka, J.T. (2006) Collagen-hydroxyapatite composites for hard tissue repair. Eur. Cell Mater., Vol. 28, No. 11, pp.43-56.

Weissman, I.L. (2000) Stem cells: units of development, units of regeneration, and units in evolution. Cell, Vol. 100, pp.157-1168.

Yoshikawa, H.; Tamai, N.; Murase, T.; Myoui, A. (2009) Interconnected porous hydroxyapatite ceramics for bone tissue engineering. J. R. Soc. Interface, Vol. 6, Suppl 3, pp.S341-S348.

Zhang Y.; Reddy V.J.; Wong S.Y.; Li X.; Su B.; Ramakrishna S.; Lim C.T. (2010) Enhanced biomineralization in osteoblasts on a novel electrospun biocomposite nanofibrous substrate of hydroxyapatite/collagen/chitosan. Tissue Eng Part A., Vol. 16, No. 6, pp.1949-1960.

Zellin, G.; Hedner, E.; Linde, A. (1996) Bone regeneration by a combination of osteopromotive membranes with different BMP preparations: a review. Connect. Tissue Res., Vol. 35, pp.279-284.

Zuk, P.A.; Zhu, M.; Mizuno, H.; Huang,J.; Futrell, J.W.; Katz, A.J.; Benhaim, P.; Lorenz, H.P., Hedrick, M.H. (2001) Multilineage cells from human adipose tissue: implications for cell-based therapies. Tissue Eng., Vol. 7, No. 2, pp.211-228.

Zuk, P.A.; Zhu, M.; Ashijan, P.; De Urgate, D.A.; Huang, J.I.; Mizuno, H.; Alfonso, Z.C., Frazer, J.I. (2002) Human adipose tissue is a source of multipotent stem cells. Mol. Biol. Cell., Vol. 13, No. 12, pp.4279-4295.

3

Oral Tissues as Source for Bone Regeneration in Dental Implantology

Dilaware Khan[1], Claudia Kleinfeld[1], Martin Winter[2] and Edda Tobiasch[1]
[1]University of Applied Sciences Bonn-Rhine-Sieg, Rheinbach
[2]Oralchirurgische Praxis, Rheinbach
Germany

1. Introduction

One of the most common problems in Regenerative Medicine is the regeneration of damaged bone with the aim of repairing or replacing lost or damaged bone tissue by stimulating the natural regenerative process. Particularly in the fields of orthopedic, plastic, reconstructive, maxillofacial and craniofacial surgery there is need for successful methods to restore bone. From a regenerative point of view two different bone replacement problems can be distinguished: large bone defects and small bone defects. Currently, no perfect system exists for the treatment of large bone defects. Autologous bone material from the hip or the split calvarial graft is the gold standard to repair bone defects, as it has osteoinductive and osteoconductive properties (Tessier, 1982; Tessier et al., 2005a; Laurencin et al., 2006). Unfortunately this method is associated with an additional invasive intervention that leads to an increase risk of infection, pain during recovery, morbidity and frequent long periods of convalescence due to surgical trauma. Besides, only a limited amount of tissue can be obtained and harvested (Younger & Chapman, 1989; Tessier et al., 2005b). Also, the outcome is not always satisfactory after surgical treatment using bone splits (Baltzer et al., 2000; Lietman et al., 2000; Sorger et al., 2001). Heterologous transplants on the other hand, bear the risk of infection and rejection of the donor material. If the required amount of implant material cannot be obtained, another source is bovine-derived xenografts. There is, however, a potential risk for prion infection that cannot be totally avoided. Last not least large bone defect replacement needs nutrient and oxygen supply via blood vessels, so angiogenesis must be considered. This is very different in small bone defects: here angiogenesis is not an issue, but most of the other problems addressed above do play a role here too. This chapter will focus on small bone defects, especially those linked to dental implants.

2. Bone structure and regulation

The skeletal system is composed of bones that support the body, protect internal organs, and allow movement. Bone itself can be described as a natural composite material that consists of minerals and collagen that are merged in a complex amalgam. It consists mainly of two structures: an organic component as a matrix that contains collagen and a mineral component that is predominantly hydroxyapatite (Rho et al., 1997). The complex mineral substances give hardness to the bone and the softer organic collagen matrix causes visco-elasticity and toughness (Hutmacher et al., 2007). Together with cartilage, connective tissue, nerves, blood vessels, and marrow, they constitute the bone.

In the mineralized organic bone matrix, living and dead cells are present. Three types are known to play a role in bone homeostasis: osteoblasts, osteocytes and osteoclasts.

Osteoblasts are derived from MSCs and are cuboidal in shape (Fig. 1). They contain prominent Golgi bodies with a well developed rough endoplasmic reticulum, which is a histological sign for prominent protein production. These cells are located on the endosteal and periosteal bone surfaces. They secrete collagen type I and the non-collagenous proteins of the organic bone matrix. These cells also synthesize the enzyme alkaline phosphatase (ALP) that regulates the mineralization of the bone matrix. Their lifetime is about three months, after which they become metabolically inactive, flattened bone lining cells (Fig. 1). Bone lining cells are found covering inactive bone surfaces where they serve as a barrier for certain ions. The osteocytes originate from metabolically inactive osteoblasts and become trapped within the newly formed bone matrix during bone formation. Osteocytes have reduced synthetic activity compared to osteoblasts but maintain their sensitivity to vitamin D while continuing to participate in calcium regulation. On the other hand osteoclasts are derived from the fusion of monocyte and macrophage lineages (Ash, 1980) (Fig. 1). They are multi-nucleated cells that resorb bone. Osteoblasts regulate the differentiation of osteoclasts and osteocytes, which secrete factors in a feedback loop that play a role in regulating the functions of osteoblasts (Hartmann, 2006) and osteoclasts (Seeman & Delmas, 2006). The formation and resorption of bone is a continuous process that is kept in balance by the regulation of these three types of cells, with emphasis on osteoblasts and osteoclasts.

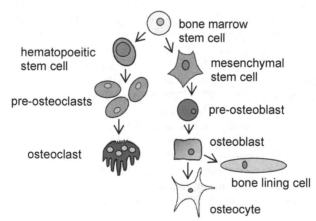

Fig. 1. Development of Bone Cells. Bone marrow stem cells give rise to hematopoietic stem cells and mesenchymal stem cells. Hematopoietic stem cells give rise to osteoclasts and mesenchymal stem cells are differentiated into osteoblasts together with other cell types. Osteoblasts further develop into bone lining cells and osteocytes.

In some diseases this balance is disrupted, as in osteoporosis, where increased osteoclast activity results in more resorption of bone than formation by osteoblasts. Along with osteoporosis, other medical conditions like bone cancer and osteogenesis imperfecta can lead to weakness of bones that can result in fractures. Bone defects can also occur due to trauma after accidents (Schäffler & Büchler, 2007). In addition, changes in recreational behavior especially in young adults lead to more need for bone replacement. Also, improved conditions of public health, nutrition and medicine have increased the life expectancy that resulted in an enhanced need for dental replacement. Taken together there is a growing need for bone regeneration and replacement.

3. Bone regeneration and replacement

3.1 The need for bone regeneration in dental defects

Studies revealed that approximately 70 % of all adults between 35 and 44 years lost at least one permanent tooth and by the age of 74 around 26 % of the adults lost all their permanent teeth (National Institutes of Health, 2001). Additionally, 45 % of the adults between 35 and 44 years and 54 % of the seniors between 65 and 74 years suffered from a middle heavy periodontitis, which is connected with a higher risk of tooth-loss (Holtfreter et al., 2010). To overcome these problems dental implants are one of the most common features to realize oral prosthetic reconstruction.

In order to guarantee a long and successful osseointegration of dental implants, they should be circumferentially covered with bone. Furthermore, it seems advantageous that the intraosseous part of the fixture is longer than the extraosseous prosthetic part. At least, the length of the implant should not be shorter than the abutment. Nowadays correct implant placement is determined by esthetic and prosthetic aspects, which often cannot be realized when only the residually available bone (restoration-driven implant placement) is being used (Garber et al., 1995). (National Institutes of Health, 2001)

There are defects of the alveolar bone which occur as a result of trauma, inflammation, resective surgical intervention such as tumor resection, bone loss after periodontal disease or athrophia after tooth loss or agenesis. In the posterior maxilla the phenomenon of pneumatization of the sinus maxillaris increases after tooth loss, which results in a vertical compromized bone level (Fig. 2A). Thus, bone reconstruction before or simultaneously to implant placement is often necessary (Fig. 2B). To do so guided, bone regeneration with autologous material such as bone graft material or other autologous or artificial grafting

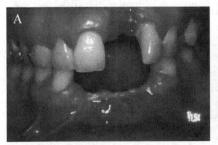 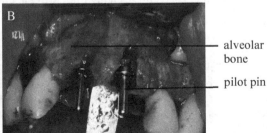

alveolar bone

pilot pin

Fig. 2. A) Bone Degeneration. After tooth loss, reduced jawbone is as a result of trauma in a 24 years old male. B) Pilot pins *in situ* demonstrate the compromized bone-situation (male, 43 years old). Stable integration of implants is dependent on a thick jawbone. Stem cells could be used to fill the gaps and increase the thickness and induce osseointegration of implants.

procedures are methods of choice. Nevertheless, there exist many unsolved problems such as a e.g. higher morbidity in conjunction with the second wound of the donor site.

Therefore the use of stem cells (SCs) as source material for bone regeneration could represent an interesting approach for dental implantology.

3.2 Stem cells for bone regeneration

A modern strategy in Regenerative Medicine is the approach to combine living cells and scaffold material to establish a biological alternative for the diseased organ or tissue that can restore the functions. (Sittinger et al., 1996; Vacanti & Langer, 1999; Khademhosseini et al., 2009). Some degradable polymers, ceramics, or a combination of both can provide desirable mechanical and osteoconductive properties as basic scaffold material for bone replacement (Zippel et al., 2010b). Different factors should be considered for the use of such a biomaterial scaffold. It should imitate the three dimensional environment of the extracellular matrix, it should provide stability until replaced by regrown bone tissue and serve as an extended surface area for migration, adhesion, and differentiation of cells to encourage the growth of new tissue (Schultz et al., 2000; Ringe et al., 2002; Moroni et al., 2008).

The proliferating cells cover the scaffold and can grow into three dimensional tissue within. They are also an important factor for forming new tissue through extracellular matrix synthesis (Bonassar & Vacanti, 1998). Due to the development of new blood vessels towards, and to some extent onto, the new tissue, the scaffold begins to degenerate from the outside and is reconstituted by new natural bone tissue. As tissue related cell types cannot always be obtained in an adequate number or quality, SCs are a useful alternative for tissue regeneration.

Stem cells are the precursors of all cells and are involved in the repair system of the body. They are defined by three characteristics: self sustainability, self renewal and the potential of differentiation into different tissue types. For example adipocytes, astrocytes, chondroblasts, or osteoblasts come from mesenchymal stem cells (MSCs) (Pittenger et al., 1999; Pansky et al., 2007). In several publications, it has been suggested that MSCs can differentiate towards lineages that are naturally derived from the endoderm (Zuk et al., 2002; Tobiasch, 2009). Thus, increasing their potential because of these properties, the use of SCs to heal or rebuild damaged organs may provide an approach in future Regenerative Medicine (Zippel et al., 2010a).

SCs have been isolated from embryonic sources and well developed tissues of adult organism such as bone marrow, skin, dental pulp and adipose tissue (Kern et al., 2006). In addition two other sources for SCs have been discovered: cancer stem cells and induced pluripotent stem cells (iPS) (Takahashi et al., 2007; Aoi et al., 2008). Since the higher potency of embryonic stem cells and iPS compared to adult stem cells goes together with a higher risk of tumor formation, and embryonic stem cells are ethically problematic. Therefore, adult stem cells present themselves as an interesting cell source for bone replacement.

Adult stem cells can be divided into two main subpopulations: hematopoietic and mesenchymal stem cells (MSCs). Hematopoietic stem cells derived from bone marrow have been investigated best and could be a source for osteoclasts (Ash, 1980) (see Fig. 1). MSCs have been found in umbilical cord blood, bone marrow, and adipose tissue among others (Zuk et al., 2002). Generally, the isolation of MSCs is accomplished by plastic adherence resulting in colonies that are heterogeneous in size and morphology might contain contaminating non-mesenchymal cells such as macrophages or fibroblasts. The purity of isolated MSCs can be investigated by using the surface markers: CD73, CD90, and CD105 (should be expressed) and CD14, CD34 and CD45 (should not be expressed). These markers serve next to the adherence to plastic as a second feature for the identification and characterization of MSCs as suggested by the 'International Society for Cellular Therapy' (Dominici et al., 2006).

Another group of adult stem cells that has attracted attention are the ectomesenchymal stem cells derived from oral tissues. This stem cell group includes the dental pulp stem cells (DPSCs) and stem cells of human exfoliated deciduous teeth (SHEDs), both deriving from the pulpa, dental periodontal ligament stem cells (DPLSCs), dental follicle cells (DFCs), and stem cells from the apical papilla (SCAPs) (see Fig. 3). These cell types have the potential to differentiate into cells of all dental tissue types and bone as well. They share common phenotypic markers of MSCs (Alipur et al., 2010).

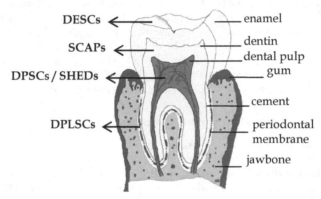

Fig. 3. Stem Cell Types in Tooth. From tooth different stem cell types namely, dental pulp stem cells (DPSCs), stem cells of human exfoliated deciduous teeth (SHEDs), dental periodontal ligament stem cells (DPLSCs), dental enamel derived stem cells (DESCs), stem cells from the apical papilla (SCAPs) and dental follicle cells (DFCs) can be obtained.

In comparison to other dental sources, dental follicle cells (DFCs) can be easily obtained in high amounts from young and healthy donors, since they are isolated from tooth extraction material collected during surgical removal of wisdom teeth. As these cells are derived from young donors, long telomeres extend their lifespan which makes them interesting cells for Regenerative Medicine (Shay & Wright, 2010). The dental follicle develops from ectomesenchyme. It surrounds the developing tooth germ before eruption (Ten Cate, 1997; Wise, 2002). During embryonic development, the ectomesenchyme is partly derived from migrating cells of the cranial neural crest. Therefore, the cells derivative from dental follicle differ from mesenchymal stem cells isolated from other sources (Chung et al., 2004; Slootweg, 2009). Due to having the more ectodermal character, these cells can have a differentiation potential diverse from MSCs. As expected these cells can differentiate into hard tissue such as the periodontal, cementoblastic, chondrocytic, and osteogenic lineages.

ATSCs and DFCs, both show osteogenic differentiation potential and are thus suitable candidates for the use in bone regeneration for stable osseointegration of dental implants. As these cells are obtained from healthy individuals, they might be used as an autograft in the future. The transplantation not only of autologous but also of allogenic sources could provide benefits in comparison to other common procedures in bone regeneration. As MSCs have low immune characteristics, they appear to be suitable for allogenic therapeutic purposes, without activating the immune response in immunocompetent patients (Jung et al., 2009). In different studies the use of MSCs has been investigated to replace lost or damaged bone (Schaefer et al., 2000; Ringe et al., 2002). After tooth loss, jawbone degenerates and stable integration of dental implant needs a thick jawbone. To overcome this problem there are two different alternatives that can be considered for using SCs in dental implants. The reconstruction after bone defects with SCs to achieve a sufficient bone thickness to insert the implants and the loading of an implant or artificial tooth-root with SCs with the aim to realize a sufficient integration in the bone.

SCs have the capability to re-establish cell function, reverse cellular damage, and heal damaged tissue (Conrad and Huss, 2005). SCs could also be a source to regenerate human teeth in the future, as these cells have been successfully used to regenerate living teeth in rabbit extraction sockets (Hung et al., 2011). In some mammals like rodents, rabbits, prairie dogs, and pikas, the teeth can grow throughout life because in these mammals as the pulp cavity remains open permanently. While on the other hand in humans tooth cannot grow continuously as pulp cavity closes when the teeth are fully grown. Therefore this study cannot be adapted easily for the regeneration of teeth or teeth related tissues in humans but it at least provides interesting basic results that can be helpful for use of SCs in dental tissues.

3.3 Bone chips for the stabilization of dental implants

Another approach next to scaffold loaded with stem cells to overcome the problem of unstable dental implants is the use of particulated non-vascularized bone autografts. The particles can be collected during the implant-bed preparation in the process of drilling the hole for the implant into the bone. An advantage of the use of these bone chips is that this material can be expected to facilitate bone regeneration. However, contradictory statements were made about the quality of this material such as if it contains living cells. In addition, it is not clear how to disinfect the bone chips, which are contaminated with bacteria of the oral cavity due to the sampling process. To address these questions bone chips were collected from two different regions of bone: carticular bone and spongy bone (see Fig. 4).

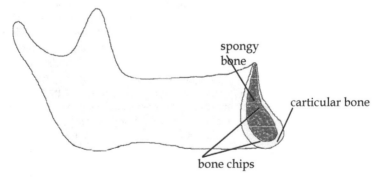

Fig. 4. Schematic Structure of Lower Jaw. Bone is composed of two tissue types mainly: spongious and carticular bone. Bone chips obtained during dental surgery for implant-bed preparation is derived from both bone tissue types.

4. Research methods

4.1 Isolation of primary cells for osteo-differentiation

4.1.1 Isolation of cells from tooth extraction material

For the isolation of ectomesenchymal stem cells, dental follicles were collected from human third molars before tooth eruption after surgical removal. The dental follicles were washed three times with 1 x PBS. Afterwards, the dental follicles were separated from the mineralized tooth and minced with a scalpel under sterile conditions. The tissue was digested in Collagenase (0.1 U / mL) and Dispase (0.8 U / mL) for 2 h at 37 °C in humidified atmosphere with 5 % CO_2. The cells were passed through a 100 μm strainer to obtain single-cell suspensions and seeded in 10 cm dishes in stem cell medium (SCM) that consisted of DMEM supplemented with 10 % FCS, 2 mM L-glutamine, 100 units / mL penicillin, 100 mg / mL streptomycin and 1 % amphotericin and cultured at 37 °C in a humidified atmosphere with 5 % CO_2. After 24 hours, non-adherent cells were removed by washing with 1 x PBS. The medium was changed and the plastic adherent cell fraction was cultured until 80 % confluent for further use.

The bone chip particles were collected with a bone filter integrated into a surgical suction pipe during the implant-bed preparation to isolate primary cells. For the isolation of bone chip derived cells (BCDCs), the same procedure as described above for DFCs was followed.

4.1.2 Isolation of adipose tissue derived stem cells

Human adipose tissue derived stem cells (ATSCs) were isolated from lipoaspirate obtained from plastic surgery. The isolation technique used during surgery was the tumescent liposuction technique. Using this particular technique, diluted epinephrine and lidocaine is infiltrated into the body fat to be removed, which leads to swelling and firmness of the targeted region, providing more accuracy during the liposuction procedure. The protocol was adjusted and modified to the procedure described by Zuk and colleagues (Zuk et al., 2001). The obtained lipoaspirate was augmented with PBS in a 1:2 ratio. After incubation for 30 minutes at room temperature (RT), two phases, a lower aqueous and upper fat phase of the lipoaspirate were obtained.

The lower phase was centrifuged at 200 x g for 10 minutes at RT. The resulting pellets, comprising the cells, were pooled and washed with 1 x PBS. Remaining erythrocytes were removed by applying 10 mL erythrolysis buffer for 10 minutes at RT. After another centrifugation step, under the same conditions as mentioned before, the cells were cultured in 60 cm^2 culture plates in SCM medium.

The upper phase comprising the fat tissue was augmented with 10 mg / mL type I collagenase in 1 x PBS and incubated for 45 minutes at 37 °C with agitation. The following steps for the treatment of the upper phase were according to the treatment of the lower phase. Cells of both phases were incubated at 37 °C with 5 % CO_2 in a humidified atmosphere. ATSCs were isolated due to their adherence to plastic and purified by washing with 1 x PBS after 24 hours, to remove undesired non-adherent cells.

4.2 Fluorescence activated cell sorting

The percentages of ATSCs or DFCs positive for the mesenchymal stem cell markers CD44, CD90 and CD105 and negative for CD14, CD45 and CD34 were measured using FACS analysis. The stem cells were trypsinized, centrifuged at 200 x g for 5 min and counted. 1 x 10^6 cells were resuspended in 1 mL 0.1 % PBSB and passed through a 100 µM cell strainer to obtain a single cell solution. 100 µL of the cell solution (100.000 cells) were incubated for 20 min in the dark with either the isotype control or the antibodies. Cells were washed with 2 mL 0.1 % (w / v) PBSB, centrifuged at 200 x g for 5 min and resuspended in 1 mL 0.1 % (w / v) PBSB. The cytometer settings and cell gates were adjusted to the isotype control, followed by measurement of the stem cell markers using the same conditions.

4.3 Adipogenic differentiation

For adipogenic induction, the isolated cells were seeded in a density of 2.8 x 10^3 cells / cm^2 in SCM. After one day, the medium was changed to adipogenic differentiation medium (AM), containing 1 µM dexamethasone, 1 µM insulin and 200 µM indomethacin. The cells were grown in AM for four weeks at 37 °C with 5 % CO_2 under humidified conditions. The AM was changed once a week. After four weeks, adipogenic differentiation was visualized with Oil Red O after fixing cells for 90 min with formalin (4 %) at 37 °C.

4.4 Osteogenic differentiation

The isolated cells were seeded in a density of 1.3 x 10^3 cells / cm^2 in 6 cm^2 and 12 well plates for osteogenic differentiation. After one day SCM was replaced with osteogenic medium (OM) containing dexamethasone, ascorbic acid and β-glycerophosphate. ATSCs were grown in OM for 4 weeks at 37 °C with 5 % CO_2 under humidified conditions. The OM medium was changed once a week. After four weeks, osteogenic differentiation was visualized by staining with Alizarin Red S after fixing cells for 5 min with formalin (4 %) at 37 °C.

4.5 Microbiological testing

Directly after surgery the obtained dental follicles were transferred into cold sodium chloride (0.9 % w / v) for determining possible microbial contaminations. The samples were kept cold until processing.

The samples were rolled over the surface of Columbia blood agar (CBA) and fastidious anaerobe agar (FAA) plates to isolate microorganisms. In addition the transport solution was put onto CBA and FAA plates. Under aerobic and anaerobic conditions the incubations were conducted over night at 37 °C. The Gas PakTM100-system was used for the incubation under anaerobic conditions. Single colonies were picked and isolated with respect to their morphological differences. Gram stainings, catalase- and oxidase-tests were used for the first characterization. API test strips were used to determine the exact bacteria species.

5. Comparison of stem cell sources

5.1 The characterization of ATSCs, DFCs and BCDCs for bone regeneration

The high plasticity of mesenchymal stem cells has resulted in an increased interest for their use in a variety of cellular therapies. However, different laboratories working with these cells isolate them from various tissue sources by following different protocols and characterizing these cells by different markers. Therefore, to set a standard, the minimal criteria for the definition of human MSCs were suggested by the 'Mesenchymal and Tissue Stem Cell Committee of The International Society for Cellular Therapy' (Dominici et al., 2006). The multipotent character of the isolated adipose tissue derived stem cells, ectomesenchymal dental follicle cells and bone chip derived cells was tested according to these criteria. MSCs were isolated from human adult adipose tissue of different aged female donors. DFCs were isolated from dental follicles and BCDCs from the bone chips collected during implant-bed preparation of male and female donors. The enrichment of specific stem cells was achieved due to their property of plastic adherence that is the first criterion for the testing of aMSCs character (Dominici et al., 2006). Isolated mesenchymal and ectomesenchymal cells of all donors showed a morphology similar to fibroblasts, which is typical for these stem cells (Yoshimura et al., 2006).

According to the above mentioned criteria the isolated cells should express the stem cell specific surface markers CD73, CD90, and CD105, and should not express CD14, CD34, and CD45. All isolated SC types expressed the expected markers (CD73, CD90 and CD105) as assessed by RT-PCR. The mesenchymal character of ATSCs and DFCs was also confirmed using FACS analysis for the presence of CD90, CD105, and in addition CD44. Furthermore, the cell types ATSCs and DFCs did not show the expression of leukocyte marker CD45 and macrophage marker CD14. ATSCs were positive and DFCs were negative for CD34. The presence of the expression of CD34 on ATSCs is controversial discussed. Some studies confirm the absence of CD34 expression on ATSCs (Zuk et al., 2002; Lee et al., 2004; Wagner et al., 2005) while other investigations showed ATSCs expressing CD34 (Mitchell et al., 2006; Yoshimura et al., 2006; De Francesco et al., 2009). These differences could be due to different stem cell isolation protocols, passage number or a different gating strategy during FACS analysis. In this study a subpopulation of ATSCs was stained positive for CD34.

Another typical MSCs character is the multilineage differentiation potential towards various lineages such as adipocytes, chondroblasts and osteoblasts. ATSCs showed a strong adipogenic differentiation potential whereas DFCs and BCDCs could not differentiate towards adipocytes. However, Kémoun and colleagues reported DFCs to differentiate towards the adipogenic lineage (Kémoun et al., 2007). The differences during isolation and precipitation in cell population might be possible reasons for this discrepancy. Also, DFCs can be different in their potency because these cells are derived from ectomesenchyme that is more committed toward hard tissue as tooth enamel.

According to all the findings mentioned above, the isolated ATSCs can be considered to belong to the population of multipotent MSCs, whereas the DFCs and BCDCs have a limited differentiation potential. Haddouti and colleagues showed that DFCs have a strong commitment towards the osteogenic lineage and show a more quantitative osteogenic differentiation (Haddouti et al., 2009). Thus, DFCs and BCDCs seem to be more committed towards osteogenic lineage.

Taken together all these stem cell types are good candidates for bone regeneration. But material from the oral cavity for isolation of primary cells such as DFCs and BCDCs cannot be obtained without microbial contamination. The question arises if this is a draw back on the use of these stem cells.

5.2 Microbial load of the oral tissue material

In order to evaluate the quality of the cells derived from oral tissues, microbiological investigations were performed. Our results revealed that all samples contained microbial species. Pre-treatment of patients with the antibiotics chlorhexidine (0.2 %), which is done anyway to decrease the chances of inflammation after surgery, reduced the number of microorganisms to less than 5 % but did not suffice to eliminate all bacteria. On the other hand pre-surgical, antibiotic treatment seemed to be negative for cell-outgrowth. To reduce contamination of the harvested cell-material, an optimized surgical procedure is more important than pre-surgical irrigation with chlorhexidine (0.2 %), and the use of a stringent dual suction pipe procedure. The predominantly found species were gram-positive cocci being either catalase-positive and oxidase-negative or catalase- and oxidase-negative. Most microorganisms belonged to the families of *Streptococcaceae* and *Staphylococcaceae*. The detected microorganisms did not interfere with cell growth and differentiation. They can be easily suppressed with standard antibiotics, applied routinely in patient treatment during the implantation procedure. Thus, these stem cells can be used for bone regeneration in dental implants.

6. Conclusion

The stability of dental implants is associated with a successful osseointegration into thick jawbone. Due to bone defects, bone regeneration is often needed before an implant can be inserted. For this stem cells can be a suitable candidates.

The stem cells isolated from adipose tissue, dental follicle and bone chips share mainly the multipotent character of mesenchymal stem cells. ATSCs can be successfully differentiated towards adipogenic and osteogenic lineages while DFCs and BCDCs did not show adipogenic differentiation. However, these cell types showed stronger commitment and differentiation towards osteogenic lineage. Therefore all three cell types are promising candidates for the treatment of various bone defects, and therefore also for the incorporation of tooth implants. They can be used to reconstruct jawbone defects to achieve enough bone thickness for the insertion of dental implants. It might be possible to load these cells on a dental implant or an artificial tooth root to increase its integration stability with the bone.

DFCs might be an ideal option if there will be a bank of donor material for these cells in the future, similar to those banks already existing as umbilical cord blood stem cells. If DFCs and BCDCs are not available for a specific patient, ATSCs are a reasonable option as they can differentiate towards the osteogenic lineage and be obtained from the patient itself as well, reducing the risk for rejection. Taken together all these tested stem cell types are suitable to improve the conditions for dental implants. Patients could preserve their dental follicle cells for later use in the future or their stem cells could be isolated from fat tissue directly before use. If a stem cell bank is arranged in the future, stem cells from other stem cell donors for dental follicle and fat tissue derived SCs could be used.

7. Acknowledgements

This work was supported by the BMBF-AIF, AdiPaD; FKZ: 1720X06 for ET and the Higher Education Commission of Pakistan, DAAD Germany for DK.

8. List of abbreviation

ALP	Alkaline phosphatase
AM	Adipogenic medium
ATSCs	Human adipose tissue derived mesenchymal stem cells
BCDCs	Bone chip derived cells
BMP2	Bone morphogenetic protien 2
°C	Degree centigrade
CBA	Columbia blood agar
CD14	Cluster of differentiation 14
CD34	Cluster of differentiation 34
CD45	Cluster of differentiation 45
CD73	Cluster of differentiation 73
CD90	Cluster of differentiation 90
CD105	Cluster of differentiation 105
cm	Centimeter
CO_2	Carbon dioxide
DESCs	Dental enamel derived stem cells
DFCs	Dental follicle cells
DMEM	Dulbecco's modified Eagle medium
DPLSCs	Dental periodontal ligament stem cells
DPSCs	Dental pulp stem cells
ECSs	Embryonic stem cells
FAA	Fastidious anaerobe agar
FACs	Fluorescence activated cell sorting
FCS	Fetal calf serum
iPS	Induced pluripotent stem cells
IGF-1	Insulin-like growth factor 1
LPL	Lipoprotein lipase
mL	Milliliter
mM	Millimolar
µL	Microliter
OM	Osteogenic medium
PBS	Phosphate buffer saline
PPARγ	Peroxisome proliferator-activated receptor gamma
RT	Room temperature
RT-PCR	Reverse transcriptase polymerase chain reaction
Runx2	Runt-related transcription factor 2
SCAPs	Stem cells from the apical papilla
SCM	Stem cell medium
SCs	Stem cells
SHEDs	Stem cells of human exfoliated deciduous teeth
w / v	Weight per volume
x g	Relative centrifugal force

9. References

Alipur, R., Sadeghi, F., Hashemi-Beni, B., Zarkesh-Esfahani, S.H., Heydari, F., Mousavi, S.B., Adib, M., Narimani, M., & Esmaeili, N. (2010). Phenotypic characterizations and comparison of adult dental stem cells with adipose-derived stem cells. Int. J. Prev. Med, 1, 164-171

Aoi, T., Yae, K., Nakagawa, M., Ichisaka, T., Okita, K., Takahashi, K., Chiba, T. & Yamanaka, S. (2008). Generation of pluripotent stem cells from adult mouse liver and stomach cells. Science, 321, 699-702

Ash, P., Loutit, J.F. & Townsend, K.M. (1980). Osteoclasts derived from haematopoietic stem cells. Nature, 283, 669-670

Baltzer, A.W., Lattermann, C., Whalen, J.D., Wooley, P., Weiss, K., Grimm, M., Ghivizzani, S.C., Robbins, P.D., & Evans, C.H. (2000). Genetic enhancement of fracture repair: healing of an experimental segmental defect by adenoviral transfer of the BMP-2 gene. Gene Ther, 7, 734-739

Bonassar, L.J. & Vacanti, C.A. (1998). Tissue engineering: The first decade and beyond. J. Cell. Biochem, 72, 297-303

Chung, U.I., Kawaguchi, H., Takato, T. & Nakamura, K. (2004). Distinct osteogenic mechanisms of bones of distinct origins. J. Orthop. Sci, 9, 410-414

Conrad, C. & Huss, R. (2005). Adult stem cell lines in regenerative medicine and reconstructive surgery. J. Surg. Res, 124, 201-208

De Francesco, F., Tirino, V., Desiderio, V., Ferraro, G., D'Andrea, F., Giuliano, M., Libondi, G., Pirozzi, G., De Rosa, A. & Papaccio, G. (2009). Human CD34+/CD90+ ASCs are capable of growing as sphere clusters, producing high levels of VEGF and forming capillaries. PLoS One, 4, e6537

Diagnosis and management of dental caries throughout Life. Consensus development conference statement, national institutes of health 2001

Dominici, M., Le Blanc, K., Mueller, I., Slaper-Cortenbach, I., Marini, F., Krause, D., Deans, R., Keating, A., Prockop, D. & Horwitz, E. (2006). Minimal criteria for defining multipotent mesenchymal stromal cells. The International Society for Cellular Therapy position statement. Cytotherapy, 8, 315-317

Garber, D.A. & Belser, U. (1995). Restoration-driven implant placement with restoration-generated site development. Compend. Contin. Educ. Dent, 16, 796-804

Haddouti, E.-M., Skroch, M., Zippel, N., Müller, C., Birova, B., Pansky, A., Kleinfeld, C., Winter, M. & Tobiasch, E. (2009). Human Dental Follicle Precursor Cells of Wisdom Teeth: Isolation and Differentiation towards Osteoblasts for Implants with and without Scaffolds. Mater. Sci. Engin. Technol, 40, 732-737

Hartmann, C. (2006). A Wnt canon orchestrating osteoblastogenesis. Trends. Cell. Biol, 16, 151-158

Holtfreter, B., Kocher, T., Hoffmann, T., Desvarieux, M., & Michaelis, W. (2010). Prevalence of periodontal disease and treatment demands based on a German dental survey (DMS IV). J. Clin. Periodontol, 37, 211-219

Hung, C.N., Mar, K., Chang, H.C., Chiang, Y.L., Hu, H.Y., Lai, C.C., Chu, R.M. & Ma, C.M. (2011). A comparison between adipose tissue and dental pulp as sources of MSCs for tooth regeneration. Biomaterial, 32, 6995-7005

Hutmacher, D.W., Schantz, J.T., Lam, C.X., Tan, K.C. & Lim, T.C. (2007). State of the art and future directions of scaffold-based bone engineering from a biomaterials perspective. J. Tissue. Eng. Regen. Med, 1, 245-260

Jung, D.I., Ha, J., Kang, B.T., Kim, J.W., Quan, F.S., Lee, J.H., Woo, E.J. & Park, H.M. (2009). A comparison of autologous and allogenic bone marrowderived mesenchymal stem cell transplantation in canine spinal cord injury. J. Neurol. Sci, 285, 67-77

Kémoun, P., Laurencin-Dalicieux, S., Rue, J., Farges, J.C., Gennero, I., Conte-Auriol, F., Briand-Mesange, F., Gadelorge, M., Arzate, H., Narayanan, A.S., Brunel, G. & Salles, J.P. (2007). Human dental follicle cells acquire cementoblast features under stimulation by BMP-2/-7 and enamel matrix derivatives (EMD) in vitro. Cell. Tissue. Res, 329, 283-294

Kern, S., Eichler, H., Stoeve, J., Kluter, H. & Bieback, K. (2006). Comparative analysis of mesenchymal stem cells from bone marrow, umbilical cord blood, or adipose tissue. Stem Cells, 24, 1294-1301

Khademhosseini, A., Vacanti, J.P. & Langer, R. (2009). Progress in tissue engineering. Sci. Am, 300, 64-71

Laurencin, C., Khan, Y. & El-Amin, S.F. (2006). Bone graft substitutes. Expert. Rev. Med. Devices, 3, 49-57

Lee, R.H., Kim, B., Choi, I., Kim, H., Choi, H.S., Suh, K., Bae, Y.C. & Jung, J.S. (2004). Characterization and expression analysis of mesenchymal stem cells from human bone marrow and adipose tissue. Cell. Physiol. Biochem, 14, 311-324

Lietman, S.A., Tomford, W.W., Gebhardt, M.C., Springfield, D.S. & Mankin, H.J. (2000). Complications of irradiated allografts in orthopaedic tumor surgery. Clin. Orthop. Relat. Res, 375, 214-217

Mitchell, J.B., McIntosh, K., Zvonic, S., Garrett, S., Floyd, Z.E., Kloster, A., Di Halvorsen, Y., Storms, R.W., Goh, B., Kilroy, G., Wu, X. & Gimble, J.M. (2006). Immunophenotype of human adipose-derived cells: temporal changes in stromal-associated and stem cell-associated markers. Stem Cells, 24, 376-385

Moroni, L., Wijn, J. & Van Blitterswijk, A. (2008). Integrating novel technologies to fabricate smart scaffolds. J. Biomater. Sci. Polymer Edn, 19, 543-572

Pansky, A., Roitzheim, B & Tobiasch, E. (2007). Differentiation potential of adult human mesenchymal stem cells. Clin Lab, 53, 81-84

Pittenger, M., Mackay, A., Beck, S., Jaiswal, R., Douglas, R., Mosca, J., Moorman, M., Simonetti, D., Craig, S. & Marshak, D. (1999). Multilineage potential of adult human mesenchymal stem cells. Science, 284, 143-147

Rho, J., Tsui, T. & Pharr, G. (1997). Elastic properties of human cortical and trabecular lamellar bone measured by nanoindentation. Biomaterials, 18, 1325-1330

Ringe, J., Kaps, C., Burmester, G.-R. & Sittinger, M. (2002). Stem cells for regenerative medicine: advances in the engineering of tissues and organs. Naturwissenschaften, 89, 338-351

Seeman, E & Delmas, P.D. (2006). Bone quality—the material and structural basis of bone strength and fragility. N. Engl. J. Med, 354, 2250-2261

Schaefer, D., Klemt, C., Zhang, X., & Stark, G. (2000). Tissue engineering with mesenchymal stem cells for cartilage and bone regeneration. Chirurg, 71, 1001-1008

Schäffler, A. & Büchler, C. (2007). Concise review: adipose tissue-derived stromal cells--basic and clinical implications for novel cell-based therapies. Stem Cells, 25, 818-827

Schultz, O., Sittinger, M., Haeupl, T. & Burmester, G.R. (2000). Emerging strategies of bone and joint repair. Arthritis. Res, 2, 433 – 436

Sengupta, A. & Cancelas, J.A. (2010). Cancer stem cells: A stride towards cancer cure? J. Cell. Physiol, 225, 7-14

Shay, J.W. & Wright, W.E. (2010). Telomeres and telomerase in normal and cancer stem cells. FEBS Lett, 584, 3819-3825

Sittinger, M., Bujia, J., Rotter, N., Reitzel, D., Minuth, W.W. & Burmester, G.R. (1996). Tissue engineering and autologous transplant formation: practical approaches with resorbable biomaterials and new cell culture techniques. Biomaterials, 17, 237-242

Slootweg, P.J. (2009). Lesions of the jaws. Histopathology, 54, 401-418

Sorger, J.I., Hornicek, F.J., Zavatta, M., Menzner, J.P., Gebhardt, M.C., Tomford, W.W. & Mankin, H.J. (2001). Allograft fractures revisited. Clin. Orthop. Relat. Res, 382, 66-74

Takahashi, K., Okita, K., Nakagawa, M. & Yamanaka, S. (2007). Induction of pluripotent stem cells from fibroblast cultures. Nat. Protoc, 2, 3081-3089

Ten Cate, A.R. (1997). The development of the periodontium - a largely ectomesenchymally derived unit. Periodontology, 13, 9-19

Tessier, P. (1982). Autogenous bone grafts taken from the calvarium for facial and cranial applications. Clin. Plast. Surg, 9, 531-538

Tessier, P., Kawamoto, H., Matthews, D., Posnick, J., Raulo, Y., Tulasne, J.F. & Wolfe, S.A. (2005a). Autogenous bone grafts and bone substitutes--tools and techniques: I. A 20,000-case experience in maxillofacial and craniofacial surgery. Plast. Reconstr. Surg, 116, 6-24

Tessier, P., Kawamoto, H., Posnick, J., Raulo, Y., Tulasne, J.F. & Wolfe, S.A. (2005b). Complications of harvesting autogenous bone grafts: a group experience of 20,000 cases. Plast. Reconstr. Surg, 116, 72-73

Tobiasch, E. (2009) Adult human mesenchymal stem cells as source for future tissue engineering, Forschungsspitzen und Spitzenforschung. Zacharias, C., Horst, KW Ter., Witt, K.-U., Sommer, V., Ant, M. Essmann, U and Mülheim, L. 329-338, Spring Verlag, ISBN: 978-3-7908-2126-0

Vacanti, J. & Langer, R. (1999). Tissue engineering: the design and fabrication of living replacement devices for surgical reconstruction and transplantation. Lancet, 354, 132-34

Wagner, W., Wein, F., Seckinger, A., Frankhauser, M., Wirkner, U., Krause, U., Blake, J., Schwager, C., Eckstein, V., Ansorge, W. & Ho, A.D. (2005). Comparative characteristics of mesenchymal stem cells from human bone marrow, adipose tissue, and umbilical cord blood. Exp. Hematol, 33, 1402-1416

Wise, G.E., Frazier-Bowers, S. & D'Souza, R.N. (2002). Cellular, molecular, and genetic determinants of tooth eruption. Crit. Rev. Oral. Biol. Med, 13, 323-334

Yoshimura, K., Shigeura, T., Matsumoto, D., Sato, T., Takaki, Y., Aiba-Kojima, E., Sato, K., Inoue, K., Nagase, T., Koshima, I. & Gonda, K. (2006). Characterization of freshly isolated and cultured cells derived from the fatty and fluid portions of liposuction aspirates. J. Cell. Physiol, 208, 64-76

Younger, E.M. & Chapman, M.W. (1989). Morbidity at bone graft donor sites. J. Orthop. Trauma, 3, 192-195

Zippel, N., Limbach C.A., Ratajski, N., Urban, C., Luparello, C., Pansky, A., Kassack, M.U., & Tobiasch, E. (2010a) Purinergic Receptors Influence the Differentiation of Human Mesenchymal Stem Cells," Stem cells & Development. Epub ahead of print doi:10.1089/scd.2010.0576.

Zippel, N., Schulze, M. & Tobiasch, E. (2010b). Biomaterials and mesenchymal stem cells for regenerative medicine. Recent. Pat. Biotechnol, 4, 1-22

Zuk, P., Zhu, M., Ashjian, P., De Ugarte, D., Huang, J., Mizuno, H., Alfonso, Z., Fraser, J., Benhaim, P. & Hedrick, M. (2002). Human adipose tissue is a source of multipotent stem cells. Mol. Biol. Cell, 13, 4279-4295

Part 2

Use of Scaffolds

4

Preparation of Deproteinized Human Bone and Its Mixtures with Bio-Glass and Tricalcium Phosphate – Innovative Bioactive Materials for Skeletal Tissue Regeneration

Magdalena Cieslik[1], Jacek Nocoń[2], Jan Rauch[3], Tadeusz Cieslik[4],
Anna Ślósarczyk[5], Maria Borczuch-Łączka[6] and Aleksander Owczarek[7]
[1]Faculty and Institute of Stomatological Materials Science,
Medical University of Silesia, Katowice, Bytom,
[2]Private Dentistry Practice, Oberhausen,
[3]NZOZ – Specialist Dentistry Clinic, Wadowice,
[4]Faculty and Clinic of Oral and Maxillofacial Surgery,
Medical University of Silesia, Katowice,
[5]Faculty of Glass Technology and Amorphous Coatings,
AGH - Krakow University of Science and Technology, Kraków,
[6]Faculty of Ceramic Technology,
AGH - Krakow University of Science and Technology, Kraków,
[7]Division of Statistics, Medical University of Silesia, Katowice, Sosnowiec,
[1,3,4,5,6,7]Poland
[2]Germany

1. Introduction

Repair of the skeletal system is one of the principal research problems in medical science is closely associated with the field of material engineering. The reasons for using bone implants and grafts include injuries, infections, neoplasms and other hard tissue lesions. Bone replacement materials are predominantly used in medical disciplines such as dentistry, dental surgery, maxillofacial surgery and plastic surgery, as well as in orthopedics and traumatology (Barradas et al., 2011; Kao & Scott, 2007; Precheur, 2007).

From a biological, immunological, and legal point of view, autogenous bone grafting still remains a very popular method in reconstruction following skeletal loss (Block, 2002; Giannoudis et al., 2005). Factors considered in the selection of the source of the bone graft include, among others, the ease of surgical access and the volume of bone mass required (Precheur, 2007). The type of autogenous bone used as a graft (cortical bone vs. cancellous bone) should also be considered. For instance, the higher content of morphogenetic proteins (BMPs) in cortical bone means that grafts of this type induce the process of bone growth more effectively than cancellous bone grafts. Nonetheless, skeletal reconstruction with autogenous bone grafts always requires additional surgical manipulations that constitute an increased burden to the patient and prolong the duration of the procedure. Another very frequent limitation of using autogenous bone is its poor quality, when there is a skeletal system disorder (e.g. osteoporosis) (Bohner, 2010; Giannoudis et al., 2005). Allogenic implants derived from the structures of human bones can be one alternative to autogenous grafts (Ferreira, 2007). Mineralized (FDBA) and demineralized (DFDBA) forms of such implants, additionally subjected to lyophilization, are most frequently used in reconstructive surgery. An advantage of demineralized bone arises from the fact that the organic bone matrix (collagen fibers) has to be exposed in order to remove its mineral components, and therefore so-called matrix proteins (e.g. morphogenetic proteins) can easily diffuse into the implantation site and work osteoinductively (Barradas et al., 2011). Xenogenic implants also play an important role in reconstructive bone surgery. These implants are made of skeletal material obtained from animals (Merkx et al., 2003), in most cases from equine, bovine or porcine bones. Animal material is processed by means of thermal treatment in order to deplete it completely of its organic components (Barakat et al., 2009). As a result, implants lose their immunogenic properties and become neutral to hosts (Liu et al., 2008). Therefore, ready to use preparations for bone replacement (Bio-Oss®, Endobone®) are most frequently available in deproteinized forms (DBBM) (Accorsi-Mendonça et al., 2008). Due to their osteoconductive properties they can serve as an inactive scaffold or platform for the maturation of bone cells present within the defect. They are used in orthopedics, dental and maxillofacial surgery, as well as in periodontology and implantology, etc. (Baldini et al., 2011; Cao et al., 2009; Jian et al., 2008; Merkx et al., 2003; Precheur, 2007; von Wattenwyl et al., 2011). The limited possibilities of modulating the resorption time of such preparations during skeletal tissue reconstruction, however, can be related to the poorer quality of bone at the site of their application.

An alternative solution, eliminating the potential complications associated with the application of materials of autogenous, allogenic or xenogenic origin, is the use of alloplastic implants for the purpose of bone replacement. Such implants can be synthesized from both natural and synthetic materials (Bohner, 2010; Giannoudis et al., 2005). Bioresorbable ceramic based on calcium phosphate plays a distinct role amongst novel synthetic materials used for bone replacement (Barradas et al., 2011). Hydroxyapatite (HAp) is the principal representative of this group, with the widest application in reconstructive surgery. Due to its calcium phosphate content and natural occurrence as an inorganic substance in bones and teeth, hydroxyapatite is characterized by the highest biocompatibility and bioactivity of all currently known implant materials. Additionally, due to the osteoconductive properties of hydroxyapatite, and (to a lesser extent) its osteoinductive properties, hydroxyapatite-based implants can bind directly to bone. Numerous clinical trials, supported by the results of histological observations, have confirmed complete biotolerance to hydroxyapatite ceramic, as well as its positive effects on the process of bone healing and reconstruction. Additionally, hydroxyapatite ceramic can initiate and stimulate various processes that are associated with bone formation (Bellucci et al., 2011; Ravarian et al., 2010; Yuan et al., 2001). Contact between bioactive ceramic and living skeletal tissue induces osteogenesis. As a result, an intermediate binding layer is formed between the living tissue and the implant, serving as a kind of biological glue. The structural similarity of calcium phosphate-based ceramic and the natural mineral components of bone is crucial for infiltration of the implant by the skeletal tissue of the host. This supports the intra-tissue application of hydroxyapatite-based implants whenever long-term remodeling of bone is required. Beta-

Preparation of Deproteinized Human Bone and Its Mixtures with Bio-Glass and Tricalcium Phosphate – Innovative
Bioactive Materials for Skeletal Tissue Regeneration

69

tricalcium phosphate (betaTCP, betaCa$_3$(PO$_4$)$_2$) is another calcium phosphate that has been used successfully in bone substitution. Its mineralogical analogue is whitlockite (TCP) (Barradas et al., 2011). Similar to HAp, TCP is characterized by high biocompatibility. In comparison to hydroxyapatite materials, it has a higher solubility *in vitro* and a resultant higher susceptibility to resorption and biodegradation in the environment of the living organism (Bohner, 2010; Henkel et al., 2006). TCP is considered an osteoinductive material, which stimulates the processes of bone reconstruction (Wang et al., 2009). Many studies, mostly dealing with the gradual, controlled resorption rate of calcium phosphate ceramic, resulted in the design of the second polymorphic variant of TCP, namely αTCP (Zima et al., 2010). Similar to beta-TCP, it is formed as a result of the non-stoichiometric heating of HAp with a well-defined temperature and defined kinetics of thermal processing. Compared to beta-TCP, αTCP has an approximately five-fold higher susceptibility to resorption in living tissues, along with higher biocompatibility (Oonishi et al., 1999). The high degree of osteointegration of αTCP-based bioceramic is plausibly the result of the higher solubility of αCa$_3$(PO$_4$)$_2$ than of HAp or βTCP. Delivered within the ceramic, calcium and phosphate ions constitute the material for synthesizing the layer composed of non-stoichiometric hydroxyapatite that binds the implant to bone (Kon et al., 1995). Some authors suggest that αTCP can be cytotoxic, probably due to pH changes that are induced *in vitro* (Santos et al., 2002). These suggestions, however, were not confirmed during *in vivo* studies, and αTCP is included in many commercially available bone cements. Since the 1990s, biphasic HAp-βTCP ceramic (BCP biphasic calcium phosphate) has also been used in the reconstruction of skeletal defects (Deculsi, 1998, Deculsi et al., 2003; Fellah et al., 2008; Schwarz et al., 2007).

Bio-glass and apatite-wollastonite glass-ceramic also play an important role amongst the bioactive materials used in the processes of bone synthesis. The biological activity of glass and glass-derived crystalline materials (glass-ceramic materials) is mostly exploited for the manufacture of surface-active implants or implants that can be resorbed in the human body (Giannoudis et al., 2005). The composition of surface-active materials is selected in order to enable interactions between the physiological environment and certain components of the implant. As a result, living tissue is bound to the implant surface. Resorbable glass is characterized by its high content of chemical elements involved in metabolic processes of the human body. In both cases, living tissues can infiltrate the implant and bind it directly to the bone. These processes result not only from the chemical composition of the implants but also from the specific nature of the contained glass substance. The binding abilities of bioactive glass and glass-ceramic implants to skeletal tissue have been the subject of many studies. These studies confirmed the usefulness of such materials in tissue engineering, where they can be used in cell culture (Ferreira, 2007; Xynos et al., 2000). Their application in reconstructive surgery is reflected by their ability to stimulate and supporting bone reconstruction. In view of their confirmed ability to directly bind to skeletal tissue, they have been used successfully in various stomatological disciplines, including implantology, dental surgery and periodontology. Moreover, modern surface engineering has allowed the coating of metal implants with bioactive glass. Such coatings either protect surfaces of metal alloys against corrosion and wear, or stimulate the processes of bone formation in their surroundings. Additionally, resorbable glass can be used as a drug carrier, providing prolonged release of an active substance. Furthermore, some attempts have been made to combine various materials with each other to manufacture glass-containing bioactive composites, used as the components of binders, among others (Bellucci et al., 2011). These experiments were aimed at obtaining biomaterials with better durability parameters and optimal biological characteristics. Various types of bio-glass and glass-ceramics may differ in terms of their biological properties, depending on the technique for their synthesis (Bellucci et al., 2011; Yuan et al. 2001). Amongst various methods of synthesis, the advantages of the chemical sol-gel method are worth noting. This technique enables material whose biological activity is greater than products manufactured using other processing methods to be obtained (Ravarian et al., 2010). Moreover, the sol-gel method does not require high temperature processing. Additionally, this technique allows the production of material with a strictly defined texture and parameters. Due to the possibility of manufacturing porous forms, bio-glass and glass-derived crystalline materials are morphologically similar to bone; this facilitates their infiltration by bone cells at the implantation site. Additionally, the porous structure of the implant enables the supply of fluids and nutrients required for growth to the newly formed bone, as well as the elimination of metabolites (Yuan et al., 2001). Finally, the resorption rate of the implant material is also determined by the degree of its porosity.

In view of the complexity of the biological environment at the implantation site, one principle problem of biomaterial engineering pertains to issues associated with the biodegradation and bioresorption of implanted biomaterials. Determination of degradation time and rate, and the kinetics of this process in the human body, constitute a significant challenge in the design of new implant materials (including bioceramic) used for the purposes of skeletal tissue substitution (Daculsi et al., 2003; Giannoudis et al., 2005). The controlled degradation rate of the implant along with the associated reconstruction of skeletal tissue should result in the formation of bone tissue resembling its natural structure as closely as possible, both at the biological and physico-mechanical levels. One of many methods allowing for the controlled biodegradation of bone replacement materials is the design of implants made of various composites or mixtures. Combining two or more different materials results in the manufacture of an absolutely new composite biomaterial, which is frequently superior in terms of biological and mechanical properties. Due to its specific properties, bioceramic is very frequently used as a basic component of ceramic-ceramic, metal-ceramic and polymer-ceramic systems (Thomas et al., 2005). Hydroxyapatite is very frequently included in bone composites, mostly due to its chemical similarity to the natural components of bone. Some studies have confirmed the positive effects of hydroxyapatite used in combination with metals, ceramic or polymers (Abu Bakar et al., 2003; Bellucci et al., 2011; Choi et al., 2004; Daculsi et al., 2003). The results of research on HAp-containing composites based on resorbable polymers, mostly polylactide (PLA), polyglycolide (PGA), co-polymer of glycolide and lactide (PLGA) or collagen [Cieślik et al., Nagata et al., 2005], seem particularly interesting. These studies confirmed the possible application of such composites as binding and reconstructive elements in reconstructive surgery, as culture media in tissue and genetic engineering, and as drug carriers (Wei & Ma, 2004; Nagata et al., 2003). Although hydroxyapatite is characterized by high biocompatibility, its reactivity with living skeletal tissue is relatively low. In view of these findings, attempts to design composites that combine this biomaterial with markedly more biologically active bio-glass propose an interesting solution. Such a composite can stimulate osteogenesis, leading to the rapid formation of new skeletal tissue around the implant (Yuan et al., 2001; Ravarian et al., 2010). Biological tests of SiO_2-CaO-Mg/natural HAp (bovine bone) composite obtained by means of thermal plasma processing have confirmed its lack of

Preparation of Deproteinized Human Bone and Its Mixtures with Bio-Glass and Tricalcium Phosphate – Innovative
Bioactive Materials for Skeletal Tissue Regeneration

71

toxicity. Moreover, the glass-ceramic contained in this composite was confirmed to stimulate the growth and proliferation of human fibroblasts (Yoganand et al., 2010). Attempts at bone replacement with materials obtained by combining autogenous bone and deproteinized bovine bone constitute another example of the potential optimization of biological conditions for new skeletal tissue growth within a skeletal defect. The inclusion of autogenous material with osteoinductive properties in such composites results in the enhanced formation of better quality bone (Kim et al., 2009; Pripatnanont et al., 2009; Thorwarth et al., 2006; Thuaksuban et al., 2010). *In vitro* cellular studies have confirmed that allogenic materials of human origin (demineralized bone matrix, deproteinized bone) may also have some osteoinductive activity. This activity was confirmed by an increase in alkaline phosphatase (ALP), osteocalcin (OC) and Ca^{2+} concentrations observed in human bone marrow stromal osteoprogenitor cells (hBMSCs) cultured for three weeks in medium based on human bone components (Zhang et al., 2009).

The increasing demand for bone replacement materials stimulated us to design original composite materials for use in the regeneration of skeletal defects, characterized by both osteoinductive and osteoconductive properties. In designing such composites, we have used well-described biomaterials that have been applied successfully to skeletal defect regeneration, namely bio-glass (BG) and tricalcium phosphate (TCP). Lyophilized human bone obtained from a tissue bank served as a base for designing three types of mixtures: 1) human bone/bio-glass; 2) human bone/TCP; and 3) human bone/bio-glass/TCP. Such variants of material combinations enabled us to analyze the effects of particular components on the process of bone formation, and specifically on its dynamics and on the quality of newly formed bone. Also, the selection of the components included among the analyzed materials (mixtures) was not accidental. We have assumed that both bio-glass and tricalcium phosphate will activate and stimulate osteoblasts to dynamically grow on a biological scaffold of lyophilized human bone, thereby providing optimal biological conditions for the formation of full value bone.

2. Material

The materials used in the study included lyophilized, deproteinized human bone (B) – group B, and its mixtures with: 1) bio-glass (BG) in a proportion of 80:20% weight ratio (B:BG) – group B+BG; 2) tricalcium phosphate (TCP) in a proportion of 80:20% weight ratio (B:TCP) – group B+TCP; 3) bio-glass and tricalcium phosphate in a proportion of 70:15:15% weight ratio (B:BG:TCP) – group B+BG+TCP. The deproteinized human bone and all other components used in the mixtures were in a granulated form with diameters ranging from 0.3 to 0.5 mm.

Human bone used in this study was obtained from the Tissue Bank of the Regional Center of Blood Donation and Treatment in Katowice (Poland). It was cancellous bone subjected to lyophilization, deep freezing and irradiation sterilization with a dose of 35 kGy.

The bio-glass was made from the $CaO\text{-}SiO_2\text{-}P_2O_5$ system with the use of the sol-gel technology, in the laboratory of the Department of Glass and Amorphous Coatings at the AGH Science and Technology University in Cracow, Poland. Its high-calcium A2 variety was used (54% mol. CaO) with a density of 2.9082 g/cm^3, a dominating glassy phase and the beginnings of apatite crystallization. The thermal treatment of the bio-glass was performed at a temperature of 800°C, and its specific surface area (calculated by BET method) amounted to 57.8166 m²/g.

Resorbable, monophasic βTCP ceramic – a salt of trialkaline orthophosphoric acid $Ca_3(PO_4)_2$ – was synthesized from powdered components obtained by means of wet synthesis in the Bioceramic Laboratory of the Department of Ceramic and Fire Resistant Material Technology at the AGH Science and Technology University in Cracow, Poland (Ślósarczyk & Paszkiewicz, 2005; Zima at al., 2010). The reagents included CaO (obtained by means of calcination of Ca(OH)₂ – pure for analysis; MERCK, Poland), and H_3PO_4 (pure for analysis; POCH, Poland).

3. *In vivo* animal experiments

The study was carried out on a group of 48 guinea pigs, with an equal number of both sexes, and weights ranging from 500 to 600 grams. The animals were divided randomly into four groups, which corresponded to 12 animals for each studied composite material (6 males and 6 females). The animal experiments were performed on the 7th, 14th, and 21st days of the study, as well as after the 4th, 8th and 12th experimental weeks. Two guinea pigs (one male and one female) were examined in each experiment. All animal surgical procedures were performed at the Central Experimental Animal Farm at the Medical University of Silesia and were granted permission by the university's Bioethical Board for Experimental Animals.

Before starting any surgical procedures, the animals received general anesthesia with thiopental (0.4 g/kg b.w.). Bone defects (6 mm in diameter and 3 mm in depth) were formed bilaterally on the external surface of the mandibular trunk, 2 mm below its lower edge (between the radices of the incisive and molar teeth) with the aid of a rosette burr placed in the straight hand-piece of a dental machine (Fig.1a). Depending on the experimental group, bone defects on the right side of the mandible were filled with: 1) a preparation of deproteinized human bone (group B), 2) a mixture of deproteinized human bone and bio-glass (group B+BG), 3) a mixture of deproteinized human bone and tricalcium phosphate (group B+TCP), or 4) a mixture of deproteinized human bone with bio-glass and tricalcium phosphate (group B+BG+TCP). Before implantation into the mandibular bone defect, each material was mixed with the animal's blood obtained from the surgical wound (Fig. 1b) in a

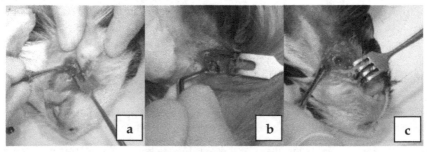

Fig. 1. Bone defect in the mandibular trunk of the experimental animal: a) defect prepared for filling with implant based on deproteinized human bone; b) defect filled with the mixture of deproteinized human bone and bio-glass with animal's blood; c) control defect filled with postoperatively clotted blood

proportion of 25:75% weight ratio (examined material to blood). Blood served as a binder, supplying the implanted material with organic components. Additionally, it prevented the displacement of the implanted granules from within the bone defect, and facilitated their insertion. The defect on the left side of the mandible was left to fill postoperatively with clotted blood and undergo spontaneous healing (Fig.1c), and was considered a control to the right mandibular defect in each animal (control group). The bilateral wounds were closed in multiple layers with Dexon 4.0 sutures.

4. Methods of examination

On each examination day, all guinea pigs were clinically evaluated for surgical wound healing and general condition. Additionally, radiographs were taken in order to assess the regeneration of mandibular bone defects. Newly formed skeletal tissue in the defects was also analyzed quantitatively and qualitatively in terms of bone mineral density at the implantation site (computed tomography and radiographic densitometry). Following euthanasia with Morbital (sodium pentobarbital 133.3 mg/mL and pentobarbital 26.7 mg/mL, 1-2 mL/kg b.w.), the operated area and surrounding tissues were examined macroscopically. Moreover, tissue specimens from the euthanized animals were subjected to histopathologic analysis of the skeletal tissue and bone marrow at the implantation site and at its periphery, including the healing rate of the skeletal tissue and the soft and hard tissue reactions to the implanted material. Histopathologic analysis also included organs involved in detoxification of the body (i.e. liver and kidneys).

Radiographs of the mandibular trunk with the sites of the bone defects were taken with a Heliodent type MD/D – 3195 nr 051692 apparatus (SIEMENS), and AGFA DENTUS M2 CONFORT films for axial pictures (75 mm x 65mm), using the following exposure conditions: 0.16 s, 7 mA and 60 kV.

The tissue specimens taken for the histopathologic examinations were preserved in a 10% solution of buffered formalin. The osseous tissue was decalcified either in a 10% solution of disodium versenate, or electrolytically in Romeis liquid (80 mL of hydrochloric acid + 100 mL of formic acid, diluted to make 1000 mL with water) using PW23 bone decalcifier and an electric current of 0.5A. Next, all the tissues were routinely processed in Technicon's Duo autotechnicon using the sequence of 96% alcohol, acetone and xylene. They were then embedded in paraplast. The obtained cubes were then shaved on a Microm HM335E rotating microtome. The shavings (4-6 microns in thickness) were put onto basic slides, deparaffinized, and stained with hematoxylin and eosin (H&E). They were subsequently mounted with Canada balsam. Histologic slides were analyzed under an Olympus BX50 light microscope equipped with a set for optical (Olympus SC35) and digital microphotography (Olympus Canmedia C-5050 Zoom), at 40 to 400 x magnification. Additionally, the slides were consulted by other histologists using a dual-head Nikon Labophot-2 microscope.

Bone mineral density (BMD) was determined by means of dual-energy X-ray absorptiometry (DXA) with a DPX-L densitometer (LUNAR Radiation Corporation, Madison, USA) using Small Animal Appendicular scanning. Total bone mineral density (BMD; g/cm^2) was determined on the basis of examination of the entire area of the transverse cross-section of the bone defect (28.26 mm^2), analyzed as 0.5 mm^2 to 3 mm^2 sections. One hundred and twenty

BMD measurements were taken in each group (corresponding to 20 measurements per experimental day). In most cases, reproducible results were not included in further analysis; only unique values and the most frequent reproducible values were analyzed, which corresponded to 10 BMD measurements for each day of examination. Additionally, the BMD of the normal mandibular trunk of the guinea pig was determined for the purpose of comparative analysis. Based on 10 consecutive measurements, this value was estimated at 0.51 $\pm$ 0.001 g/cm^2. During the measurements, the densitometer was regularly calibrated and controlled according to the manufacturer's recommendations. Both DXA measurements and BMD result analysis were performed by the same investigator.

Additionally, computed tomography (CT) was used to determine the bone mineral density, expressed in Hounsfield units (HU). These measurements were taken using a Somatom Emotion 6 scanner (Siemens; exposure parameters: 13.4 s, 14 mA, 130 kV). Transverse cross-sections of the mandible were visualized in 2 mm slices. Then, cross-sections including the area of the bone defect were selected and analyzed using Volume Viewer software. In each experimental group, six measurements were taken for each examination day. Additionally, six measurements of the normal mandible were taken for the purpose of comparative analysis. Based on these measurements, the normal bone mineral density was determined to be 1218 $\pm$ 15.2 HU.

The results of bone density are presented as mean values $\pm$ standard deviation. Variables distribution was evaluated by the Shapiro-Wilk test. Homogeneity of variance was assessed by the Levene test. ANOVA for repeated measurements with contrasts analysis were done to assess time and preparation of deproteinized human bone type interaction. The Mauchley test was done to check sphericity. Differences were considered to be statistically significant at $p<0.05$. All calculations were performed using the commercially available statistical package Statistica 9.0.

5. Results

5.1 Clinical observations

Throughout the entire study period, no complications in surgical wound healing were observed in animals of any experimental group. The guinea pigs were calm, which suggested a lack of pain. The animals ate and drank water normally, and neither scraped against the cage nor scratched their wounds during the entire postoperative period. Also, wound dehiscence was not observed in any of the groups.

Tissue edema over the surgical skin wounds resolved 3 to 5 days following surgery and was replaced by protrusions of the tissue. There were no signs of excessive fluid accumulation around the wound or of hematoma formation, but in some animals skin redness was observed around the stitches. In most animals, tissue protrusions persisted until the 21st day after surgery. The stitches were removed 10 to 14 days after surgery. Over the entire study period, the animals gained weight gradually (in a statistically insignificant manner).

5.2 Macroscopic examination

Up to 14th experimental day, the sites of the implanted bone defects were clearly distinguishable from the surrounding tissues as clear, oval protrusions covered with delicate tissue, which could be compressed elastically. Additionally, clearly distinguishable white granulation was visible throughout the superficial tissue in animals of the B+BG and B+BG+TCP groups. Probably, these granules corresponded to the bio-glass particles included in the material implanted in these groups. In the control group, the site of the bone defect was visible as a clear protrusion up to the 7th experimental day. On the next day of examination (the 14th day), however, the site was covered with a tissue whose coloration was darker in comparison to the surrounding tissues.

After the 3rd experimental week, the protrusion visible over the implantation site in groups B+BG, B+TCP and B+BG+TCP was markedly smaller in size, and covered with a hard tissue of more compact texture. Coloration of the tissues covering the implantation site still differed from the color of normal bone. In group BG, white granulation was still visible throughout the superficial tissue. On the 21st day after surgery, the coloration of the bone defect implanted with deproteinized human bone (group B) resembled the color of the surrounding tissues more closely than in previous periods. In both group B and in the control group, clearly distinguishable small areas in the form of a dark-colored spot were visible within the defects. Additionally, tissue protrusion observed over the defects in the control group increased in size when compared to previous periods.

Four weeks following implantation, the area of the bone defect in group B+BG was slightly smaller in size but still clearly distinguishable and differed in color from the surrounding tissues. Similar changes were observed in the B+TCP group; the implantation site in this group was concave, but still appeared hard when compressed. The tissue visible over the implantation site in group B+BG+TCP resembled the surrounding normal tissues the most closely when compared to the other groups. In group BG, white granulation was still visible throughout the superficial tissue covering the bone defect. In the control group, on the other hand, a large protrusion was still visible over the implantation site, with a small dark-colored spot at its center.

After the 8th and 12th weeks of experiment, the implantation sites of the group B animals were still clearly distinguishable on macroscopic examination; they were protruding and differed in color from the surrounding tissues. Protrusions over the implantation sites were also visible in group B+BG, but only up to the 8th week of the study. After this time, the implantation site was hardly distinguishable from the normal tissues, and only the presence of granulation, which was hardly visible throughout the superficial tissue, enabled its visual identification. In group B+BG+TCP, the implantation site could also only be localized due to the subtle appearance of white granulation as early as after 8 weeks of the experiment. In group B+TCP, no concavity was observed over the implantation site beginning from the 8th week of the study, and the tissue covering the defect only slightly differed in color from the surrounding normal bone. After 12 weeks of observation, the tissue over the bone defects in this group had an identical appearance to the surrounding tissues. On the last examination day, the site of the bone defect was distinguishable only in the control group. Although the implantation site was covered with hard tissue, minute concavities and dark spots were still visible on its surface.

5.3 Radiological examinations

Material-related differences in the rates of new skeletal tissue formation were revealed as early as after the 7th day of the study. In group B, spherical translucencies with regular edges were observed on radiographic images, with a size corresponding to the size of the bone defect. The initial process of bone reconstruction, manifested by a foggy appearance of the implantation site, was observed no earlier than after the second experimental week (Fig. 2a). At that same time point, initial signs of bone formation were also observed on radiographic images taken in group B+BG+TCP (Fig. 5a), while in group B+BG this phenomenon was already visible after 7 days (Fig. 3a). Irregular translucencies at the implantation site were seen in this group, but a small shadow was observed in the central zone, whose area and intensity increased with time. Radiologic findings suggested that the beginning of new tissue formation was most delayed in group B+TCP (Fig. 4a) and in the controls (Fig. 6a). In these groups, a distinct shadow was observed no earlier than after the 3rd week of the experiment; this shadow was larger and more intense in B+TCP group.

After the 4th week of the study, radiographic images taken in group B revealed the nearly complete formation of new skeletal tissue. At this point in time, indistinct translucencies were seen only at the periphery of the skeletal defect, suggesting osteogenesis was ongoing in this area. After 8 weeks of the experiment, bone reconstruction was complete in this group. The whole defect was excessively shadowed, suggesting that tissue with greater mineralization was present in this area when compared to normal bone (Fig. 2b). As with group B, in group B+TCP the mineralization of the implantation site was complete after the 8th week of the study, as suggested by a fully shadowed area of the bone defect visible on radiographic images (Fig. 4b). At the same time, a small translucency was visible in the superior-medial aspect of the bone defect in group B+BG. In this group, the process of bone formation was completed no earlier than after the 12th week of the experiment. This was confirmed by the excessive mineralization of skeletal tissue, manifested radiographically as a distinct shadow at the implantation site (Fig. 3b). In the B+BG+TCP group, a homogenous shadow was visible at the implantation site as early as after the 8th week of the experiment, and an incomplete process of skeletal tissue regeneration was suggested only by the presence of spotted translucencies. However, the site of the bone defect could not be distinguished from the surrounding tissues until at least the 12th week of the study (Fig. 5b). In the control group, the process of bone formation was markedly delayed, and after the 8th week of the study a distinct, longitudinal translucency could still be seen at the site of the bone defect. Moreover, non-calcified areas were still visible on the last examination day despite newly formed skeletal tissue present within the entire area of the bone defect (Fig. 6b).

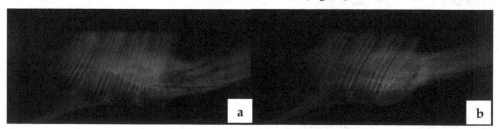

Fig. 2. Radiographic images of the mandible in experimental animals. Bone defect healing in the presence of deproteinized human bone: a) 14th day of the study; b) 8th week of the study

Preparation of Deproteinized Human Bone and Its Mixtures with Bio-Glass and Tricalcium Phosphate – Innovative
Bioactive Materials for Skeletal Tissue Regeneration

77

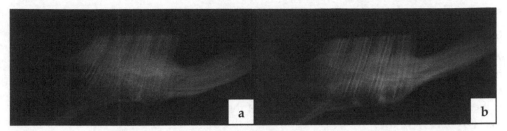

Fig. 3. Radiographic images of the mandible in experimental animals. Bone defect healing in the presence of the mixture of deproteinized human bone with bio-glass: a) 7th day of the study; b) 12th week of the study

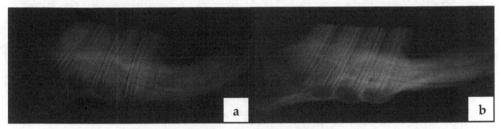

Fig. 4. Radiographic images of the mandible in experimental animals. Bone defect healing in the presence of the mixture of deproteinized human bone with tricalcium phosphate: a) 21st day of the study; b) 8th week of the study

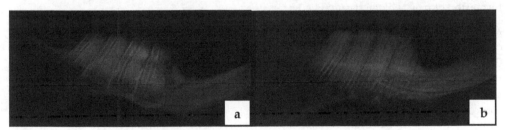

Fig. 5. Radiographic images of the mandible in experimental animals. Bone defect healing in the presence of the mixture of deproteinized human bone with bio-glass and tricalcium phosphate: a) 14th day of the study; b) 12th week of the study

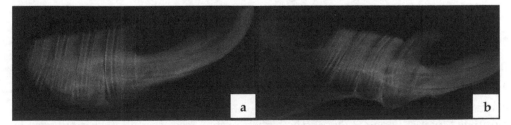

Fig. 6. Radiographic images of the mandible in experimental animals. Bone defect healing on the basis of clotted blood: a) 21st day of the study; b) 12th week of the study

5.4 Bone Mineral Density

5.4.1 Radiographic densitometry

A gradual increase in BMD was observed in all experimental groups and in the controls. The highest BMD value was observed after the 8th week of the study in bone defects implanted with B+TCP (0.40 ± 0.05 g/cm²) and B+BG+TCP (0.39 ± 0.05 g/cm²) (Table 1). However, these values were still lower than the normal BMD of the mandibular trunk determined in guinea pigs (0.51 ± 0.001 g/cm²).

	BMD [g/cm²]					
Group	1st week	2nd week	3th week	4th week	8th week	12th week
B	0.25 ± 0.01	0.27 ± 0.01	0.28 ± 0.01	0.33 ± 0.02	0.35 ± 0.03	0.35 ± 0.03
B+BG	0.27 ± 0.02	0.30 ± 0.03	0.30 ± 0.03	0.31 ± 0.02	0.31 ± 0.03	0.33 ± 0.01
B+TCP	0.22 ± 0.03	0.24 ± 0.03	0.33 ± 0.01	0.32 ± 0.04	0.40 ± 0.05	0.36 ± 0.02
B+BG+TCP	0.23 ± 0.03	0.28 ± 0.02	0.32 ± 0.03	0.35 ± 0.04	0.39 ± 0.05	0.38 ± 0.02
Control	0.24 ± 0.01	0.25 ± 0.01	0.22 ± 0.02	0.34 ± 0.01	0.33 ± 0.04	0.32 ± 0.02

Table 1. Bone mineral density (BMD) of skeletal defects implanted with various materials and in control defects determined radiographically at various time points in the study

The most regular increase in BMD was observed in defects implanted with B+BG+TCP, followed by B and B+BG. Some irregularities in the time profiles of BMD changes were noted, however, in animals of group B+TCP and in the controls, suggesting inhomogeneous formation of new skeletal tissue (Fig. 7).

Additionally, statistical analysis revealed intergroup differences in the time profiles of BMD changes. The most pronounced differences were observed between groups B and B+BG – 0.98, followed by B+BG vs. B+TCP – 0.79, and B vs. B+TCP – 0.78. Slight differences in the time profiles were noted between the B+BG+TCP group and other material groups, and no significant differences were observed when experimental groups were compared to the control group (Table 2).

Profile comparison (p-values)				
Group	Control	B	B+BG	B+TCP
B	<0.05	–	–	–
B+BG	<0.05	0.98	–	–
B+TCP	<0.05	0.78	0.79	–
B+BG+TCP	<0.01	0.20	0.21	0.32

Table 2. The p-values for comparison of bone mineral density (BMD) changes in time (profiles) between the tested material and control groups

Moreover, a relative increase in BMD between the 1st and 12th experimental weeks was calculated for each group (Table 3). The highest relative increase in BMD was observed in bone defects in group B+BG+TCP (25.49) but the increase in the B+TCP group was only slightly lower (24.14). The lowest relative increase in BMD between the 1st and 12th experimental weeks was observed in animals of group B+BG (9.98); the time plot of BMD changes in this group was closest to a vertical line.

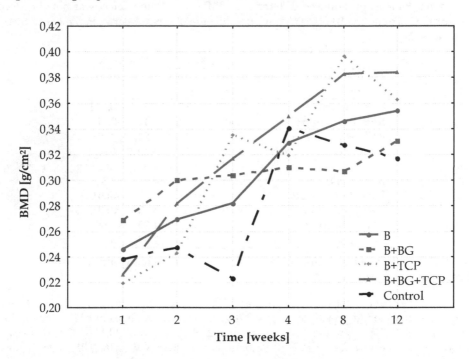

Fig. 7. Time profile of changes in bone mineral density (BMD) determined radiographically in bone defects implanted with various materials and in control defects

Due to non-sphericity (Mauchley test: 0.42; $p < 0.001$) only multivariable tests were used. We confirmed that there were statistically significant changes in BMD with time (F = 894.17; $p < 0.001$). Moreover, the interaction between time and the type of material used (group) was also statistically significant (F = 35.59; $p < 0.001$).

Group	$|t|$	p
12th vs. 1st week		
B	17.11	<0.001
B+BG	9.98	<0.001
B+TCP	24.14	<0.001
B+BG+TCP	25.49	<0.001
Control	13.58	<0.001

Table 3. Comparison of bone mineral density (BMD) values between the 12th and 1st weeks with regard to the tested material and control groups

Finally, statistical analysis revealed several significant intergroup differences in BMD values determined in experimental weeks 1 and 12 (Table 4). In the earlier period, the most pronounced difference was observed between groups B+BG and B+TCP (4.33), while the lowest difference pertained to groups B+TCP and B+BG+TCP. After 12 weeks of the experiment, the most pronounced difference in BMD of the bone defect was noted between the control group and the B+BG+TCP group, while the difference between the B and B+TCP groups was the lowest.

	1st week		12th week	
Groups	|t|	P	|t|	p
B vs. Control	0.70	0.48	3.63	<0.001
B+BG vs. Control	2.48	<0.05	1.41	0.17
B+TCP vs. Control	1.85	0.07	4.54	<0.05
B+BG+TCP vs. Control	1.27	0.21	6.40	<0.001
B vs. B+BG	1.78	0.08	2.22	<0.05
B vs. B+TCP	2.55	<0.05	0.91	0.37
B vs. B+BG+TCP	1.98	0.05	2.78	<0.01
B+BG vs. B+TCP	4.33	<0.001	3.13	<0.01
B+BG vs. B+BG+TCP	3.75	<0.001	4.99	<0.001
B+TCP vs. B+BG+TCP	0.57	0.57	1.87	0.07

Table 4. Comparison of bone mineral density (BMD) values in the 1st and 12th weeks between the tested material and control groups

We have also observed statistically significant differences in the growth of BMD with time between the analyzed groups ($F=8.15$; $p<0.001$). The smallest changes in BMD were yielded by B+BG (0.06 ± 0.01), then the control group (0.08 ± 0.01) and B (0.11 ± 0.02). The largest changes were observed for B+TCP (0.14 ± 0.01) and B+BG+TCP (0.16 ± 0.01). For all paired comparisons, statistically significant differences were noted ($p<0.01$).

5.4.2 Computed tomography

Table 5 summarizes the values of bone density in the experimental groups and in the controls as determined by CT. A gradual increase in the density of healing bone defects was observed in all studied groups. After 12 weeks of the experiment, the highest values of CT bone density were observed in the B+BG (1014.8 ± 53.9 HU) and B+BG+TCP (941.2 ± 28.9 HU) groups, while the lowest values were noted in the controls (812.3 ± 21.8 HU). However, the highest determined values of CT bone density were still lower compared to the bone density of the normal mandible (1218 ± 15.2 HU).

CT Bone Density [HU]					
Group	1st week	2nd week	3th week	4th week	8th week	12th week
B	647.7 ± 79.1	784.0 ± 82.3	863.2 ± 13.3	763.8 ± 136.1	954.3 ± 56.3	902.8 ± 13.5
B+BG	597.2 ± 48.8	730.5 ± 9.8	814.3 ± 38.1	822.5 ± 99.8	933.3 ± 22.0	1014.8 ± 53.9
B+TCP	410.3 ± 34.0	468.2 ± 59.1	606.7 ± 41.8	804.0 ± 51.7	826.3 ± 39.3	879.2 ± 24.6
B+BG+TCP	454.7 ± 17.1	526.3 ± 35.6	523.2 ± 27.7	725.7 ± 36.3	923.7 ± 31.8	941.2 ± 28.9
Control	256.0 ± 20.4	510.3 ± 28.7	539.0 ± 38.3	597.8 ± 35.3	681.8 ± 19.4	812.3 ± 21.8

Table 5. CT bone density (expressed in Hounsfield units, HU) in bone defects implanted with various materials and in control defects at various time points in the study

The most homogeneous increase in CT bone density values was observed in groups B+BG and B+TCP, and in the controls. Some irregularities in the time profile of bone density were, by contrast, noted in animals of the B and B+BG+TCP groups (Fig. 8).

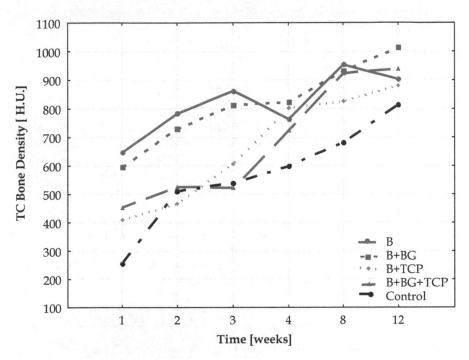

Fig. 8. Time profile of changes in CT bone density (expressed in Hounsfield units, HU) in bone defects implanted with various materials and in control defects

Due to non-sphericity (Mauchley test: 0.0030; p<0.001) only multivariable tests were used. We confirmed that there were statistically significant changes in Hounsfield Units with time (F = 1244.88; p<0.001). Moreover, the interaction between time and the type of material used (group) was also statistically significant (F = 65.35; p<0.001).

When the time profiles of CT bone density changes were compared between the studied groups, the only significant differences observed were between groups B and B+BG – 0.86, and B+TCP and B+BG+TCP – 0.30 (Table 6).

	Profile comparison (p-values)			
Group	Control	B	B+BG	B+TCP
B	<0.001	–	–	–
B+BG	<0.001	0.86	–	–
B+TCP	<0.001	<0.001	<0.001	–
B+BG+TCP	<0.001	<0.001	<0.001	0.30

Table 6. The p-values for comparison of CT bone density (expressed in Hounsfield units, HU) with changes in time (profiles) between the tested material and control groups

The most evident intragroup differences in CT bone density determined in the 1st and 12th experimental weeks were observed in the control group (29.77), but the differences were only slightly less pronounced in groups B+TCP (24.10) and B+BG+TCP (22.94). The least evident differences between the two analyzed time points were noted in the B (10.67) and B+BG (16.77) groups (Table 7).

	12th vs. 1st week	
Group	|t|	p
B	10.67	<0.001
B+BG	16.77	<0.001
B+TCP	24.10	<0.001
B+BG+TCP	22.94	<0.001
Control	29.77	<0.001

Table 7. Comparison of CT bone density values (expressed in Hounsfield units, HU) between the 12th and 1st weeks with regard to the tested material and control groups

After seven days of the experiment, the most pronounced intergroup differences in CT bone density were observed between the control group and groups B and BG. The least pronounced intergroup differences noted in this period pertained to groups B and B+BG. After 12 weeks of the study, the most evident intergroup differences in CT bone density were again observed between the controls and group B+BG, while the lowest differences were noted between groups B and B+TCP.

	1st week		12th week	
Groups	|t|	p	|t|	p
B vs. Control	16.63	<0.001	4.91	<0.001
B+BG vs. Control	15.23	<0.001	10.29	<0.001
B+TCP vs. Control	8.48	<0.001	3.67	<0.05
B+BG+TCP vs. Control	10.36	<0.001	6.83	<0.001
B vs. B+BG	1.56	0.1325	6.01	<0.001
B vs. B+TCP	9.11	<0.001	1.39	0.1779
B vs. B+BG+TCP	7.00	<0.001	2.14	<0.05
B+BG vs. B+TCP	7.55	<0.001	7.40	<0.001
B+BG vs. B+BG+TCP	5.44	<0.001	3.87	<0.001
B+TCP vs. B+BG+TCP	2.11	<0.05	3.53	<0.01

Table 8. Comparison of CT bone density (expressed in Hounsfield units, HU) values in the 1st and 12th weeks between tested material and control groups

We have also observed statistically significant intergroup differences in the relative increase in CT bone density (expressed in Hounsfield units, HU) (F = 39.22; p<0.001). The smallest changes in CT bone density were yielded by group B (255.2±67.6). Larger changes were observed for B+BG (417.7±25.7), B+TCP (468.8±43.3) and B+BG+TCP (486.5±16.5). The largest change was noted in the control group (556.2±34.4). For all paired comparisons, statistically significant differences (with p<0.05) were observed, with the only exception being a comparison between B+TCP and B+BG+TCP.

Preparation of Deproteinized Human Bone and Its Mixtures with Bio-Glass and Tricalcium Phosphate – Innovative
Bioactive Materials for Skeletal Tissue Regeneration

83

5.5 Histopathologic analysis

In all analyzed groups, after 7 days of the study, mandibular bone defects had filled with immature fibrous tissue. Numerous, minute granules of deproteinized human bone (with no signs of activity) were seen in this tissue (group B). Additionally, depending on the implant composition, foggy fractions of bio-glass or linearly cracked deposits of tricalcium phosphate could be seen (in groups B+BG, B+TCP and B+BG+TCP). At the same time, active reconstruction of skeletal tissue was observed at the entire periphery of the bone defects implanted with B, B+TCP and B+BG+TCP, as suggested by the presence of ground substance (osteoid) containing numerous immature bone trabeculae covered with osteoblasts. In controls, as well as in groups B and B+BG, blood clots along with the remnants of necrotic bone trabeculae could be seen in the bone marrow at the base of the bone defect. In groups where bio-glass was implanted into the bone defect (B+BG and B+BG+TCP), fragments of this material formed pseudocystic structures that were covered with a thin connective tissue capsule comprised of fibroblasts, fibrocytes and single giant polynuclear cells.

After two weeks of the experiment, the implanted bone defects were filled with mature fibrous connective tissue that contained collagen fibers. Only in group B could immature connective tissue with numerous blood vessels be seen at the periphery of the defect. Immature bone trabeculae were visible in this tissue, surrounded with osteoblasts. Depending on the implant composition, fragments of deproteinized bone granules, bio-glass and/or tricalcium phosphate were seen in the fibrous connective tissue. Around BG and TCP particles, distinct, thick-walled pseudocystic structures could be observed, containing numerous giant polynuclear cells. Additionally, giant polynuclear cells were frequently visible on the surface of deproteinized bone but they did not form distinct capsule-like linear structures in this location. Fragmentation of some TCP particles could be observed due to infiltration by cells composing the previously mentioned cystic structures. Active osteogenesis was evident in all analyzed groups, as manifested by the pronounced growth of numerous immature bone trabeculae covered with osteoblasts. This process was particularly intensive around the particles of implanted material.

In group B, advanced reconstruction of bone defects was observed after three weeks of the study. Most bone trabeculae filling the defect were mature with either no or very little osteoblastic activity. Linearly placed osteoblasts, or even osteoclasts, could be seen on the surface of remaining trabeculae (Fig. 9). A similar advancement in the bone formation process was observed in B+TCP specimens: osteoid was formed on the base of connective fibrous tissue along with the intensive growth of numerous bone trabeculae. Some of these trabeculae were mature already and showed no signs of cellular activity. Skeletal tissue regeneration in this group was particularly enhanced around the fragments of deproteinized bone and tricalcium phosphate (Fig. 10). In contrast to B particles, TCP particles showed signs of dilution and structural fragmentation. Only a few giant polynuclear cells could be seen around the implants, and the previously observed cystic structures of TCP had only residual character. After three weeks of the study, slightly less advanced processes of skeletal defect healing were observed in histologic specimens from groups B+BG and B+BG+TCP. Growth of immature skeletal tissue was observed in these groups on the "scaffold" of deproteinized bone, giving the impression of the implant being "incorporated" into the growing bone trabeculae. Only single giant polynuclear cells could be seen on the surface of specimens from group B+BG. Additionally, thin, linearly placed cells could be observed around some bio-glass particles, forming pseudocystic structures. These structures were visible mostly in areas directly adjacent to fibrous connective tissue. Numerous bone trabeculae were observed around the B+BG+TCP mixture particles, as well as in the fibrous connective tissue between the particles (Fig. 11). Some trabeculae were mature and showed no signs of osteoblastic activity on their surfaces. Some implant particles in this group were covered with giant polynuclear cells forming structures resembling foreign body granulomas. In the control group, all osteoid trabeculae were surrounded by osteoblasts still showing signs of osteoblastic activity.

After four weeks of the study, only the bone defects in group B were nearly completely filled with mature, compact skeletal tissue. This tissue contained numerous "incorporated" granules of deproteinized human bone. Growing bone trabeculae with surface signs of osteoblastic activity could only be seen in a narrow layer of fibrous connective tissue located between the newly formed bone and the bottom of the defect. At the same time, mature cancellous skeletal tissue could only be observed at the periphery of bone defects in groups B+TCP and B+BG+TCP. "Incorporated" fragments of the implanted material, mostly human bone, were visible in this tissue. The central part of the defects was still filled with fibrous connective tissue, showing signs of the ongoing process of bone formation. This area also contained B particles and a few particles of TCP ceramic. These fragments of tricalcium phosphate were covered with a pseudo-capsule comprised of giant polynuclear cells, and were gradually fragmented and resorbed. After four weeks of the experiment, numerous mature bone trabeculae with no signs of cellular activity were observed in specimens from group B+BG (Fig. 12). Some of these trabeculae developed around B and BG particles, giving the impression of "incorporating" implanted material into the structure of reconstructed bone. Some bone defects were still partially filled with mature fibrous connective tissue containing numerous collagen fibers along with particles of implanted material. Additionally, pseudocystic structures could be observed around the BG particles, comprised of linearly placed giant polynuclear cells.

Histopathologic examination performed after eight weeks of the study revealed the completed process of bone healing in group B. Bone structure was fully regenerated, and mature compact bone and cancellous bone could be observed at the defect site, along with normal bone marrow (Fig. 13). Observations made in the B+BG+TCP group after the 8th and 12th weeks of the experiment gave similar findings. In this group bone defects were also filled with mature compact and cancellous skeletal tissue, with "incorporated" particles of bio-glass and deproteinized bone still visible (Fig. 14). These particles showed no signs of activity, and were covered with thin fibrous capsules. In the 8th experimental week, these particles could also be observed in fibrous connective tissue. After the 8th week of the study, the process of osteogenesis was still incomplete in B+BG and B+TCP specimens. In defects implanted with bio-glass, some areas, usually peripheral ones, were still filled with fibrous connective tissue containing numerous collagen fibers. This connective tissue showed signs of ongoing bone formation: maturing or mature bone trabeculae, along with bio-glass particles forming pseudocystic structures (Fig. 15). Particles of deproteinized bone were more rarely evidenced. At the same time, continued bone formation was observed in the central part of bone defects in group B+TCP (Fig. 16). This process was particularly

Preparation of Deproteinized Human Bone and Its Mixtures with Bio-Glass and Tricalcium Phosphate – Innovative
Bioactive Materials for Skeletal Tissue Regeneration

85

intensive around the B particles, giving the characteristic impression of "incorporating" this material into newly formed bone. After eight weeks of the study, only some bone trabeculae in the control group showed signs of osteoblastic activity, while other areas of the defect contained mature trabeculae.

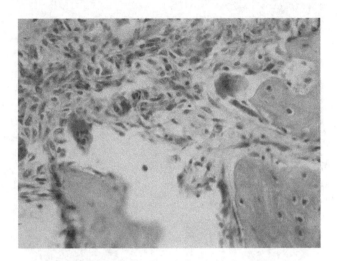

Fig. 9. Histopathologic specimen – 3rd week, group B – single osteoclasts on the surface of bone trabeculae (H&E staining, magnification 400 x)

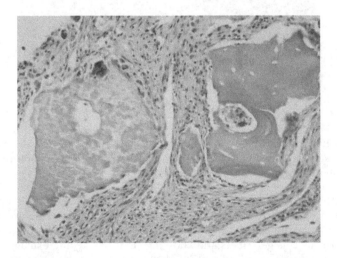

Fig. 10. Histopathologic specimen – 3rd week, group B+TCP – regeneration of skeletal tissue around fragments of deproteinized human bone and tricalcium phosphate (H&E staining, magnification 200 x)

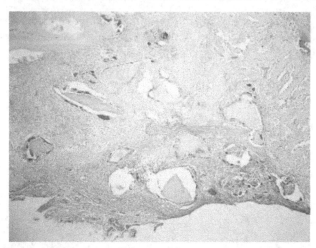

Fig. 11. Histopathologic specimen – 3rd week, group B+BG+TCP – numerous bone trabeculae around the implanted material visible within fibrous connective tissue (H&E staining, magnification 40 x)

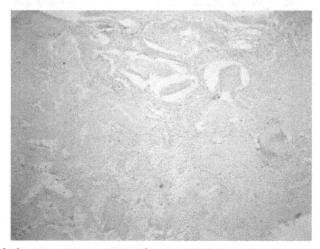

Fig. 12. Histopathologic specimen – 4th week, group B+BG – mature bone trabeculae with no signs of cellular activity, along with particles of deproteinized human bone and bio-glass visible within fibrous connective tissue (H&E staining, magnification 40 x)

After 12 weeks of the study, the process of skeletal tissue regeneration in specimens from groups B+BG and B+TCP was still not complete. Although the defects were nearly filled in their entirety with mature compact and cancellous bone, mature fibrous connective tissue containing numerous collagen fibers and showing signs of ongoing osteogenesis could still be seen in the superficial zone (Fig. 17). This superficial layer contained remnants of deproteinized bone, covered with capsules comprised of giant polynuclear cells, which formed inactive, fibrous foreign body granulomas. Additionally, cystic structures containing foggy remnants of incompletely resorbed TCP (group B+TCP) or BG particles (group B+BG)

Preparation of Deproteinized Human Bone and Its Mixtures with Bio-Glass and Tricalcium Phosphate – Innovative
Bioactive Materials for Skeletal Tissue Regeneration

87

were revealed in fibrous connective tissue (Fig. 18). In the control group, specimens obtained in the 12th week of the study contained completely matured and fully mineralized bone.

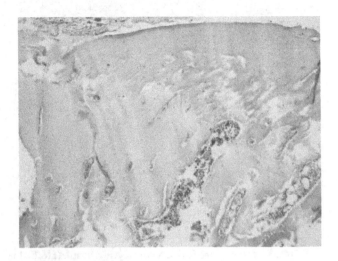

Fig. 13. Histopathologic specimen – 8th week, group B – mature skeletal tissue and bone marrow (H&E staining, magnification 100 x)

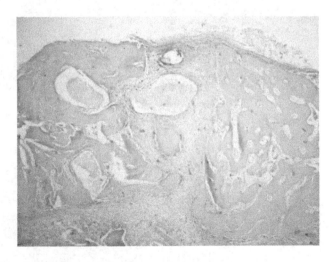

Fig. 14. Histopathologic specimen – 8th week, group B+BG+TCP – mature compact and cancellous skeletal tissue with "incorporated" particles of bio-glass and human bone (H&E staining, magnification 100 x)

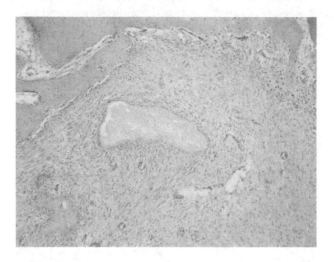

Fig. 15. Histopathologic specimen – 8th week, group B+BG – bio-glass particle forming pseudocystic structure within the mature fibrous connective tissue (H&E staining, magnification 100 x)

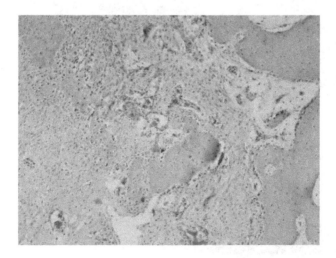

Fig. 16. Histopathologic specimen – 8th week, group B+TCP – fibrous connective tissue with massive osteogenesis (H&E staining, magnification 100 x)

Preparation of Deproteinized Human Bone and Its Mixtures with Bio-Glass and Tricalcium Phosphate – Innovative
Bioactive Materials for Skeletal Tissue Regeneration

89

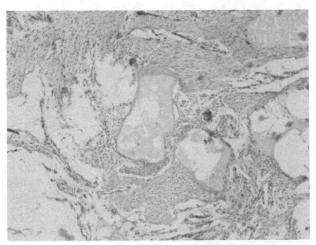

Fig. 17. Histopathologic specimen – 12th week, group B+BG – mature fibrous connective tissue
with numerous cystic spaces filled with foggy deposits of bio-glass (H&E staining, 100 x)

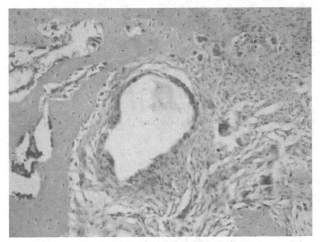

Fig. 18. Histopathologic specimen – 12th week, group B+TCP – cystic structures within
fibrous connective tissue containing foggy remnants of tricalcium phosphate (H&E staining,
200 x)

6. Discussion

Due to the limited regenerative ability of skeletal tissue, bone grafting or the implantation of
bone derivatives or bone replacement materials is required for the complete healing of large
bone defects, whether the result of surgical removal of skeletal cysts or tumors, or caused by
other skeletal disorders (Precheur, 2007). The most satisfactory results in stimulating skeletal
tissue regeneration have been reported after using autogenous grafts. After being implanted
into the bone defect, autogenous grafts can induce all the basic mechanisms responsible for
bone reconstruction, i.e. osteogenesis, osteoinduction and osteoconduction (Giannoudis et

al., 2005; Merkx et al., 2003). Osteogenic activity is associated with the presence of osteoprogenitor cells in the periosteum, endosteum and bone marrow. In the case of free bone grafts, some of the cells located most superficially may survive and are involved in regeneration processes. The results of bone healing stimulation are definitely most satisfactory when autogenous cancellous bone chips are implanted, since this type of bone contains a high number of osteoprogenitor cells. Osteogenic activity can only be observed in fresh bone grafts. Osteoinduction is associated with the presence of so-called bone morphogenetic proteins (BMP) in the bone matrix. These proteins are released during bone remodeling, and can stimulate minimally differentiated connective tissue cells surrounding the graft to transform into osteoblasts (Barradas et al., 2011). Both fresh autogenic bone grafts and the allogenic grafts obtained from tissue bank (especially when frozen and partly decalcified) have osteoinductive properties. Additionally, BMP preparations can be obtained by extraction from bones, and as of recent, also by biotechnological synthesis in recombinant form. Allogenic bones are very frequently lyophilized, which depletes them of BMP. Additionally, such grafts lose their immunogenic properties due to irradiation sterilization and deep freezing (Bohner, 2010; Liu et al., 2008). This process of sterilization results in decreased durability of the material, and the preserved bone matrix has only osteoconductive properties. It is degraded by osteoclasts with the simultaneous formation of woven bone, which is further transformed into lamellar bone through the process of osteoclasia. Such grafts have been shown to undergo revascularization and remodeling – similar to autogenous grafts, but at a slower rate. Apart from bone implants, organic and inorganic alloplastic bone replacement materials also have osteoconductive properties. Combined with growth factors and autogenous barrier membranes, they are frequently used as basic elements in the process of guided bone regeneration (GBR) (Kao & Scott, 2007; Schwarz et al., 2007).

For various reasons, different bone materials are frequently combined with each other or with alloplastic biomaterials. As a result, biologically improved material compositions are obtained, some of which positively influence the bone formation processes. Combination of natural hydroxyapatite with chitosane resulted in a composite with osteoconductive properties. In the presence of this composite, tibial consolidation in rabbits was observed as early as 12 weeks after implantation, and complete healing was observed after 16 weeks of the study (Yuan et al., 2008). In another study, a composite based on bovine bone with the addition of bio-glass showed no cytotoxicity to human fibroblasts. Moreover, a crystalline carbonated apatite phase was developed on the sample surface as early as 12 days after immersion in simulated body fluid (Yoganad e al., 2010). Another example of the positive effects of combining deproteinized bovine bone with autogenous bone comes from a study in which such a material was used for the regeneration of bone defects in the frontal part of the porcine skull. The presence of autogenous bone in the mixture was the basis for the osteoinductive properties of the material and the more favorable biological conditions for bone growth when compared to deproteinized bovine bone alone (Thorwarth et al., 2006). Similarly, more satisfactory clinical results were reported when deproteinized bovine bone was used in combination with autogenous bone in the management of alveoschisis in humans, instead of bone autograft alone (Thuaksuban et al., 2010). Experiments on rabbits have also given interesting results. It was revealed that the addition of deproteinized bovine bone to autogenous grafts increased the mean optical density of newly formed skeletal tissue, with a simultaneous decrease in its content in bone defects (skullcap). The opposite

Preparation of Deproteinized Human Bone and Its Mixtures with Bio-Glass and Tricalcium Phosphate – Innovative
Bioactive Materials for Skeletal Tissue Regeneration

91

effects were observed when autogenous bone graft was used alone (Pripatnanont et al., 2009). Using a mixture of allogenic bone and deproteinized bovine bone (BioOss®/Orthoblast II®) for the purposes of maxillary sinus lift did not have results as satisfactory as with the application of deproteinized animal bone or synthetic bone (Osteon®) alone. The individual use of one of these two implant materials was associated with a higher percentage of newly formed osseous fraction collected from the lateral sinus at 4 and 6 months post-operatively (Kim et al., 2009).

In this study we have combined allogenic bone with artificially obtained biomaterials (bio-glass – BG, and/or beta-tricalcium phosphate – TCP) in order to form bone replacement material with improved biological characteristics. Reference materials for comparative analysis of the studied mixtures (B+BG, B+TCP, B+BG+TCP) included lyophilized human bone (B) and the clotted blood of experimental animals. Both clinical observations and further macroscopic, radiographic and histopathologic examinations confirmed that bone defects healed normally in the presence of all studied biomaterials. However, the type of implanted mixture modulated the kinetics of bone formation and the quality of newly formed bone. Bone regeneration was induced markedly earlier whenever biologically active bio-glass was included in the implanted mixture (B+BG, B+BG+TCP). In groups where bio-glass was implanted, irregular shadows were observed on radiographic images of the bone defect sites as early as after two weeks of the study. Probably, these radiographic changes resulted from ongoing reparative processes within the bone. This was additionally confirmed on histopathologic analysis, which revealed intense bone formation processes as early as three weeks after the implantation of BG-containing material. However, bone density measurements (BMD and CT bone density) taken in the early period of this study confirmed the superior quality of newly formed bone only in case of the B+BG mixture. It is plausible that the lower bone densities determined for B+BG+TCP implants resulted from the low content of bio-glass in this mixture. Moreover, as confirmed by histopathologic analysis, resorption of beta-tricalcium phosphate contained in B+BG+TCP already began in the early period of this study. Nonetheless, in the later period of this study, increases in BMD and CT bone density of B+BG implanted bone were markedly lower. As a result, after 12 weeks of the experiment, the defects filled with this mixture were characterized by the lowest BMD values, and histopathologic examination confirmed ongoing bone formation. The final result of bone regeneration was markedly better in the case of defects implanted with B+BG+TCP. In the 12th week, histopathologic analysis revealed mature skeletal tissue (both compact and cancellous bone) at the implantation sites, and this finding was confirmed on radiographic examination. Additionally, new bone formed using B+BG+TCP implantation was characterized by the highest BMD and relatively high CT bone density. Therefore, this regenerated bone most closely resembled the normal skeletal tissue of experimental animals of all mixtures examined. In the 12th week of this study, bone formation processes were still observed in B+TCP implanted defects. Although the BMD of tissue formed on the basis of this implant was higher than in the B+BG implanted bone, it was still lower than in the B+BG+TCP group. Notably, in both the 1st and 12th experimental weeks, only slight differences in BMD and CT bone density were observed between the B+TCP and B+BG+TCP mixtures. Undoubtedly, the process of bone defect regeneration was completed the earliest in group B. Histopathologic studies confirmed that bone defects in this group were filled with mature skeletal tissue with no signs of osteoblastic activity as early as after eight weeks of the study. Early completion of skeletal healing was also confirmed by the radiographic images taken in this group. In the 12th experimental week, BMD of bone defects implanted with human bone alone was higher in comparison to defects filled with B+TCP and B+BG+TCP, in contrast to the early period of this study when BMD and CT bone density in group B were among the highest.

Results of this study suggest that the quality of bone formed in the late period of the experiment was poorest in the control group, as suggested by the low bone density of defects healing on the basis of clotted blood. Since histopathologic studies confirmed that bone formation in controls was complete in week 12, one should not expect further increases in bone density in this group. It is likely that bone density would increase further, however, with prolonged observation of the B+BG and B+TCP groups, since the last densitometric measurements in these groups were taken on incompletely matured bone.

7. Conclusion

This *in vivo* animal study revealed that both lyophilized human bone (B) and mixtures formed on its basis (B+BG, B+TCP, B+BG+TCP) are fully biocompatible materials. We have confirmed that, in the presence of these materials, there is a possibility of forming normal, mature skeletal tissue in mandibular bone defects of guinea pigs. This was possible mostly thanks to the inclusion of deproteinized human bone in analyzed mixtures. Due to its osteoconductive properties, the presence of human bone resulted in favorable biological conditions that promoted skeletal regeneration. Therefore, deproteinized bone formed a scaffold to support the growth of osteogenic cells within the defects. Furthermore, the addition of alloplastic materials, bio-glass and beta-tricalcium phosphate, markedly influenced the rate of bone formation and the quality of newly formed bone. The most satisfactory results were observed in the case of lyophilized human bone mixed with bio-glass and beta-tricalcium phosphate (B+BG+TCP). The group implanted with this material was the only one in which fully matured compact and cancellous bone was observed on histopathologic examination performed after 12 weeks of the study. The particles of bio-glass and beta-tricalcium phosphate included in the mixture induced the processes of bone formation and stimulated the growth of osteogenic cells. As a result of these initiated biological processes, defragmented and resorbed β-TCP was gradually replaced with newly formed skeletal structures. Such a course of bone formation process modulated the quality of newly formed bone, as confirmed by high BMD and CT bone density values determined after 12 weeks in B+BG+TCP implanted defects. As confirmed on histopathologic examination, throughout the three-month period of this study, skeletal regeneration was not completed in defects implanted with B+BG and B+TCP mixtures. This incomplete regeneration was reflected by the lower bone density values observed in these groups when compared to the B+BG+TCP group. In conclusion, the results of this study confirmed our initial assumptions. We have revealed that, in addition to a proper course of bone formation processes, another important outcome in the presence of various bone replacement materials is the high quality of newly formed bone. In our opinion, these two aforementioned results were positively achieved by the mixture of lyophilized human bone with bio-glass and tricalcium phosphate.

8. References

Abu Bakar, M.S., Cheng, M.H.W., Tang, S.M., Yu, S.C., Liao, K., Tan, C.T., Khor, K.A. & Cheang, P. (2003). Tensile Properties, Tension–tension Fatigue and Biological

Response of Polyetheretherketone–hydroxyapatite Composites for Load-bearing Orthopedic Implants. *Biomaterials,* Vol.24, No.13, (July 2003), pp. 2245-2250, ISSN 0142-9612

Accorsi-Mendonça, T., Conz, M.B., Barros, T.C., de Sena, L.Á., de Almeida Soares, G. & Granjeiro, J.M. (2008). Physicochemical Characterization of Two Deproteinized Bovine Xenografts. *Brazilian Oral Research,* Vol.22, No.1, (January-March 2008), pp. 5-10, ISSN 1806-8324

Baldini, N., De Sanctis, M. & Ferrari, M. (2011). Deproteinized Bovine Bone in Periodontal and Implant Surgery. *Dental,* Vol.27, No.1, (January 2011), pp. 61-70, ISSN 1879-0097

Barakat, N.A.M., Khil, M.S., Omran, A.M., Sheikh, F.A. & Kim, H.Y. (2009). Extraction of Pure Natural Hydroxyapatite from the Bovine Bones Bio Waste by Three Different Methods. *Journal of Materials Processing Technology,* Vol.209, No.7, (April 2009), pp. 3408-3415, ISSN 0924-0136

Barradas, A.M.C., Yuan, H., van Blitterswijk, C.A. & Habibovic, P. (2011). Osteoinductive Biomaterials: Current Knowledge of Properties, Experimental Models and Biological Mechanisms. *European Cell and Materials,* Vol.21, (2011), pp. 407-429, ISSN 1473-2262

Bellucci, D., Cannillo, V. & Sola, A. (2011). A New Highly Bioactive Composite for Scaffold Applications: A Feasibility Study. *Materials,* Vol.4, (January 2011), pp. 339-354, ISSN 1996-1944

Block, M.S., Finger, I. & Lytle, R. (2002). Human Mineralized Bone in Extraction Sites Before Implant Placement. *The Journal of the American Dental Association,* Vol.133, No.12, (December 2002), pp. 1631-1638, ISSN 0002-8177

Bohner, M. (2010). Resorbable Biomaterials as Bone Graft Substitutes. *Materials Today,* Vol.13, No.1-2, (January-February 2010), pp. 24-30, ISSN 1369-7021

Cao, K., Huang, W., An, H., Jiang, D., Shu, Y. & Han, Z. (2009). Deproteinized Bone with VEGF Gene Transfer to Facilitate the Repair of Early Avascular Necrosis of Femoral Head of Rabbit. *Chinese Journal of Traumatology (English Edition),* Vol.12, No.5, (October 2009), pp. 269-274, ISSN 1008-1275

Choi, J.W., Cho, H.M., Kwak, E.K., Kwon, T.G., Ryoo, H.M., Jeong, Y.K., Oh, K.S. & Shih, H.I. (2004). Effect of Ag-doped Hydroxyapatite as a Bone Filler for Inflamed Bone Defects. *Key Engineering Materials,* Vol.254-256, (2004), pp. 47-50, ISSN 1013-9826

Cieślik, M., Mertas, A., Morawska-Chochół, A., Sabat, D., Orlicki, R., Owczarek, A., Król, W. & Cieślik, T. (2009). The Evaluation of the Possibilities of Using PLGA co-polymer and Its Composites with Carbon Fibers or Hydroxyapatite in Bone Tissue Regeneration Process – In Vitro and In Vivo Examinations. *International Journal of Molecular Science,* Vol.10, No.7, (July 2009), pp. 3224-3234, ISSN 1422-0067

Daculsi, G., Laboux, O., Malard, O. & Weiss, P. (2003). Current State of the Art of Biphasic Calcium Phosphate Bioceramics. *Journal of Materials Science Materials in Medicine,* Vol.14, No.3, (March 2003), pp. 195-200, ISSN 0957-4530

Deculsi, G. (1998). Biphasic Calcium Phosphate Concept Applied to Artificial Bone, Implant Coating and Injectable Bone Substitute. *Biomaterials,* Vol.19, No.16, (August 1998), pp. 1473-1478, ISSN 0142-9612

Fellah, B.H., Gauthier, O., Weiss, P., Chappard, D. & Layrolle, P. (2008). Osteogenicity of Biphasic Calcium Phosphate Ceramics and Bone Autograft in a Goat Model. *Biomaterials*, Vol.29, No.9, (March 2008), pp. 1177-1188, ISSN 0142-9612

Ferreira, J.M.F. (2007). Development and In Vitro Characterization of Sol–gel Derived CaO–P_2O_5-SiO_2–ZnO Bioglass. *Acta Biomaterialia*, Vol.3, No.2, (March 2007), pp. 255-262, ISSN 1742-706

Giannoudis, P.V., Dinopoulos, H. & Tsiridis, E. (2005). Bone Substitutes: An Update. Injury, Vol.36, No.3, Supp.1, (November 2005), pp. 20-27,ISSN 0020-1383

Henkel, K.O., Gerber, T., Gundlach, K.K.H. & Bienengräber, V. (2006). Macroscopical, Histological, and Morphometric Studies of Porous Bone-Replacement Materials in Minipigs 8 Months After Implantation. *Oral Surgery, Oral Medicine, Oral Pathology, Oral Radiology, and Endodontology*, Vol.102, No.5, (November 2006), pp. 606-613, ISSN 1079-2104

Jian, Y., Tian, X., Li, B., Qiu, B., Zhou, Z., Yang, Z. & Li, Q. (2008). Properties of Deproteinized Bone for Reparation of Big Segmental Defect in Long Bone. *Chinese Journal of Traumatology (English Edition)*, Vol.11, No.3, (June 2008), pp. 152-156, ISSN 1008-1275

Kao, S.T. & Scott, D.D. (2007). A Review of Bone Substitutes. *Oral and Maxillofacial Surgery Clinics of North America*, Vol.19, No.4, (November 2007), pp. 513-521, ISSN 1042-3699

Kim, Y.K., Yun, P.Y., Kim, S.G. & Lim, S.C. (2009). Analysis of the Healing Process in Sinus Bone Grafting Using Various Grafting Materials. *Oral Surgery, Oral Medicine, Oral Pathology, Oral Radiology, and Endodontology*, Vol.107, No.2, (February 2009), pp. 204-211, ISSN 1076-2104

Kon, M., Ishikawa, K., Miyamoto, Y. & Asaoka, K. (1995). Development of Calcium Phosphate Based Functional Gradient Bioceramics. *Biomaterials*, Vol.16, No.9, (June 1995), pp. 709-714, ISSN 2079-4983

Liu, L., Pei, F., Tu, C., Zhou, Z. & Li, Q. (2008). Immunological Study on the Transplantation of an Improved Deproteinized Heterogeneous Bone Scaffold Material in Tissue Engineering. *Chinese Journal of Traumatology (English Edition)*, Vol.11, No.3, (June 2008), pp. 141-147, ISSN 1008-1275

Merkx, M.A.V., Maltha, J.C. & Stoelinga, P.J.W. (2003). Assessment of the Value of Anorganic Bone Additives in Sinus Floor Augmentation: A Review of Clinical Reports. *International Journal of Oral and Maxillofacial Surgery*, Vol.32, No.1, (February 2003), pp. 1-6, ISSN 1548-1336

Nagata, F., Miyajima, T. & Yokagawa, Y. (2003). Preparation of Porous Composites Consisting of Apatite and Poly(D,L-lactide). *Key Engineering Materials*, Vol.240-242, (2003), pp. 167-170, ISSN 1013-9826

Nagata, F., Miyajima, T., Teraoka, K. & Yokogawa, Y. (2005). Preparation of Porous Poly(lactic acid)/Hydroxyapatite Microspheres Intended for Injectable Bone Substitutes. *Key Engineering Materials*, Vol.284-286, (2005), pp. 819-822, ISSN 1013-9826

Oonishi, H., Hench, L.L., Wilson, J., Sugihara, F., Tsuji, E., Kushitani, S. & Iwaki, H. (1999). Comparative bone growth behavior in granules of bioceramic materials of various sizes. *Journal of Biomedical Material Research*, Vol.44, No.1, (January 1999), pp. 31-43, ISSN 0021-9304

Precheur, H.V. (2007). Bone Grafts Materials. *Dental Clinics of North America*, Vol.51, No.3, (July 2007), pp. 729-746, ISSN 0011-8532

Pripatnanont, P., Nuntanaranont, T. & Vongvatcharanont, S. (2009). Proportion of Deproteinized Bovine Bone and Autogenous Bone Affects Bone Formation in the Treatment of Calvarial Defects in Rabbits. *International Journal of Oral and Maxillofacial Surgery*, Vol.38, No.4, (April 2009), pp. 356-362, ISSN 1399-0020

Ravarian, R., Moztarzadeh, F., Solati Hashjin, M., Rabiee, S.M., Khoshakhlagh, P. & Tahriri, M. (2010). Synthesis, Characterization and Bioactivity Investigation of Bioglass/Hydroxyapatite Composite. *Ceramics International*, Vol.36, No.1, (January 2010), pp. 291-297, ISSN 0272-8842

Santos, L.A., Carrodeguas, R.G., Rogero, S.O., Higa, O.Z., Boschi, A.O. & Arruda, A.C.F. (2002). α-Tricalcium phosphate cement: "in vitro" cytotoxicity. *Biomaterials*, Vol.23, No.9, (May 2002), pp. 2035-2042, ISSN 2079-4983

Schwarz, F., Herten, M., Ferrari, D., Wieland, M., Schmitz, L., Engelhardt, E. & Becker, J. (2007). Guided Bone Regeneration at Dehiscence-type Defects Using Biphasic Hydroxyapatite + Beta Tricalcium Phosphate (Bone Ceramic®) or a Collagen-coated Natural Bone Mineral (BioOss Collagen®): An Immunohistochemical Study in Dogs. *International Journal of Oral and Maxillofacial Surgery*, Vol.36, No.12, (December 2007), pp. 1198-1206, ISSN 0901-5027

Ślósarczyk, A. & Paszkiewicz, Z. (2005). Method of obtaining highly reactive calcium phosphate powder. Pl Patent 1900486 B1, App. No. 331907, Int. Cl.{7} : C01B 25/32, (December 2005)

Thomas, M.V., Puleo, D.A. & Al-Sabbagh, M. (2005). Bioactive Glass Three Decades on. *Journal of Long-Term Effects of Medical Implants*, Vol.15, No.6, (February 2005), pp. 585-597, ISSN 1050-6934

Thorwarth, M., Schlegel, K.A., Wehrhan, F., Srour, S. & Schultze-Mosgau, S. (2006). Acceleration of de Novo Bone Formation Following Application of Autogenous Bone to Particulated Anorganic Bovine Material *In Vivo*. *Oral Surgery, Oral Medicine, Oral Pathology, Oral Radiology, and Endodontology*, Vol.101, No.3, (March 2006), pp. 309-316, ISSN 1076-2104

Thuaksuban, N., Nuntanaranont, T. & Pripatnanont, P. (2010). A comparison of Autogenous Bone Graft Combined with Deproteinized Bovine Bone and Autogenous Bone Graft Alone for Treatment of Alveolar Cleft. *International Journal of Oral and Maxillofacial Surgery*, Vol.39, No.12, (December 2010), pp. 1175-1180, ISSN 1399-0020

Von Wattenwyl, R., Siepe, M., Arnold, R., Beyersdorf, F. & Schlensak, C. (2011). Sternum Augmentation with Bovine Bone Substitute in the Neonate. *The Annals of Thoracic Surgery*, Vol.91, No.1, (January 2011), pp. 311-313, ISSN 0003-4975

Wang, S., Zhang, Z., Zhao, J., Zhang, X., Sun, X., Xia, L., Chang, Q., Ye, D. & Jiang, X. (2009). Vertical Alveolar Ridge Augmentation with β-tricalcium phosphate and Aautologous Osteoblasts in Canine Mandible. *Biomaterials*, Vol.30, No.13, (May 2009), pp. 2489-2498, ISSN 0142-9612

Wei G. & Ma P.X. (2004). Structure and Properties of Nano-Hydroxyapatite/Polymer Composite Scaffolds for Bone Tissue Engineering. *Biomaterials*, Vol.25, No.19, (August 2004), pp. 4749-4757, ISSN 0142-9612

Xynos, I.D., Hukkanen, M.V., Batten, J.J., Buttery, L.D., Hench, L.L. & Polak, J.M. (2000). Bioglass 45S5 Stimulates Osteoblast Turnover and Enhances Bone Formation *In*

Vitro: Implications and Applications for Bone Tissue Engineering. *Calcified Tissue International*, Vol.67, No.4, (October 2000), pp. 321-329, ISSN 1432-0827

Yoganand, C.P., Selvarajan, V., Cannillo, V., Sola, A., Roumeli, E., Goudouri, O.M., Paraskevopoulos, K.M. & Rouabhia, M. (2010). Characterization and In vitro-bioactivity of Natural Hydroxyapatite Based Bio-glass–ceramics Synthesized by Thermal Plasma Processing. *Ceramics*, Vol.36, No.6, (August 2010), pp.1757-1766, ISSN 0272-8842

Yuan, H., Chen, N., Lü, X. & Zheng, B. (2008). Experimental Study of Natural Hydroxyapatite/Chitosan Composite on Reconstructing Bone Defects. *Journal of Nanjing Medical University*, Vol.22, No.6, (November 2008), pp. 372-375, ISSN 1007-4376

Yuan, H., de Bruijn, J.D., Zhang, X., van Blitterswijk, C.A. & de Groot, K. (2001). Bone Induction by Porous Glass Ceramic Made from Bioglass (45S5). *Journal of Biomedical Materials Research*, Vol.58, No.3, (May 2001), pp. 270-276, ISSN 1549-3296

Zhang, B., Zhao, J. & Liu, M. (2009). Osteoinductive Activity of Demineralized Bone Matrix and Deprotenized Bone Derived from Human Avascular Necrotic Femoral Head. *Chinese Journal of Traumatology (English Edition)*, Vol.12, No.6, (December 2009), pp. 379-383, ISSN 1008-1275

Zima, A., Paszkiewicz, Z. & Ślósarczyk, A. (2010). TCP Bioceramics (αTCP, βTCP, BTCP) for Orthopaedic and Stomatological Applications – Preparation and *In Vitro* Evaluation. *Ceramic Materials*, Vol.62, No.1, (2010), pp. 51-55, ISSN 1644-3470

5

Tissue Engineering in Low Urinary Tract Reconstruction

Chao Feng and Yue-min Xu

Department of Urology, Shanghai Jiaotong University-Affiliated 6th People's Hospital,
Shanghai,
China

1. Introduction

Acquired and congenital abnormalities of the lower urinary tract often require eventual reconstruction. Traditionally, different types of autologous tissue can be chosen for surgery, depending on which organ requires reconstruction. Bladder reconstruction, for example, is usually performed with intestinal tissue while urethral reconstruction can us buccal mucosa, lingual mucosa, colonic mucosa or prepuce skin. However, the problems of a shortage of patients' own tissues, and of nmany complications related to surgery, have not yet been resolved. There is therefore an effort to obtain sufficient tissue resources, to involve fewer complications, to reduce surgery to relatively minor invasion and to achieve better surgical outcomes. These goals may be attainable by the use of tissue engineering techniques.

Over the last 50 years, tissue engineering techniques for low urinary tract regeneration have been applied successfully in a variety of animal models and clinical patients. Rapid advancement has been made in this field, which has broadened the theoretical options for the future of low urinary tract reconstruction. These developments include improvements in cell culture techniques, such as the development of cell resources and identification of markers to isolate and characterize specific cell types. Many new types of natural and synthetic biomaterials for use as scaffold components have been created (1). In addition to these, the applications of nanotechnology and bioreactors have been strengthened within recent decades. Here, we review the literature on the basic principles and latest developments of tissue engineering technologies in lower urinary tract reconstruction.

2. Basic knowledge of tissue engineering in low urinary tract

2.1 Cell sources

2.1.1 Autologous stromal cells

Because epithelial cells are one of the most important components of the lower urinary tract, optimizing sources for them have always been a popular focus of investigators. Traditionally, urothelial cells obtained from bladder or urethra have often been used in previous studies (Fig 1a) (2,3). Although this technique exploits homotypy between the graft cells and host, it involves injury to the genitourinary tract and the operation is complicated.

Fu, *et al.* chose epidermal cells as graft cells because of its abundant resources; they can be obtained by a less invasive method than the traditional method of bladder or urethral biopsy followed by dissection of transitional cells. The results suggest that the epidermal cells can transform to transitional epithelial cells under the influence of the urethral or bladder environment (4). From our experience, we suggest using the oral keratinocytes, such as buccal keratinocytes and lingual keratinocytes, as a source of epithelial cells, (Fig 1b,c). Such cells express the β-defensin, IL-8, which can mediate an innate immune response against microbes (5). Therefore, compound grafts were easily resisted infection both in vitro and in vivo. In addition, these oral keratinocytes expressed AE1/AE3, which is similar to epidermal cells or urothelial cells in a previous report (6). However, 3T3 cells are usually needed as a feeder layer when culturing oral keratinocytes. The purification of oral keratinocytes therefore needs to be should be improved before clinical application.

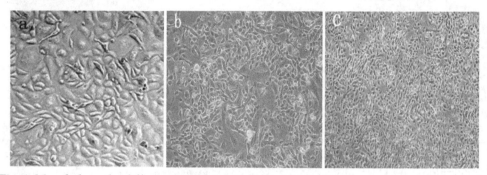

Fig. 1. Morphology the different kinds of epithelial seeding cells.
a. Bladder urethelial cells; b. buccal keratinocytes; c. lingual keratinocytes

To construct 3D bladder or urethral tissue, smooth muscle cell is also necessary. Previously, bladder smooth muscle cells were used for tissue engineering bladder reconstruction (Fig2a). The corpora cavernosa smooth muscle cells were used for constructing the corpora spongiosum, which is one of the most important components of the penile urethra (Fig2b). The advantage of using those cells is that some angiogenic growth factors and their receptors, such as Flk-1 and VEGF, are present in smooth muscle cells. They might contribute to the angiogenesis of bladder or urethral tissue (7). Since contamination by fibroblast cells is a

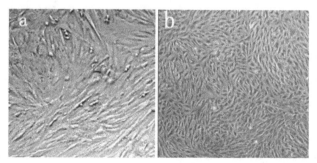

Fig. 2. Morphology the different kinds of smooth muscle cells.
a. Bladder smooth muscle cells; b. corpora cavernosa smooth muscle cells

problem during culturing of these, we advise that a velocity sedimentation method be used to evaluate the purification of smooth muscle cells. Of course, obvious trauma after the procedure is also the shortcoming of this method. As a result of these problems, smooth muscle cells are being replaced by muscle stem cells in urinary reconstruction.

2.1.2 Bone marrow and adipose derived stem cells

Stem cells from bone marrow (BMSC) have been characterized as being either hematopoietic or mesenchymal. They are easily isolated due to their affinity with and adherence to plastic dishes. Their ability to proliferate ensures that even a small number of BMSC multiply into millions of cells under the right culture conditions. Another merit of these cells is that they do not express MHC II, rendering them nonimmunogenic and thereby eliminating possible graft rejection (8). Previous studies showed that BMSCs contained higher concentrations of α-SM actin than did bladder SMC. Meanwhile, BMSCs showed strong response to the Ca^{2+}-ionophore, whereas fibroblasts did not contract their baseline even in the presence of calcium. Those results indicate that BMSCs and smooth muscle cells from low urinary tract are very similar (9). Therefore, BMSCs may serve as an alternative cell source in lower urinary tract tissue engineering.

Stem cells from adipose tissue (ADSCs) have also been popular in tissue engineering research. Adipose tissue is derived from embryonic mesodermal precursors and it contains multipotent progenitor cells that are capable of differentiating into mesenchymal tissue. Since adipose tissue contains 100-1,000 times more pluripotent cells per cubic centimeter

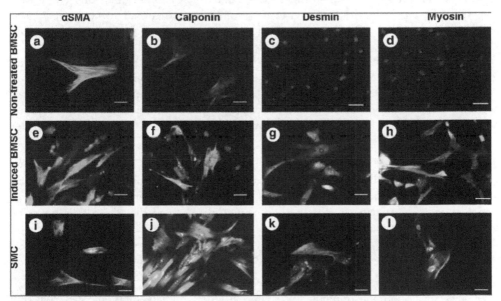

Fig. 3. Myogenic differentiation of human BMSCs using SMC-derived CM. Human BMSCs (p4) were stained with a-SMA (a, e, i), calponin (b, f, j), desmin (c, g, k), and myosin (d, h, l) antibodies without induction as negative control (a–d) and with induction for 14 days (e–h). SMCs were also stained with the same antibodies as a positive control (i–l). (Picture from ref 11)

than does bone marrow, it is easier to obtain ADCSs than other kinds of adult stem cells. Of course, immunoprivilege is also the advantage of this kind of cell. For these reasons, many investigators have selected ADSCs as an ideal source of seeding cells in lower urinary reconstruction, such as repair of bladder and urethra (10).

In many studies, mesenchymal cells have been found to differentiate into many different lineages, such as chondrocytes, osteoblasts, adipocytes, neurons and myoblasts. To urologists, the most interesting thing is the possibility for differentiation of BMSCs or ADSCs into smooth muscle cells and keratinocytes. According to previous reports, these stem cells can acquire a smooth muscle cell phenotype, staining positively for α-SMA, myosin and calponin after being cultured in conditioned medium. Also, culturing in the presence of other myogenic growth factors, such as PDFF-BB,HGF,TGF-β, can also lead to a phenotypic profile of smooth muscle cells (Fig 3) (8,11). Another group has demonstrated the differentiation of marked BMSC into urothelial cells on a seeded scaffold in porcine bladder augmentation, suggesting that mesenchymal stem cells can be made into urothelial cells. However, few additional reports support this result. Since the BMSCs and ADSCs are derived from the mesodermal lineage, more evidence is needed to support that ectodermal lineage cells can be induced from mesenchymal stem cells, such as BMSCs and ADSCs.

2.1.3 Other seeding cells

As well as the autologous stromal cells, BMSCs and ADSCs, other kinds of seeding cells have also shown possibilities for lower urinary tract reconstruction. Drewa (12) *et al.* used hair follicle stem cells for bladder regeneration in rats. This type of cell is CD34 positive, which facilitates the isolation of live epithelial cells with stem cell characterisitcs. In their study, Drewa *et al.* concluded that pluripotent stem cells within rodent hair follicle can differentiate into neurons, glia, keratinocytes and smooth muscle cells. They used an acellular matrix seeded with those cells and achieved a successful bladder wall reconstruction. Further research should be focused on better characterization of these cell populations and on the exact mechanism by which these cells enhance bladder regeneration.

Zhang's study focused on a subpopulation of cells isolated from naturally voided urine (13). This kind of cell demonstrated features typical of progenitor/stem cells, including expression of MSC and pericyte cell surface markers and clonogenic, multipotential, and plastic adhensive capacity. Furthermore, recent study showed that these cells have the capability to differentiate into the urothelial and smooth muscle cells (Fig 4)(14). The latest study has demonstrated the feasibility of forming a tissue-engineered conduit for use in urinary diversion by generating scaffolds seeded with human urine-derived stem cells.

Other cells, such as human amniotic fluid stem cells (AFS), human embryonic stem cells (ES) and human induced pluripotent stem cells (iPS), have also shown a potential for application in lower urinary reconstruction. However, most reports have been rather preliminary investigations. Several key points still need to be studied in depth before the cells can be used in patients.

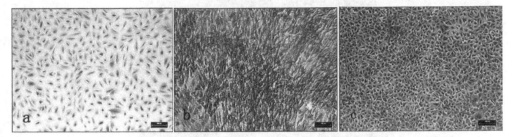

Fig. 4. Morphology of urine-derived stem cells obtained from upper urinary tract (USC-UUT) with differentiation. a. non-treated USC; b. The shape of -UUT changed from an oval to a spindle shape with the addition of myogenic medium; c. a cuboidal shape with the addition of uro-epithelial medium. Scale bar shown is 100 mm (Picture from ref 14).

2.2 Biomaterials

Creating an ideal biomaterial for lower urinary tract reconstruction has been an aspiration of urologists for over a century. An excellent biomaterial for tissue engineering should possess optimal mechanical properties, good biocompatibility, suitable three dimensional structures and degradation rates (15).

2.2.1 Traditional biomaterials

Traditionally, biomaterials can be classified into naturally derived materials, including chitosan, collagen; acellular matrix , such as small intestine submucosa (SIS), bladder acellular matrix (BAMG), acellular corpous spongious matrix (ACSM) and urethral extra matrix (UEM) , as well as synthetic materials, such as PGA and PLGA. Most of them have been used in animal models and human subjects, which will be discussed in the later section. Brehmer provides a useful classification of scaffolds into carrier-, fleece- and sponge-types, according to the structure of biomaterials (16) Carrier-type scaffolds are fiber meshes with very small pore sizes (<15 μm). The pore size of the sponge-type scaffolds is greater than 15 μm. Fleece-type scaffolds have huge interfilamentary spaces (200 μm). In our previous study, we compared the dimensional structures of SIS, BAMG, handmade PGA mesh and ACSM. SEM demonstrated that the pore size of the PGA (>200 μm) was the largest among all biomaterials. The surface pore sizes in SIS were significantly larger than BAMG (58.32 ± 10.31 μm vs 6.77 ± 0.49 μm; $P < 0.05$). Although a looser structure of BAMG could be seen with H&E staining, its pore sizes in surface views were smaller than those of ACSM (6.77 ± 0.49 μm vs 11.12 ± 1.43 μm; $P < 0.05$). An obvious difference of pore diameters in ACSM could be distinguished between urethral surface and cavernosal surface. (2.04 ± 0.32 μm vs 11.12± 1.43 μm; $P < 0.05$)(Fig 5)(17). This data can guide the following cell seeding procedure, since cellular growth and infiltration are strongly related to the scaffold's pore sizes. Of course, it should be noted that the structure of PGA or PLGA can be controlled now with the development of electrospin techniques. Therefore, the dimensional structure of synthetic materials is becoming more similar to the naturally derived scaffolds, and even to the original organs.

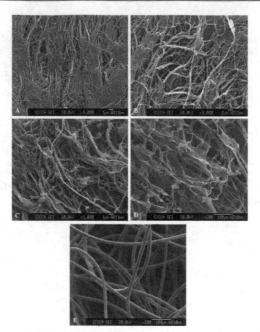

Fig. 5. EMS examination of different materials' surface. (A) urethral surface of ACSM, EMS×5,000, (B) cavernosal surface of ACSM,EMS×5,000 (C) surface of BAMG, EMS×5,000. (D) surface of SIS, EMS_200. (E) surface of PGA, EMS×200.

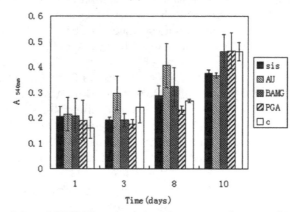

Fig. 6. Metabolic activity of CCSMCs cultured with extracts of various biomaterials or cultured directly in normal medium at 1, 3, 8, and 10 days, as determined by MTT assays. The difference between biomaterials and negative controls was not statistically significant

To address the issue of biocompatibility, our study used the MTT assay technique to evaluate cytotoxicity of different kinds of biomaterials. There were no statistically significant differences in MTT results between the cells cultured with biomaterial extracts and with controls (Fig 6). Thus, we may suggest that all scaffolds could be used safely for lower urinary tract reconstruction.

The mechanical properties of biomaterials are also key to successful reconstruction of the lower urinary tract. For urethral reconstruction, a uniaxial mechanical test is necessary to evaluate the scaffold. In our previous study, all biomaterials exhibited the classic biological nonlinear stress - strain response (Fig. 7) in a mechanical test. The ACSM showed good response in Young's modulus and breaking stress, these being better than in other scaffolds, even the normal rabbit urethra. For the bladder, physiological loading of the tissue involves compressive loads perpendicular to the bladder surface, induced by urine and surrounding pelvic tissues, so biaxial mechanical testing is more realistic. In addition, a burst experiment should also be considered (18) (Fig 8)

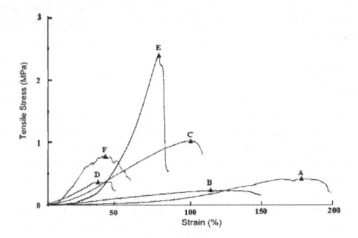

Fig. 7. Stress–Strain curves of various biomaterials. (A) Normal rabbit urethra; (B) SIS; (C) 4-layer SIS; (D) BAMG; (E) ACSM; (F) PGA

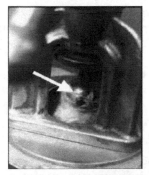

Fig. 8. Picture of ball-burst test with a ruptured test material. Arrow points at the rupture site from (ref 18)

2.2.2 Modified & advanced biomaterials

Since inherit weaknesses always exist in traditional biomaterials, many modified biomaterials have been studied to avoid them.

To enhance angiogenesis, some investigators have modified traditional matrices by incorporating heparin and subsequently loading the heparinized matrices with VEGF. Preliminary studies have shown that this loading of the matrices with VEGF increases the induction of microvessels in both heparinized and non-heparinized matrices, the effect being largest in the case of the heparinized matrices (19).

In order to control the three dimensional structure and degradation rate of synthetic scaffolds such as PGA or PLGA, electrospin techniques are often considered for tissue engineering in lower urinary tract reconstruction. Various materials have been examined for their ability to support cellular adhension, proliferation and formation of a multilayerd urothelium. The results provide the evidence that electrospinning scaffolds show significant benefitsa over commonly used acellular materials in vitro, and suggest that they should be further examined in vivo (20).

2.3 Advanced technique

2.3.1 Bioreactor

The bioreactor is a device that provides a fluid environment for the growth of cells for various applications, such as industrial fermentation and cell culturing. Bioreactors should be introduced in tissue engineering to optimize, through fluid shear, oxygenation and the supply of nutrients, the growth of cells on a 3D scaffold. This approach has been shown to result in better tissue-like constructs than do conventional static culture conditions (21). It is possible to use in vivo graft sites as 'bioreactors' that feature flowing fluids (blood). An example that is commonly used in tissue engineering for lower urinary reconstruction is the greater omentum. Baumert et al (21) used urothelial and smooth muscle cells to seed a sphere-shaped small intestinal submucosa matrix, which was transferred into the omentum after 3wk of cell growth. By this approach, they obtained tissue engineered bladder with a wall thickness was 4 mm. The construct presented a multilayer urothelium on the lumial aspect and deeper fascicles of organized tissue composed of differentiated smooth muscle cells and mature fibroblasts. There was no evidence of inflammation or necrosis (Fig 9). Gu et al (22) implanted 8Fr silastic tubes into the peritoneal cavity of a rabbit. Those tubes were harvested and the tubular tissue covering the tubes was reverted. A pendulous urethral segment of 1.5 cm long was totally excised and urethroplasty was performed with the reverted tubular tissue in an end-to-end fashion. Finally, the results of study showed that the recipients' peritoneal cavity can be used as bioreactor for tissue engineering urethral reconstruction.

More manufactured bioreactors have been designed for tissue engineering bladder. In order to mimic the dynamics of the urinary bladder, bioreactors that imitate the filling and emptying of a normal bladder have been suggested. A bladder bioreactor built this way should be able to recapitulate those dynamics while providing a cellular environment that facilitates cell-cell and cell-matrix interactions. Under the mechanical stimulation from bioreactor, the physiological and mechanical properties of the bladder can be improved. The growth behavior of urothelial cells and bladder smooth cells can be changed, resulting in the cells undergoing adaptive changes in mechanically-stimulated environment (23, 24).

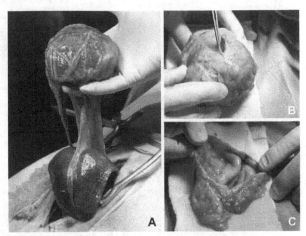

Fig. 9. Harvesting of the matured construct 3 wk after implantation in the omentum (ref 21)

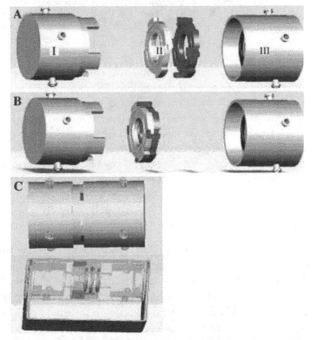

Fig. 10. a. Disassembled urinary bladder bioreactor. I. This chamber will be subjected to controlled pressure and hence would mimic in vitro the urinary bladder chamber. II. Tissue engineered construct ring. III. Compliance chamber (cell culture medium will be recirculated to accommodate the expansion of the scaffold upon pressure generation). b Interlocking discs for cell-seeded scaffold. c Assembled bioreactor (ref 23)

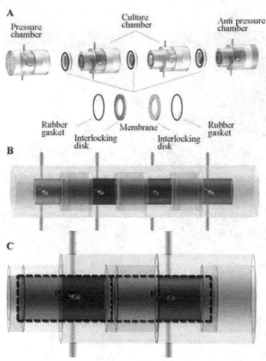

Fig. 11. The bioreactor system. A: A diagram of the disassembled bioreactor, showing the 2 pressure chambers and 2 culture chambers, separated by 3 interlocking rings with elastic membrane. Every interlocking ring was 2 interlocking disks that hold the cell-seeded membrane, which was glued by α-cyanoacrylate. B: The assembled bioreactor with the ports, to which tubing would be attached for medium flow and pressure monitoring. The red parts are culture chambers, blue parts are pressure chambers. C: The assembled culture chambers, the dashed frame showing the pressure P1 and P2 on both sides of cell-seeded membrane. the elastic membrane deformation was driven by pressure difference (P1-P2). (ref 24)

2.3.2 Nanotechnology

Nanotechnology has largely emerged in the last decade of the 20th century as a potential new enabling technology for medicine. For bladder reconstruction, this technology provides a new set of tools to solve many problems that may encountered during the reconstructive procedure. Especially, the incorporation of nanotechnology into bladder tissue engineering materials provides for better bladder materials. Recent published work has demonstrated that increasing of material surface roughness at the nanoscale can improve the adsorption of select proteins important for bladder cell functions (25). Furthermore, some reports showed more bladder smooth muscle cell attachment and growth on polystyrene nanofiber scaffolds fabricated, using an electrospinning technique, to possess surface features at the nanoscale. Cellular adhesive and proliferative ability of keratinocytes were also improved in the nanoscaled scaffold (26).(Table1)

As well as the electrospinning technique mentioned above, another useful nanotechnique is the use of nanoparticles as a delivery system. Mondalek et al (27) investigated the use of PLGA nanoparticles to alter the permeability of SIS scaffolds. Preliminary results indicated that particles ranging from 200 to 500 nm would become imbedded in the SIS scaffold. Particles below this size range would pass through the graft and not become entrapped, and particles above this size range could not penetrate the scaffold. Those results provided the possibility of using nanoparticles to deliver growth factors into seeded cells and scaffolds, to enhance the regeneration of lower urinary tract.

	Bladder Cell Adhesion	Bladder Cell Proliferation	Bladder Cell Synthesis of Proteins	Other Important Functions
Nanostructured PLGA	Highly increased (SMC)[27]	Increased (SMC)[45]	Increased synthesis of elastin and collagen[46]	Decreased formation of calcium stones[29]
	Highly increased (UC)[29]	Highly increased (UC)[29]		
Nanostructured PU	Increased (SMC)[27]	Small increased (SMC)[45]		Decreased formation of calcium stones[29]
	Increased (UC)[29]	Increased (UC)[29]		
Nanostructured PCL	Highly increased (SMC)[27]	Increased (SMC)[45]		
Polymer nanofibers		Increased (SMC)[51]	Production of collagen[51]	Increased cell migration[51]

JC, urothelial bladder cells; SMC, smooth muscle bladder cells.

Table 1. Nanotechnology Approaches to Increase Bladder Cell Functions (ref 26)

2.3.3 Oxygen generating scaffolds

The limitation of oxygen diffusion has led to the general concept that cell or tissue components may not be implanted in large volumes. Many efforts have been made to overcome this limitation. Recently, implantable oxygen releasing biomaterials have been developed in order to provide a sustained release of oxygen to cells and tissues with the goal of prolonging tissue survival and decreasing necrosis (28). In those studies, an oxygen rich compound of sodium percarbonate or calcium peroxide was incorporated into films or 3D constructs of PLGA and used for in situ production of oxygen. In vitro, release of oxygen could be observed from the film more than 24h. Furthermore, these biomaterials were able to extend cell viability growth under hypoxic conditions. Those findings indicate that the use of oxygen generating biomaterials may enhance the scaffold neovascularization after implantation (29). All results suggested that oxygen generating scaffolds can be used for lower urinary tract reconstruction in the future.

3. Applications of tissue engineering in the lower urinary tract

3.1 Bladder reconstruction

Congenital disorders, cancer or trauma can lead to obvious bladder damage. For patients with these problems, bladder reconstructive procedures may be considered. Although gastrointestinal segments are commonly used for bladder augmentation or replacement, multiple complications cannot yet be completely avoided; they include infection, metabolic disturbance and ureolithiasis. A number of animal studies and even clinical experiences have, however, shown the possibility of using tissue engineering techniques to reconstruct bladder tissue. In the laboratory, tissue could be engineered to have function equivalent to the original tissue. In the clinic, patients provided with engineered bladder tissue have obtained satisfactory results.

3.1.1 Animal experiments

Since 1955, many investigators have tried to use different kinds of scaffold for bladder reconstruction in animal models; these have included polyvinyl sponges, polyethylene moulds, Teflon, gelatin sponges, and decellularized pericardial tissue. The outcomes in most studies were unsatisfactory (30). One really successful experiment was reported by Kropp BP et al. (31) in 1995. In this study, the rat underwent partial cystectomy with immediate bladder augmentation with SIS. Host cellular infiltration into the scaffold could be seen 2 weeks after operation. By the end of 48 weeks, the SIS graft presented the three-layered structure of normal bladder, which was indistinguishable from the original bladder. This preliminary study demonstrated the feasibility of using an optimal tissue engineering scaffold for bladder reconstruction. Further study has shown that muscarinic, purinergic and functional cholinergic innervation occurred in rats (32). More recently, bladder regeneration has shown to be more reliable when the SIS was derived from the distal ileum (33). However, graft contraction could be observed in large animal models after using SIS for bladder augmentation, which means that pre-seeding cells may be necessary for tissue engineering-based bladder reconstruction in humans.

Zhang et al. first seeded human bladder urothelial cells and smooth muscle cells onto the SIS by a sandwich culture method (34). This kind of seeding method resulted in organized cell sorting, formation of a well-defined pseudostratified urothelium and multilayered smooth muscle cells with enhanced matrix penetration (Fig 12). The initial study demonstrated that using SIS combined with cell culture could be a valuable model for the study of tissue engineering in bladder reconstruction. To address the problem of graft contraction, Brown et al. showed that opposite-side co-culture of smooth muscle cells and epithelial cells produced a less pronounced matrix contraction than same-side co-culture (20) (Fig 13). The other problem to be addressed in tissue engineering bladder in vitro is cellular infiltration. Recently, Liu et al used preacetic acid (PAA) and Triton X-100

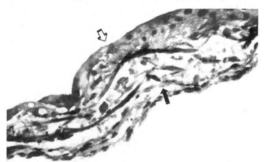

Fig. 12. Sandwich coculture at 28 days shows similar growth pattern to layered coculture technique except that urothelial cells and smooth muscle cells are on opposite sides of small intestinal submucosa membrane. Pseudostratified layer of urothelium is on mucosal surface (open arrow) while multiple layers of smooth muscle cells are on serosal surface and are penetrating into matrix of small intestinal submucosa membrane (solid arrow)(ref 34)

(A) group A   group C   group D   (B)   group A   group C   group D

(C)   (D)

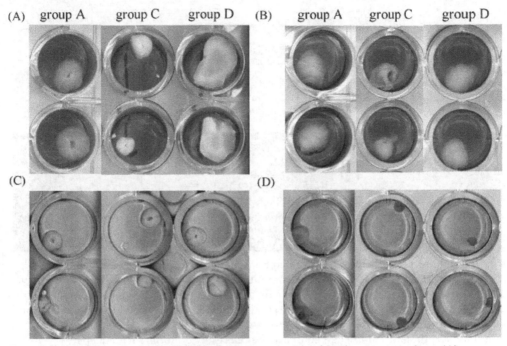

Fig. 13. Gross appearance of cell seeded constructs at 7 and 28 days post seeding. (A) Collagen Gels, 7 days. (B) BAM, 7days. (C) Collagen Gels, 28 days. (D) BAM, 28 days. Group A: SMCs only. Group C: same side co-culture. Group D: opposite side co-culture (ref 20)

to treat the acelluar matrix for bladder tissue engineering reconstruction in vitro (35). This method led to high porosity on the surface of the matrix with about 75% of normal strength. After 3-D dynamic culture, cells could penetrate deeper into the lamina propria of the matrix compared to untreated matrix. (Fig 14). The authors believe that treated scaffold might be more suitable for bladder tissue engineering reconstruction. In order to enhance the vascularization of tissue engineered bladder scaffold in vitro, Baumert et al. transferred the compound matrix into the greater omentum, which has been mentioned above (21).

After meticulous investigation in vitro, Yoo, et al. used scaffold seeded with multiple cell types to reconstruct bladder tissue in 10 beagle dogs, which on which a partial cystectomy had been performed. As a result, 99% a increased in capacity was achieved in the reconstructed bladder. Immunocytochemical analyses confirmed the urothelial and muscle cell phenotypes and showed the presence of nerve fibers (36). Compared to the the technique of seeding with stromal cells, mesenchymal stem cell-seeded scaffold is becoming much more popular in bladder reconstruction. Chung et al. first performed bladder reconstruction using a BMSCs-seeded SIS in rats. At the level of gene expression, regenerated bladder was similar to the control bladder (37). Compared with the BMSCs, ADSCs can be procured more easily. Therefore, we chose ADSCs-seeded scaffolds for bladder reconstruction. At the end of 24 weeks after the operation, the reconstructed bladders reached a mean volume of 94.68±3.31% of the pre-cystectomy bladder capacity in our study. Smooth muscle cells, urothelium and nerve bundles could be detected by

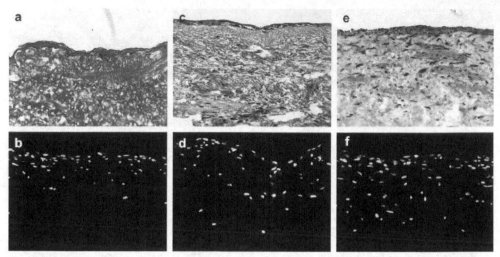

Fig. 14. Cell penetration in 5% PAA-treated BSM in different speeds (0, 10 and 40 rpm) in three-dimensional dynamic culture. Smooth muscle cells and urothelial cell were seeded as layers and co-cultured on the submucosa side of 5% PAA-treated BSM using static culture (left column; a,b) and 3-D rotation culture conditions at 10 (middle column; c,d) and 40 rpm (right column; e,f). H&E staining (a,c,e) and DAPI staining (b,d,f) are shown at 200. Compared with static culture (left column), the cells grew uniformly with deeper penetration in the matrix using 3-D dynamic culture (middle and right column). The cells grown at 40 rpm had deeper penetration of cells within the matrix (e,f) compared to cells cultured at 10 rpm rotation speed (c,d) (ref 35)

immunohistochemical assays. On the contrary, the mean bladder volume was 69.33±5.05% in the control group, made using unseeded scaffolds, and in these there was no evidence of organized muscle or nerve tissue (10) (Fig 15,16). In our study, we also noted that the optimal area for bladder regeneration using seeded scaffold is more than 40-60%, since smaller areas can be regenerated by native bladder tissue. These data provide a useful reference for further clinical application. Other stem cell-seeded scaffolds have also been reported for bladder reconstruction, such as hair-follicle stem cell-seeded scaffolds and urine-derived stem cell-seeded scaffolds (12). However, the number of reports is limited and the actual effectiveness of those scaffold need to be further studied.

As well as traditional cell seeded scaffolds, many modification techniques have been used for tissue engineered bladder reconstructions in animal models. Gregory et al. seeded human adipose stem cells onto PLGA (85:15) bladder dome composites and grafted the result into rat hosts. Results showed that bladder capacity and compliance were maintained in the cell-seeded group throughout the 12 weeks (38) (Fig 17). SIS, modified by hyaluronic acid nanoparticles, has been used for bladder reconstruction. Urinary bladder augmentation has been performed in beagle dogs following hemi-cystectomy using nanoparticle-modified SIS. The results showed that the modified scaffold had significantly higher vascularity compared to unmodified one. This report demonstrated that the nanotechnology can represent a new approach for modifying biomaterials in bladder reconstruction (39). Wei et al.

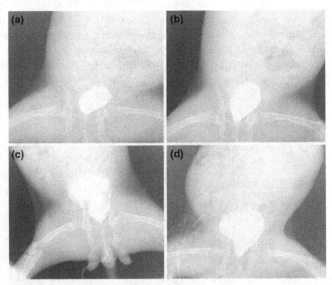

Fig. 15. Cystographies of bladders reconstructed 4 weeks postoperatively. a The control group, b the experimental group 24 weeks postoperatively, c the experimental group and d the experimental group. Cystography demonstrated an improvement in both the shape and capacity of bladders reconstructed with seeded matrices

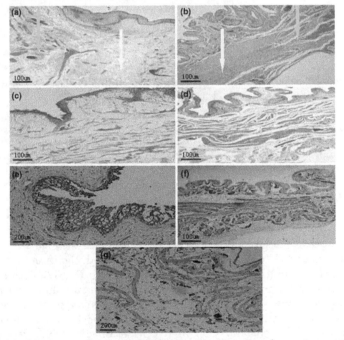

Fig. 16. Histological features of the transplanted grafts. Four weeks postoperatively, native bladder tissue (blue arrow) and in the graft (yellow arrow). a The control group, b the

experimental group 24 weeks postoperatively, c in the control group there is no evidence of organized bladder tissue regeneration, d in the experimental group, the grafts had formed a multilayer epithelium with organized smooth muscle cells. Immunohistochemistry of the transplanted grafts. e Staining with cytokeratin AE1/AE3. α-SM actin. g S-100 (arrows).

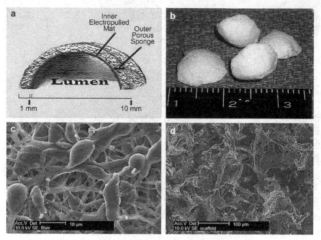

Fig. 17. Construction of the three dimensional synthetic bladder composite. a: Schematic and b: gross micrograph of the three dimensional bladder composite. c:PLGA electropulled microfibers comprising the luminal layer. d: PLGA porous sponge was used as the outer layer (ref 38).

designed a bioreactor to simulate the mechanical properties of bladder. This system successfully generated appropriate pressure waveforms. The viability of cells and tissue structures observed after culture in simulated conditions showed that mechanical stimulation improved the arrangement of cells on scaffold (24).

3.1.2 Clinical application

Although the reports about bladder reconstruction using tissue engineering techniques are few, they are the landmarks in tissue engineered lower urinary tract reconstruction. In Atala's famous study, seven patients with myelomeningocele with high-pressure or poorly compliant bladders enrolled. Urothelial and muscle cells were seeded on a biodegradable bladder-shaped scaffold made of collagen and PGA. Then the biomaterial was used for reconstruction with an omental wrap (40). (Fig 18) After the operation, none of the ultrasounds showed any abnormalities. The cystogram showed the regular shape of bladder after the reconstruction. Urodynamic studies demonstrated significant improvement in volume and compliance in the composite engineered bladders (Fig 19). Postoperatively, it is difficult to distinguish the margin between the composite matrix and the native bladders grossly. All biopsies showed a trilayered structure, consisting of a urothelial cell-lined lumen surrounded by submucosa and muscle. During the post-operative follow-up period all patients had a stable renal function in which serum creatinine was similar to the preoperative status. No metabolic abnormalities were noted. There was no evidence of urinary calculi during the study.

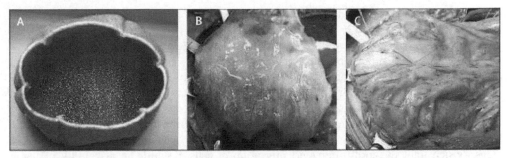

Fig. 18. Construction of engineered bladder scaffold seeded with cells (A) and engineered bladder anastamosed to native bladder with running 4–0 polyglycolic sutures (B). Implant covered with fibrin glue and omentum (C) (Ref 40)

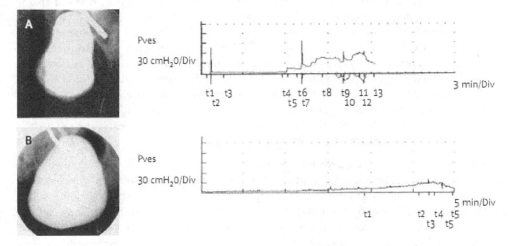

Fig. 19. Preoperative (A) and 10-months postoperative (B) cystograms and urodynamic findings in patient with a collagen-PGA scaff old engineered bladder (Ref 40)

In another clinical study reported in the 2008 AUA, patients, who had received tissue engineered bladder showed increasing capacity and reduced intravesicular pressure. According to these reports, there is a clear reason to hope that the tissue engineered bladder can be utilized for a fully functioning neurogenic bladder. More indications about using this kind of biomaterial might be obtained in the near future.

3.2 Urethral reconstruction

The application of tissue engineering techniques for urethral reconstruction has been developed in recent years and the potential market for a tissue engineered solution for urethral stricture and abnormality will continue to increase in the near future.

3.2.1 Animal experiments

In animal experiments addressing urethral reconstruction, the first attempts used biomaterials alone. Among these experiments, most papers reported the application of SIS in animal urethroplasty. Many results were encouraging. Regenerated urethra contained a well-differentiated epithelium, underneath which was circular smooth muscle and abundant collagen and fibrous connective tissue. The only difference between the SIS-reconstructed urethra and normal urethra was the amount and size of the circular bundles of smooth muscle. However, several key points should be considered before using this kind of biomaterial. First, El-Assmy mentioned that locally prepared SIS and commercially available SIS may lead to the different results (41).This might be related to different pore sizes, which limit the infiltration and migration of cells. Second, the feasibility of using tabularized matrix for urethroplasty is still controversy although SIS has been proven to be useful for onlay urethroplasty. In Shokeir's study, a 3cm segment of the whole urethral circumference was excised and replaced by a tube matrix of the same length and width in 14 dogs. However, all dogs suffered a urethral fistula and/or stricture after the stent removal. This result demonstrated that a tube formed of matrix without seeded cells was not able to replace the long segment including the whole circumference of the canine urethra (42). Third, the length of urethral defect is another key point that should be considered during the urethroplasty. In order to investigate the maximum distance for normal tissue regeneration, Dorin et al. performed the tabularized urethroplasty in 12 male rabbits using acellular scaffold at varying lengths (0.5,1,2 and 3cm). The final result indicated that the maximal defect distance suitable for normal tissue formation using acellular grafts that rely on the native cells for tissue regeneration appears to be 0.5cm (43). Although other reports showed that the synthetic scaffold alone could be used for urethroplasty, the need ror a move to using cell-seeded scaffold is obvious.

In 2003, Bhargava has developed tissue-engineered buccal mucosa for use in substitution urethroplasty. Histologically, the matrix closely resembled the native oral mucosa after culturing for 2 weeks. A gradually increasing thickness of the epidermis and remodeling of the dermis could also be seen (44) (Fig 20). Subsequently, more cell-seeded scaffolds were used for urethral reconstruction in our center. Li et al. replaced urinary epithelial cells with oral keratinocytes seeded on BAMG to reconstruct a tissue-engineered urethra. Histological results showed that multiple layers of keratinocytes had formed at 2 and 6 months after the operation. Obvious margins between graft oral keratinocytes and host epithelium could be noticed in H&E sections (Fig 21b). Fu et al. used foreskin epidermal cell-seeded scaffolds to repair a urethra defect in a rabbit model. During following up, several layers of epidermal cells with abundant vessels in the submucosa were noticed. Moreover, immunofluorescence confirmed the survival of implanted epidermal cells at 1 month after procedure (45,46) (Fig 21a).

Recently, we have investigated the feasibility of constructing 3D structure urethra using multiple seeding cell types. It has also been hypothesized that building three-dimensional constructs in vitro prior to implantation would facilitate matrix vascularization in vivo and minimize the inflammatory response towards the matrix. Therefore, we seeded autologus corporal smooth muscle cells (CSMCs) and lingual keratinocytes into ACSM, using a static-dynamic seeding method. After being cultured 14 days, 6 scaffolds with two kind of cells

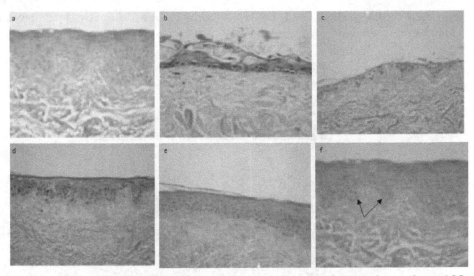

Fig. 20. buccal mucosa culture at a, the air–liquid interface; b, submerged; c, at day 1 ALI; d, at day 5 ALI; e, at day 8 ALI and with f, Protocol 2 (cells on same surface) (Ref 44)

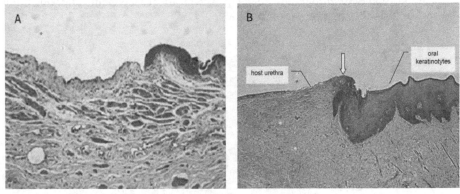

Fig. 21. Histological results of tissue engineering urethral after reconstruction. a. tissue engineering urethra using foreskin seeded scaffold; B, tissue engineering urethra using oral keratinocytes seeded scaffold. (Ref 44,45)

(Group C), 6 scaffolds with only lingual keratinocytes (Group B) and 6 matrices without cells (Group A) were used to repair a rabbit urethral defect. H&E staining of seeded ACSM showed several epithelial layers and well distributed CSMCs in the matrix. The maintenance of wide urethral caliber could be observed in Group C, while strictures were observed in groups A and B (Fig 22). Histologically, the retrieved urethra in group A showed fibrosis and inflammation during 6 months. A simple epithelial layer regenerated in group B but there was still no evidence of CSMCs growing into grafts during study period. A stratified epithelial layer and organized muscle fiber bundles were evident 6 months after implantation in group C (Fig 23). Our results demonstrated that lingual keratinocytes and CSMCs could be used as a source of seed cells for urethral tissue engineering. Using the dynamic-static seeding method, a 3-D urethra could be constructed in vivo. It can provide us an alternative method to treat the urethral disease using tissue engineering techniquea.

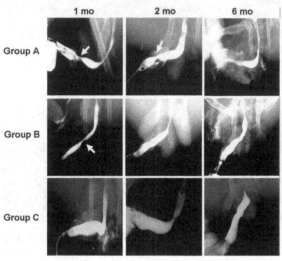

Fig. 22. Comparision of urethrography image in each group at 1,2,6 month after operation. The arrow indicates the stricture site of urethra

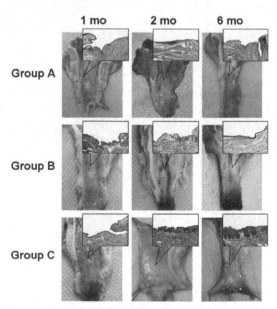

Fig. 23. Macroscopic inspection and H&E staining (inset) of retrieved urethrae in each group at 1,2,6 month after operation. In group A, a urethral stricture existed at every study time point. H&E staining did not show continuous epithelial layers but did show severe inflammation. In group B, strictures could be noticed by gross inspection. Only 1-2 epithelial layers were formed at 6 months after implantation. In group C, patent lumens without

strictures could be observed by the end of 6 months. Meanwhile, multilayer squamous epithelial layers covered the surface of the urethra.

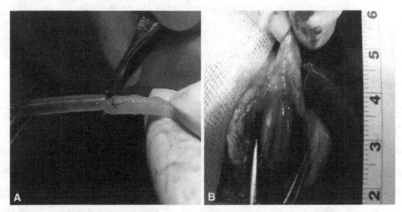

Fig. 24. a. Tubular tissue was gently everted so that the mesothelium lined the lumen. b The everted tubular tissue was interposed and anastomosed as urethral graft (Ref 48)

According to this result, the authors concluded that autologous tissue grown within the recipients' peritoneal cavity can be used successfully for tabularized urethral reconstruction (48). In addition, synthetic matrix combined with seeded cells has also been used for urethroplasty. In Selim's study, the optimal sterilization and cell seeding method for synthetic biomaterials in urethral reconstruction has been investigated. In their study, both PAA and γ-irradiation appear to be suitable methods for sterilizing PLGA scaffolds. And the sterilized PLGA 85:15 is a promising material for tissue engineering urethral reconstruction (49).

3.2.2 Clinical application

Up till now, many urologists have reported successful outcomes of urethral reconstruction using tissue engineering techniques. Most reports have been focused on treating urethral strictures using SIS. Among them, most results were satisfactory (Table 2) (50-56). In the report of Fiala et al., fifty patients with urethral strictures received urethroplasty using SIS. During post-operative follow-up, clinical, radiological, and cosmetic findings were excellent in 80% patients. No complications, such as fistulae, wound infections, or rejection were observed. This is so far the largest reports about using SIS for urethral reconstruction, in terms of numbers of patients. Their results were more satisfacory even than traditional urethral reconstruction using buccal or lingual mucosa for such low complication rate. In our center, we have also used SIS patch to undergo in 16 male patients with urethral strictures. The average length of strictures was 4.6 cm, ranging from 3.5-6 cm (Fig 25). After the operation, urethrography showed a wide patent urethra in all patients. The mean Qmax increased obviously from 3.8ml/s to 25ml/s. Only one patient needed urethral dilation due to the decreasing of Qmax at the end of 5 months. During follow-up, routine urethroscopy was performed in all patients. At the end of 4 weeks after operation, SIS could be easily noticed in the urethral lumen. However, the implanted graft could not be identified from the normal urethra 38 weeks after operation (Fig 26). The HE staining of biopsy showed that stratified squamous epithelial layers had grown on the SIS implanted site, which was similar to normal urethral mucosa (Fig 27). According to these clinical experiences, the use of an acellular matrix SIS for urethroplasty should only be done when the length of urethral stricture is short. Patients with a bulbar urethral stricture are more suitable than those with a urethral stricture in other sites. Of course, the condition of urethral plate should also be considered before using SIS. We believe that urethroplasty using tissue engineered scaffold can achieve a satisfactory outcome that is similar to the gold-standard procedure *provided optimal patients are selected.*

Author	Date	Patient number	SIS type	SIS layer	Stricture length	Recurrence
Mantovani F, et al	2003	1	patch	1	>10cm	none
Le Roux JP	2005	9	tube	1	2-4cm	66.7%(6/9)
Hauser D, et al.	2005	5	patch	4	3.5-10cm	80%(4/5)
Sievert KD, et al.	2005	13	patch	4	4-10cm	30.7%(4/13)
Donkov II,et al	2006	9	patch	4	4-6cm	11.1%(1/9)
Palminteri E,et al	2007	20	patch	4	3-7.7cm	15%(3/20)
Fiala R,et al	2007	50	patch	4	4-14cm	20%(10/50)
Farahat,YA	2009	10	patch	1	0.5-2cm	20%(2/10)

Table 2. Recoder of using SIS for urethral reconstruction in clinic

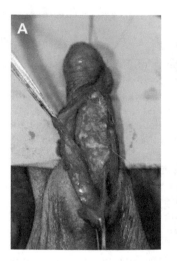
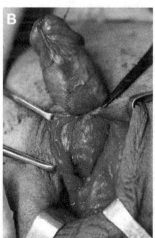
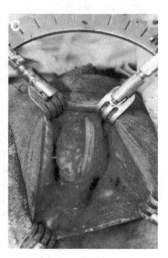

Fig. 25. Application of SIS in urethroplasty.
a. penile urethral stricture; b.bulbopenile urethral stricture; c.bulbar urethral stricture.

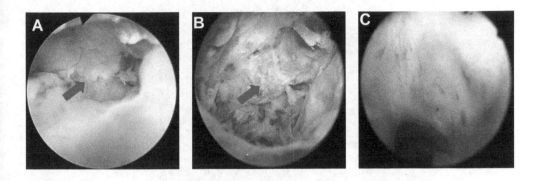

Fig. 26. Urethroscopy after the urethral reconstruction using SIS graft.Arrow headed the implanted site. a:4 weeks after op; b: 6 weeks after op; c: 38 weeks after operation.

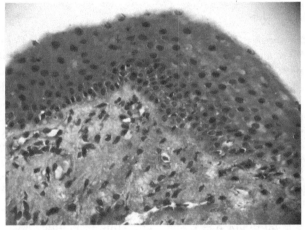

Fig. 27. The HE staining of biopsy showed that stratified squamous epithelial layers have grown on the SIS implanted site.

Cell-seeded scaffolds have also been used for urethral reconstruction in some patients. Based on the previous reports mentioned above, Bhargava et al. useed autologous tissue-engineered buccal mucosa to treat five patients with urethral strictures secondary to lichen sclerosis. After the intimal operation, one patient had complete excision of the grafted urethra and one required partial graft excision. The other three patients required some form of instrumentation although endoscopic appearance showed a patent urethra with the implanted graft in situ (57). Recently, Atala et al. reported that using cell-seeded synthetic tubularized scaffolds to repair urethral defects in five boys. At the end of follow-up, some satisfactory results were obtained. The median end Qmax was 27.1 ml/s, and serial urethrographic and endoscopic studies showed the maintenance of wide calibres without strictures (Fig 28) (58).

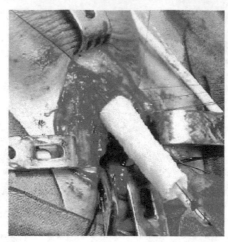

Fig. 28. A cell-seeded graft sutured to the normal urethral margins(Ref 59)

4. Challenges and risks

Based on previous studies, the potential market for a tissue-engineered solution for dysfunctional bladders and small contracted or inflamed bladders is probably far too small for commercial exploitation. The only two potential indications for commercial-scale tissue engineering lower urinary tract tissue are bladder carcinoma and urethral stricture. Cell-seeded scaffolds will probably be further investigated and applied in clinics. hree-dimensional structures and the use of bioreactors will also be more and more popular in tissue engineering research for lower urinary tract reconstruction.

However, several problems need to be solved. For example, the ethical problems about the implanted matrix (and where it is obtained) needs to be further discussed. The potential for carcinogenic problems arising form the use of stem cells is not clear. Optimal methods of cell labeling (for research) still needs to be improved.

Nevertheless, there is no doubt that tissue engineering techniques for lower urinary tract reconstruction will themselves become the gold-standard in the near future. A substantial commercial market will continue to grow and more patients will obtain benefit from this technique.

5. References

[1] Atala A. Tissue engineering for the replacement of organ function in the genitourinary system. Am J Transplant. 2004;4:58-73.
[2] Brown AL, Brook-Allred TT, Waddell JE, White J, Werkmeister JA, Ramshaw JA, et al. Bladder acellular matrix as a substrate for studying in vitr bladder smooth muscle–urothelial cell interactions. Biomaterials. 2005;26:529-543.
[3] De Filippo RE, Yoo JJ, Atala A. Urethra replacement using cell seeded tabularize collagen matrices. J Urol 2002; 168: 1789–1792; discussion 1792–1793

[4] Fu Q, Deng CL, Song XF, Xu YM. Long-term study of male rabbit urethral mucosa reconstruction. Asian J Androl. 2008;10:719-722.

[5] Kimball JR, Nittayananta W, Klausner M, Chung WO, Dale BA. Antimicrobial barrier of an in vitro oral epithelial model. Arch Oral Biol. 2006;51:775-783

[6] Li C, Xu Y, Song L, Fu Q, Cui L, Yin S. Preliminary experimental study of tissue-engineered urethral reconstruction using oral keratinocytes seeded on BAMG. Urol Int. 2008;81:290-295.

[7] Rajasekaran M, Kasyan A, Allilain W, Monga M. Ex vivo expression of angiogenic growth factors and their receptors in human penile cavernosal cells. J Androl. 2003;24:85-90

[8] Drzewiecki BA, Thomas JC, Tanaka ST. Bone marrow-derived mesenchymal stem cells: current and future applications in the urinary bladder. Stem Cells Int. 2011,3; 765-767

[9] Zhang Y, Lin HK, Frimberger D, Epstein RB, Kropp BP. Growth of bone marrow stromal cells on small intestinal submucosa an alternative cell source for tissue engineered bladder. BJU Int. 2005;96:1120-1125.

[10] Zhu WD, Xu YM, Feng C, Fu Q, Song LJ, Cui L. Bladder reconstruction with adipose-derived stem cell-seeded bladder acellular matrix grafts improve morphology composition. World J Urol. 2010;28:493-498.

[11] Tian H, Bharadwaj S, Liu Y, Ma PX, Atala A, Zhang Y. Differentiation of human bone marrow mesenchymal stem cells into bladder cells: potential for urological tissue engineering. Tissue Eng Part A. 2010;16:1769-1779.

[12] Drewa T, Joachimiak R, Kaznica A, Sarafian V, Pokrywczyńska M. Hair stem cells for bladder regeneration in rats: preliminary results. Transplant Proc. 2009;41:4345-4351.

[13] Zhang Y, McNeill E, Tian H, Soker S, Andersson KE, Yoo JJ, et al. Urine derived cells are a potential source for urological tissue reconstruction. J Urol 2008;180:2226-2233

[14] Bodin A, Bharadwaj S, Wu S, Gatenholm P, Atala A, Zhang Y. Tissue-engineered conduit using urine-derived stem cells seeded bacterial cellulose polymer in urinary reconstruction and diversion. Biomaterials. 2010;31:8889-8901.

[15] Nakanishi Y, Chen G, Komuro H, Ushida T, Kaneko S, Tateishi T,Kaneko M. Tissue-engineered urinary bladder wall using PLGA mesh-collagen hybrid scaffolds: A comparison study of collagen sponge and gel as a scaffold. J Pediatr Surg 2003;38:1781–1784

[16] Brehmer B, Rohrmann D, Becker C, Rau G, Jakse G. Different types of scaffolds for reconstruction of the urinary tract by tissue engineering. Urol Int 2007;78:23–29.

[17] Feng C, Xu YM, Fu Q, Zhu WD, Cui L, Chen J. Evaluation of the biocompatibility and mechanical properties of naturally derived and synthetic scaffolds for urethral reconstruction. J Biomed Mater Res A. 2010;94:317-325.

[18] Freytes DO, Badylak SF, Webster TJ, Geddes LA, Rundell AE. Biaxial strength of multilaminated extracellular matrix scaffolds. Biomaterials. 2004 May;25:2353-2361.

[19] Yao C, Prével P, Koch S, Schenck P, Noah EM, Pallua N, et al. Modification of collagen matrices for enhancing angiogenesis. Cells Tissues Organs. 2004;178:189-196.

[20] Kundu AK, Gelman J, Tyson DR. Composite thin film and electrospun biomaterials for urologic tissue reconstruction. Biotechnol Bioeng. 2011;108:207-215.

[21] Baumert H, Simon P, Hekmati M, Fromont G, Levy M, Balaton A, et al. Development of a seeded scaffold in the great omentum: feasibility of an in vivo bioreactor for bladder tissue engineering. Eur Urol. 2007;52:884-890.

[22] Gu GL, Zhu YJ, Xia SJ, Zhang J, Jiang JT, Hong Y, et al.Peritoneal cavity as bioreactor to grow autologous tubular urethral grafts in a rabbit model. World J Urol. 2010;28: 227-232.

[23] Farhat WA, Yeger H. Does mechanical stimulation have any role in urinary bladder tissue engineering. World J Urol. 2008;26:301-305.

[24] A novel bioreactor to simulate urinary bladder mechanical properties and compliance for bladder functional tissue engineering

[25] Khang D, Lu J, Yao C, Haberstroh KM, Webster TJ.The role of nanometer and sub-micron surface features on vascular and bone cell adhesion on titanium.Biomaterials 2008, 29:970–983.

[26] Chun YW, Lim H, Webster TJ, Haberstroh KM. Nanostructured bladder tissue replacements.Wiley Interdiscip Rev Nanomed Nanobiotechnol. 2010 Aug 20.

[27] Mondalek FG, Lawrence BJ, Kropp BP, Grady BP, Fung KM, Madihally SV,et al. The incorporation of poly(lactic-co-glycolic) acid nanoparticles into porcine small intestinal submucosa biomaterials. Biomaterials 2008,29:1159–1166

[28] Harrison BS, Eberli D, Lee SJ, Atala A, Yoo JJ. Oxygen producing biomaterials for tissue regeneration. Biomaterials. 2007;28:4628-4634.

[29] Oh SH, Ward CL, Atala A, Yoo JJ, Harrison BS. Oxygen generating scaffolds for enhancing engineered tissue survival. Biomaterials. 2009;30:757-762.

[30] Kropp BP.Small-intestinal submucosa for bladder augmentation:a review of preclinical studies. World J Urol. 1998;16:262-267.

[31] Kropp BP, Eppley BL, Prevel CD, Rippy MK, Harruff RC, Badylak SF, et al. Experimental assessment of small intestinal submucosa as bladder wall substitute. Urology. 1995;46:396-400.

[32] Kropp BP, Sawyer BD, Shannon HE, Rippy MK, Badylak SF, Adams MC, et al. Characterization of small intestinal submucosa regenerated canine detrusor: assessment of reinnervation, in vitro compliance and contractility. J Urol. 1996;156:599-607.

[33] Kropp BP, Cheng EY, Lin HK, Zhang Y. Reliable and reproducible bladder regeneration using unseeded distal small intestinal submucosa. J Urol. 2004;172:1710-1713.

[34] Zhang Y, Kropp BP, Moore P, Cowan R, Furness PD 3rd, Kolligian ME, et al. Coculture of bladder urothelial and smooth muscle cells on small intestinal submucosa: potential application for tissue engineering technology. J Urol. 2000;164:928-934; discussion 934-935

[35] Liu Y, Bharadwaj S, Lee SJ, Atala A, Zhang Y. Optimization of a natural collagen scaffold to aid cell–matrix penetration for urologic tissue engineering. Biomaterials. 2009;30:3865-3873.

[36] Yoo JJ, Meng J, Oberpenning F, Atala A. Bladder augmentation using allogenic bladder submucosa seeded with cells. Urology. 1998;51:221-225.

[37] Chung SY, Krivorov NP, Rausei V, Thomas L, Frantzen M, Landsittel D, et al. Bladder reconstruction with bone marrow derived stem cells seeded on small intestinal submucosa improves morphological and molecular composition. J Urol. 2005;174:353-359.

[38] Jack GS, Zhang R, Lee M, Xu Y, Wu BM, Rodríguez LV.Urinary bladder smooth muscle engineered from adipose stem cells and a three dimensional synthetic composite. Biomaterials. 2009;30:3259-3270.

[39] Mondalek FG, Ashley RA, Roth CC, Kibar Y, Shakir N, Ihnat MA, et al. Enhanced angiogenesis of modified porcine small intestinal submucosa with hyaluronic acid-poly(lactide-co-glycolide) nanoparticles: From fabrication to preclinical validation. J Biomed Mater Res A. 2010 ;94:712-719.

[40] Atala A, Bauer SB, Soker S, Yoo JJ, Retik AB. Tissue-engineered autologous bladders for patients needing cystoplasty. Lancet. 2006;367:1241-1246.

[41] El-Assmy A, El-Hamid MA, Hafez AT.Urethral replacement: a comparison between small intestinal submucosa grafts and spontaneous regeneration. BJU Int. 2004;94:1132-1135.

[42] Shokeir A, Osman Y, Gabr M, Mohsen T, Dawaba M, el-Baz M.Acellular matrix tube for canine urethral replacement:Is it fact or fiction. J Urol. 2004;171:453-456.

[43] Dorin RP, Pohl HG, De Filippo RE, Yoo JJ, Atala A. Tubularized urethral replacement with unseeded matrices: what is the maximum distance for normal tissue regeneration. World J Urol. 2008;26:323-326.

[44] Bhargava S, Chapple CR, Bullock AJ, Layton C, MacNeil S.Tissue-engineered buccal mucosa for substitution urethroplasty. BJU Int. 2004;93:807-811.

[45] Fu Q, Deng CL, Liu W, Cao YL.Urethral replacement using epidermal cell-seeded tubular acellular bladder collagen matrix. BJU Int. 2007;99:1162-1165.

[46] Li C, Xu YM, Song LJ, Fu Q, Cui L, Yin S.Urethral reconstruction using oral keratinocyte seeded bladder acellular matrix grafts. J Urol. 2008 ;180:1538-1542.

[47] Guan Y, Ou L, Hu G, Wang H, Xu Y, Chen J, et al. Tissue engineering of urethra using human vascular endothelial growth factor gene-modified bladder urothelial cells. Artif Organs. 2008;32:91-99.

[48] Gu GL, Zhu YJ, Xia SJ, Zhang J, Jiang JT, Hong Y, et al. Peritoneal cavity as bioreactor to grow autologous tubular urethral grafts in a rabbit model. World J Urol. 2010;28:227-232.

[49] Selim M, Bullock AJ, Blackwood KA, Chapple CR, MacNeil S. Developing biodegradable scaffolds for tissue engineering of the urethra. BJU Int. 2011;107:296-302.

[50] Mantovani F, Trinchieri A, Castelnuovo C, Romanò AL, Pisani E. Reconstructive urethroplasty using porcine acellular matrix. Eur Urol. 2003;44:600-602.

[51] Le Roux JP. Endoscopic urethroplasty with unseeded small intestinal submucosa collagen matrix grafts: a pilot study. J Urol. 2005 ;173:140-143.

[52] Schlote N, Wefer J, Sievert KD. Acellular matrix for functional reconstruction of the urogenital tract. Special form of "tissue engineering"?. Urologe A. 2004;43:1209-1212

[53] Donkov II, Bashir A, Elenkov CH, Panchev PK. Dorsal onlay augmentation urethroplasty with small intestinal submucosa: modified Barbagli technique for strictures of the bulbar urethra. Int J Urol. 2006;13:1415-1417.

[54] Palminteri E, Berdondini E, Colombo F, Austoni E. Small intestinal submucosa (SIS) graft urethroplasty: short-term results. Eur Urol. 2007;51:1695-1701

[55] Fiala R, Vidlar A, Vrtal R, Belej K, Student V. Porcine small intestinal submucosa graft for repair of anterior urethral strictures. Eur Urol. 2007;51:1702-1708;

[56] Farahat YA, Elbahnasy AM, El-Gamal OM, Ramadan AR, El-Abd SA, Taha MR. Endoscopic urethroplasty using small intestinal submucosal patch in cases of recurrent urethral stricture: a preliminary study. J Endourol. 2009;23:2001-2005

[57] Bhargava S, Patterson JM, Inman RD, MacNeil S, Chapple CR. Tissue-Engineered Buccal Mucosa Urethroplasty—Clinical Outcomes. Eur Urol. 2008;53:1263-1269.

[58] Raya-Rivera A, Esquiliano DR, Yoo JJ, Lopez-Bayghen E, Soker S, Atala A. Tissue-engineered autologous urethras for patients who need reconstruction: an observational study. Lancet. 2011;377:1175-1182

6

Endochondral Bone Formation as Blueprint for Regenerative Medicine

Peter J. Emans, Marjolein M.J. Caron,
Lodewijk W. van Rhijn and Tim J.M. Welting
Department of Orthopaedic Surgery, Maastricht University Medical Center,
The Netherlands

1. Introduction

During our life moving, walking, sport, etc., are essential for our health and quality of life. Both bones and cartilage enable us to do so. Bones support us, allow muscles to move them, and protect vital internal organs. At the end of most bones articular joints are situated. The side where 2 bones form an articular joint, the ends of these bones are covered with hyaline cartilage. This articular cartilage is able to withstand very high mechanical forces with very low friction and thereby enables easy movement. A large number of bones are formed by a process called endochondral ossification. During this process a cartilage template is replaced by bone, in contrast with the cartilage in newly formed joints which remains cartilage. Both articular cartilage and bone mature and this leads to a well organised architecture and specialisation. The arcade-like architecture of cartilage is capable to withstand an enormous amount of intensive and repetitive forces during life. However, the British surgeon William Hunter made the now famous statement that *"From Hippocrates to the present age it is universally allowed that ulcerated cartilage is a troublesome thing and that once destroyed it is not repaired"* (Hunter 1743). In contrast, bone has a very high regenerative capacity. This difference in self-healing capacity may partially be explained by the access to progenitor cells which contribute to tissue repair. For bone repair, progenitor cells of three different sources have been identified. These sources are: (i) progenitor cells form the blood stream since bone is a highly vascularised tissue, (ii) progenitor cells from the overlying periosteum and (iii) progenitor cells from the bone marrow. Cartilage is not vascularised, is not covered by periosteum, nor has a specialized tissue such as bone marrow and this might be part of the explanation for the limited self-repair capacity of cartilage. Although both tissues start from the same mesenchymal cell condensations, the contrast in self-repair is striking (Hunziker, Kapfinger et al. 2007).

From a clinical point of view there is a need for repair of both bone and cartilage. Bone and cartilage were both identified as tissues for which it was thought to be possible to recreate them in a laboratory setting, using the combination of cell isolation culture techniques and carrier materials. The science of combining cells with carrier materials to reproduce tissues in the laboratory is called Tissue Engineering (TE). The collaboration of scientists of different disciplines such as cell biology, biomaterials, biomechanics, engineering and translational medicine has already led to fruitful scientific achievements. However, initial expectations of tissue engineering have not been reached completely. Although some treatments which apply to the principles of TE have reached clinical practice, TE-created tissues are not generated on a large scale (Brittberg, Lindahl et al. 1994; Oberpenning, Meng et al. 1999; Macchiarini, Jungebluth et al. 2008). In addition, time consuming and expensive culture procedures and logistics, multiple operations and quality of the repair that is initiated by TE constructs remain important drawbacks.

Upon implantation of a TE-created construct the introduction of cells, biomaterials, growth factors, etc. in the body will have an effect on the local environment and natural repair mechanisms at the implant site. Since it is largely unknown what this local effect is and how these factors contribute to it, a clear shift is observed in the attempts to repair tissue. This shift includes more specific natural stimuli which trigger and enhance the regenerative capacity of the tissue itself. Injection of stem cells or progenitor cells (cell therapies), and the induction of regeneration by biologically active molecules can all be regarded as an example of Regenerative Medicine (RM). For both TE and RM it becomes more and more evident that studying the underlying natural and developmental processes of cartilage and bone can serve as a blueprint to identify important cell sources, biochemical, biomechanical, structural stimuli and timing thereof. It is expected that insight in these biological mechanisms and the process of endochondral ossification will enhance the progress in the field of both TE and RM.

This chapter describes the first phases of endochondral ossification, bone and cartilage (defects) and current approaches in TE and RM. Parallels with RM and endochondral ossification are identified from where endochondral ossification can serve as a blueprint for future RM approaches.

2. Endochondral ossification

Endochondral ossification is a multistage process that determines the major part of mammalian skeletal development and starts in embryogenesis with condensation of mesenchymal stem cells. The formation of cartilage, a process called chondrogenesis, is a key event in developing limb buds beginning in the center of the condensed mesenchyme. The earliest form of cartilage development is suggested to be 300 million years ago (Urist 1976). In humans, the first skeletal rudiments develop during the 5th week of gestation. In the eight week of the embryological life relatively cell-poor intermediate zones begins to develop, which will form the joint cavities (Gray and Gardner 1950; Anderson 1962; Aydelotte and Kuettner 1992). The diaphyseal cartilage, which is located at the center of the shaft of future long bones, is replaced by bone before birth (primary ossification). However most of the cartilaginous epiphysis at the end of long bones turns into bone after birth (secondary ossification). The remaining cartilage between the primary and secondary ossification centers is called the epiphyseal plate, more commonly known as the growth plate, and it continues to form new cartilage, which is replaced by bone, a process that results in increased length of the bones. Eventually all the cartilage in the growth plate will be converted into bone leaving cartilage only at the articulating surfaces of joints. Although bone and cartilage develop from the same mesenchyme, they have completely different structures, compositions and functions.

Chondrogenesis in both the primary and secondary ossification center and growth plates is characterized by highly proliferative chondrocytes, vectorially dictated to differentiate into hypertrophic chondrocytes before dying from apoptosis. The remaining mineralized extra cellular matrix provides a scaffold for infiltrating blood vessels and for bone cells to adhere to and remodel, setting the stage for *de novo* bone deposition (Kronenberg 2003) (Figure 1). The bone forming cells, osteoblasts, arise from progenitor cells from the overlying periosteal tissue and will form the bone collar (later the cortex) and primary spongiosa (later trabecular bone). In the adult, bone and overlying articular cartilage are attached by an interface of calcified cartilage (Schenk, Eggli et al. 1986). This interface distributes forces and stresses applied during load bearing and acts as a barrier to nutrients. Nutrients for the growing epiphyseal cartilage are supplied by two sources: (i) the synovial cavity and (ii) the vascularized cartilage canals (McKibbin and Maroudas 1979; Kuettner and Pauli 1983). Cartilage and synovium merge at a transitional zone which persists in the adult and is the site of osteophyte formation (Blaney Davidson, Vitters et al. 2007). This osteophyte formation is one of the first examples of endochondral ossification which takes place after growth. Another example is endochondral ossification during fracture healing where a cartilage callus is formed which will be remodelled into new bone. Studying endochondral ossification in normal growth and in healing processes will improve our understanding of both chondrogenesis and osteogenesis and as such may serve as a blueprint for Regenerative Medicine purposes of these tissues.

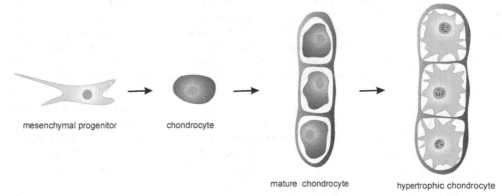

mesenchymal progenitor   chondrocyte   mature chondrocyte   hypertrophic chondrocyte

Fig. 1. The different steps of endochondral ossification; mesenchymal progenitor cells condense and undergo chondrogenesis. After maturation these chondrocytes undergo hypertrophy and die by apoptosis leaving a scaffold as a template for bone formation (these last steps are not illustrated nor discussed in this chapter).

2.1 Bone and bone defects

Bone can be formed by 2 different processes, while endochondral bone formation drives most of the skeletal bone formation, bone can also be formed by another process called intramembranous bone formation. During intramembranous bone formation, no cartilage phase is found and progenitor cells directly differentiate into bone. Intramembranous bone formation is largely responsible for the formation of flat bones as can be found in the skull and pelvis. Endochondral bone formation is largely responsible for the formation of bones of the axial skeleton. While in cartilage only one type of cell (chondrocyte) can be found, multiple cell types can be found in bone. Generally the bone forming cells are called osteoblasts and the cells which resorb bone are called osteoclasts. Osteoblasts produce the bone matrix (osteoid) which consists mainly of the organic collagen type I which is mineralized by inorganic hydroxyapatite (calcium phosphate). This gives bones a high compressive strength combined with significant elasticity. When osteoblasts become entrapped in their matrix they become osteocytes; the mature bone cells (Harada and Rodan 2003). Osteoclasts, on the other hand, are multinucleated cells that arise from the monocyte stem-cell lineage and are located at bone surfaces in Howship's lacunae. The cells are equipped with phagocytic-like mechanisms and are characterized by high expression of tartrate resistant acid phosphatase (TRAP) and cathepsin K which are able to break down bone matrix (Boyle, Simonet et al. 2003). The process of bone formation and bone resorption is able to adapt to mechanical forces and as such remodel into the desired architecture (Wolff's law). This process is mostly found in trabecular bone and while no evidence has been found that cartilage adapts/remodels after growth, bone is replaced constantly (Hunziker, Kapfinger et al. 2007). Another important function of bone resorption and formation is controlling homeostasis of important minerals such as calcium and phosphate.

Different specialized structures can be identified in bone; the bone attached to the joint cartilage is called subchondral bone. The zone directly beneath the subchondral bone is called the metaphysis. The metaphysis is characterized by a thin cortex and a highly vascularised trabecular bone. Within this trabecular bone bone marrow can be found. Bone marrow is also present at the inside of long bones where it enables hematopoiesis. In the center of long bones lies the diaphysial bone. Here, trabeculi become more sparse and the cortex thickens. The outer site of all bones is covered by periosteum. This periosteum is largely responsible for appositional growth of long bones as it contains a lining of osteoprogenitor cells. **Bone defects.** In the field of Orthopaedic and Trauma Surgery a large demand exists for autologous or allogenic bone. Clinical problems which fuel this demand are; large segmental bone defects (after infection, trauma or tumor resection), fracture non-unions (e.g. tibia, femur, humerus, carpal bones, and talus), bone defects in the increasing field of prosthesis related revision surgery, and spinal fusions (e.g. spondylolisthesis, discopaty, etc)(Glowacki 1998; Stevenson 1998; Huitema, van Rhijn et al. 2006). Although bone from the iliac crest is the golden standard, it is limited in source and donor site morbidity is a major concern. Alternatively, allografts are expensive and pose the risk of viral infection. While the inorganic part of bone (e.g. TriCalcium Phosphate (TCP), Hydroxyapatite (HA)) is widely explored as ceramics and combined with cells in the field of TE, this approach is not successful in generating a satisfying bone substitute (Petite, Viateau et al. 2000; Kim, Park et al. 2006; Zhao, Grayson et al. 2006). Main drawbacks are mechanical features and handling properties of these ceramics. Combining ceramic with polymers may overcome this problem, but toxic degradation products often affect healing and remodeling of the bone defect (Martin, Shastri et al. 2001; Kim, Park et al. 2006; Zhao, Grayson et al. 2006). In addition, these materials are often inert for Matrix Metallo-Proteins (MMPs) and often interfere with biomechanical signaling which is essential for repair and remodeling of loaded structures such as bone (Wolff's law). Furthermore, increased infection risk in implanted tissue-engineered devices is recently described (Kuijer, Jansen et al. 2007) and supply of oxygen and nutrients is the final aspect of concern when treating bone defects (Shastri 2006). Cells in autologous bone are transplanted from a highly vascularized environment to a hypoxic environment while cells residing in allografts are frozen and stored before transplantation, it is therefore likely that these cells do not contribute to the repair process (Emans, Pieper et al. 2006). Seeding of these materials with bone marrow cells is promising, however also costly, time consuming and infection prone during isolation and expansion (Shastri 2006). Among the disadvantages listed here lies the reason why this topic is currently studied extensively by many groups worldwide.

2.2 Cartilage and cartilage defects

Joint motion is possible by a both structurally and functionally truly remarkable material called hyaline cartilage (Buckwalter and Mankin 1998; Hasler, Herzog et al. 1999; Poole, Kojima et al. 2001). Hyaline cartilage is predominantly found in articular cartilage. Next to hyaline cartilage, two other types of cartilage can be found in the human body; elastic and fibrocartilage. Elastic cartilage is found in the ear, nose-tip and respiratory tract, whereas the menisci and intervertebral discs contain fibrocartilage.

The only cell type found in articular cartilage is the chondrocyte. In contrast to other tissues, the chondrocyte contributes to a relatively low percentage of the cartilage volume in human (1-5 percent). Articular chondrocytes are formed by chondrogenic differentiation of chondroprogenitor cells as described above and in Figure 1, however these cells arrest in the mature chondrocyte phase and normally do not become hypertrophic cells. Each chondrocyte is a metabolically active unit which expands and maintains the extracellular matrix (ECM) in its immediate vicinity (Aydelotte, Greenhill et al. 1988). In adults chondrocytes lack cell-cell contact; therefore communication between cells has to occur via ECM. Furthermore, cartilage is characterized by the absence of blood vessels, lymphatics and nerve fibers. Due to the lack of vascularisation in cartilage the environment is dominated by low oxygen levels and therefore the chondrocytes have an anaerobic metabolism (Schenk, Eggli et al. 1986). This also implicates that chondrocytes have to obtain their nutrients and oxygen via diffusion from the synovial fluid, through the ECM and from the underlying bone.

Structure. In articular cartilage four zones can be distinguished (see Figure 2), based on collagen type II orientation and chondrocyte shape and distribution (Buckwalter and Mankin 1998; Mankin, Mow et al. 2000; Poole, Kojima et al. 2001). In the superficial or tangential zone, chondrocytes are disc shaped and form a layer of several cells thick. The long axis of the cells are parallel to the joint surface and the cells are surrounded by a thin layer of ECM. Thin collagen fibers are oriented parallel with the articular surface. This orientation and the relatively low content of proteoglycans results in high tensile stiffness and the ability to distribute load over the surface. The cells in the transitional or middle zone are more spherical and appear dispersed randomly (Aydelotte and Kuettner 1992; Hunziker 1992), also collagen fibers in this zone are organized randomly. At this zone and at the deep zone, high concentrations of proteoglycans enable the tissue to bear compressive forces. In the radial or deep zone, chondrocytes are ellipsoid, grouped radially in columns of 2-6 cells with their long axes perpendicular to the joint surface. The thicker collagen fibres are also arranged perpendicular to the articular surface. In the calcified zone, chondrocytes are distributed sparsely and remain surrounded by a calcified matrix. The calcified cartilage is less stiff than the subchondral bone. At this calcified zone shear stresses are converted into compressive forces which are in turn transmitted to the subchondral bone (Radin, Martin et al. 1984). The junction between uncalcified and calcified cartilage is called the "tidemark", a line which can be seen on histology (Figure 2). Therefore mechanical forces also change at the tidemark which provides a definite boundary for the uncalcified layer (Donohue, Buss et al. 1983; Aydelotte and Kuettner 1992).

Cartilage defects can arise due to trauma or cartilage degeneration. Although patient's history may differentiate between traumatic and degenerative lesions, the exact cause of cartilage defects often remains difficult to diagnose. Since cartilage has no nerve fibers, cartilage lesions often present with only (minor) effusion of the affected joint or without symptoms. Diagnosis of structures likely to be damaged upon trauma (e.g. subchondral bone, ligaments or menisci), may reveal a cartilage lesion. An X-ray indicates a cartilage lesion in the minority of the cases and Magnetic Resonance Imaging (MRI) is the best non-invasive technique available for diagnosis of cartilage lesions. Important developments are new protocols such as delayed Gadolinium Enhanced MRI of Cartilage (dGEMRIC) and sodium MRI which can visualize cartilage on the Collagen and GAG content level (Gold, Burstein et al. 2006). Overall the MRI is expected to diagnose cartilage lesions in an early stage and will become more important in evaluation of progression of cartilage degeneration and cartilage repair techniques.

As early as 1743 it was recognized that articular cartilage, once destroyed, does not heal spontaneously (Hunter 1995; Hunziker 1999). Whereas the progenitor cells of bone marrow and periosteum contribute to bone formation during fracture healing, articular cartilage is deprived of these progenitors. Although it has been shown that the superficial layer of cartilage and the synovium contain progenitor cells (Dowthwaite, Bishop et al. 2004; Park, Sugimoto et al. 2005), cartilage has a limited ability for self repair (Mankin, Mow et al. 2000; Emans, Surtel et al. 2005). Therefore cartilage and tissue engineering approaches are studied in an attempt to overcome the inability of cartilage to repair itself.

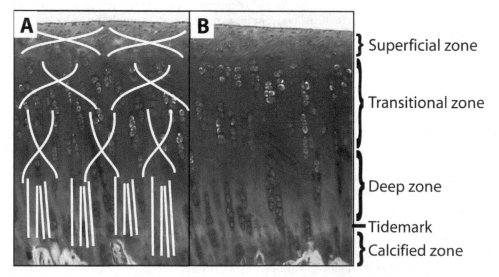

Fig. 2. Architecture of articular cartilage. Four zones can be distinguished with respect to (A) orientation of collagen fibers and (B) cell shape and orientation

3. Tissue engineering and regenerative medicine

Combining technologies from material science, cell biology, and clinical needs has led to the rise of the field of TE and RM. In the 1960's researches proposed the idea of creating tissues in a laboratory which may replace damaged or diseased tissues and cell biologists observed that cells could sort themselves *in vitro* to populations with tissue-like characteristics (Steinberg 1962). Adding a structure (material) such as a collagen gel to fibroblast cultures was shown to further resemble structural characteristics of skin. Later the work of Brittberg and co-workers showed that chondrocytes could be cultured and successfully be transplanted for the repair of cartilage defects (Brittberg, Lindahl et al. 1994). This technique is entitled Autologous Chondrocyte Transplantation or Implantation (ACT or ACI). The combination of specific tissue features and the early findings of culturing and transplanting chondrocytes and fibroblasts, skin, cartilage and bone were identified as tissues which potentially could be repaired by engineering these tissues in the laboratory by combining cells and supporting scaffolds. In the beginning of ACT no artificial structures were used to keep the chondrocytes in the cartilage defect. Optimization of ACT has led to the introduction of collagen meshes to support and maintain chondrocytes which were transplanted into the defect. Already earlier, in the mid-1980s, Langer and co-workers proposed that biodegradable polymers could serve as a scaffold for the organisation and maturation of cells into the desired tissues. As such it was proposed that this approach would enable engineering of thicker and hard tissues such as cartilage. Although cell therapies based on TE for skin are commercially available, which apply to the definition of TE such as Carticel® and Epicel® of Genzyme, the initial expectations of TE and RM have not been met. Although some examples of successful treatment by engineered tissues such as bladder and trachea can be found in the clinic, engineering tissues is not performed on a large scale (Oberpenning, Meng et al. 1999; Macchiarini, Jungebluth et al. 2008).

In the approach to engineer tissues in a laboratory setting and subsequently transplanting them into the body lies the key question; *"until what level should we engineer tissue and when should nature take over?"*. It is often the aim of many researchers to engineer a mature tissue which is directly able to take over the function of the diseased tissue or organ. Per example it is often a goal that engineered cartilage and bone should be able to bear mechanical forces directly after implantation. In contrast, in nature a cascade of interactions occur during the process of tissue repair. During this process both the environment as well as the reparative tissue adapt to each other and the biomechanical requirements. In such a manner both integration of repair tissue and tissue remodelling is achieved. The capacity of a mature TE tissue to adapt to the local needs such as integration, remodelling, etc. is lower than a relatively less mature tissue. In addition, in order to create a robust and thicker tissue, the use of scaffolds, growth factors and more differentiated cells may be inevitable. However the question remains whether the local environment is able to adapt in an appropriate manner to all non-physiological stimuli which are introduced. Per example how does the normal tissue remodelling, repair and integration respond to a scaffold which alters local biomechanical stimuli which are known to be essential for tissue remodelling? How do transplanted and environmental cells respond to material properties such as material surface, breakdown products, architecture etc? How does the normal fine-tuned orchestra of tissue repair respond to transplanted cells which are normally not present at a certain phase of tissue repair? Finally, the use of cells in RM and TE approaches often implies the use of two surgical procedures as well as costly and time consuming culture procedures and logistics.

3.1 Bone repair

Natural bone healing. As described above, endochondral ossification drives skeletal growth. Similar sequential steps of endochondral ossification are largely responsible for fracture healing of long bones (Bostrom, Lane et al. 1995; Einhorn 2005). Periosteum is the main source of progenitor cells capable of creating large volumes of non-vascularized cartilage surrounding a fracture (Hall and Jacobson 1975). This first phase of endochondral bone formation is called soft callus. During the second phase chondrocytes become hypertrophic, mineralize (hard callus) (Figure 1), secrete pro-angiogenic factors such as VEGF and finally bone is deposited. In the final phase the newly formed bone is vascularized and will remodel under influence of mechanical forces. Bone healing by endochondral ossification is influenced by many regulatory mechanisms. However, while interaction of Indian hedgehog (Ihh) and Parathyroid hormone related protein (PTHrP) is one of the best known regulatory mechanism in the growth plate, such an interplay is yet unknown for fracture healing (Wu, Ishikawa et al. 1995; Vortkamp, Lee et al. 1996; Volk and Leboy 1999). The role of growth factors during bone healing processes is better studied. Chondrocytes at different stages of maturation release cytokines and growth factors such as Fibroblast Growth Factor (FGF), Transforming Growth Factor (TGF)-β, Bone Morphogenetic Proteins (BMPs) and Vascular Endothelial Growth Factor (VEGF) (Gibson 1998; Gerber, Vu et al. 1999; Blunk, Sieminski et al. 2002). For instance FGF-2 and TGF-β control endochondral ossification by inhibition of chondrocyte proliferation, hypertrophy and apoptosis (Gibson 1998) and in addition from our own findings we know that TGF-β is important for osteo- and chondrogenesis both in *ex vivo* and *in vivo* models (Kuijer, Emans et al. 2003). *In vivo*, in the Osteoarthritic (OA) joint TGF-β is produced. Under the influence of this TGF-β osteophytes are formed which are derived from periosteum adjacent to the joint via endochondral bone formation (van der Kraan and van den Berg 2007). BMPs are also positively involved in ectopic cartilage and bone formation, partly by opposing the actions of the FGF pathways (Yoon and Lyons 2004; Miyazono, Maeda et al. 2005; Yoon, Pogue et al. 2006). Neo-vascularization under influence of VEGF ensures blood vessel formation which supply oxygen and nutrients to osteoblast and osteoclasts. The latter produce MMP-9 and -13 which degrade the matrix surrounding terminally hypertrophic chondrocytes (Gerber, Vu et al. 1999). Blocking VEGF in the hypertrophic zone of the growth plate prevents degradation of this zone which in turn enlarges (Gerber, Vu et al. 1999).

Current approaches for bone repair. Multiple causes may lead to impaired healing of large bone defects. As mentioned before, nature has a good regenerative capacity for fractures, however from a clinical perspective the need for bone is not in fracture repair but mostly for the filling of large bone defects after revision arthroplasty and spondylodesis. These bone defects can be regarded as "non-natural" occurring bone defects and bone healing or filling is impaired at these sites because endochondral ossification does not occur. To deal with this problem a scaffold is introduced as a template for bone ongrowth, ingrowth and remodelling. Currently many bone fillers (scaffolds) and growth factors are available for treatment of bone defects. Taking the scaffold which is formed during endochondral ossification (also see chapter "scaffolds") as a blueprint, bone fillers need to be further optimized; next to being expensive, these aids only address one or a few aspects of the cascade of tissue responses which are necessary for bone repair. Most bone fillers are osteoconductive (supportive) and they lack the timing and onset of essential growth factors to be osteoinductive (stimulating bone growth). Growth factors by themselves have been shown to be osteoinductive but addition of one of the essential growth factors does not necessarily recapitulate the physiological, initial tissue response which leads to fracture/bone repair.

Inflammation is the first and essential phase of tissue repair in general and bone repair in particular. Mimicking this inflammatory response may be a method to enhance bone fracture healing. Several clinical examples such as spondylodesis after infection of the intervertebral disc (e.g. after discography) and the method described by Masquelet confirm that inflammatory responses contribute to osteogenesis (Guyer, Collier et al. 1988; Masquelet and Begue 2010). However, in contrast, from an engineering perspective, the aim is often to create bone which has comparable mechanical features as native bone. The initial mechanical properties of currently used bone chip auto or allografts are incapable of withstanding the mechanical forces to which they are exposed. During impaction of these chips the mechanical properties of the impacted bone as a whole are capable to withstand mechanical forces in a non-loadbearing environment. After vascularisation, bone ingrowth and remodelling of the repaired bone defect adapts to finally bear full loading. As such surgical handling properties, osteoconduction, and most important osteoinduction are features one should aim for rather than engineering mature bone with biomechanical properties comparable to native bone. As mentioned before during endochondral ossification large amounts of cartilage are generated. This cartilage does not have the required mechanical features of the bone it should repair, but does have strong osteoconductive and osteoinductive features. Another challenge when aiming for creation of bone is the scale to which should be generated. During fracture healing bone defects can be repaired by deposition of large amounts of bone which is formed by endochondral ossification. In the pre-remodelling phase of endochondral ossification, the generated bone histologically resembles the metaphysial bone chips which are used on a large scale for bone impaction grafting. In conclusion, regarding endochondral ossification as a blueprint for engineering or regeneration of bone, it has the potential to generate vast amounts of bone, with good handling properties, and is osteoinductive and osteoconductive.

3.2 Cartilage repair

Treatment of damaged cartilage can be grouped to four concepts of principle: the four R's (O'Driscoll 1998). The joint surface can be: (i) resected, (ii) relieved, (iii) replaced or (iv) restored. A joint prosthesis is an example of joint replacement; joint distraction and osteotomies can induce joint relieve. Osteotomies are used to re-align the axis of loading in patients with a malalignment of the leg. By transferring the load to the less affected cartilage (e.g. previously less loaded/damaged cartilage) the damaged part is relieved. Arthodesis is an example of joint resection. For TE and RM techniques the focus is on cartilage restoration.

Restoration implies methods to heal or regenerate the joint surface with or without the subchondral bone into healthy hyaline articular cartilage. Three strategies can be considered when attempts are made to heal or restore cartilage.

i.   Subchondral Drilling, Abrasion or Microfracture are techniques to allow penetration of
     bone marrow through the subchondral bone into the damaged cartilage (Meachim and
     Roberts 1971; Insall 1974; Mitchell and Shepard 1976; Furukawa, Eyre et al. 1980;
     Vachon, Bramlage et al. 1986; Bradley and Dandy 1989; Rae and Noble 1989; Kim,
     Moran et al. 1991; Altman, Kates et al. 1992; Aglietti, Buzzi et al. 1994). These techniques
     improve the clinical well being of the patient and the joint surface defect may be healed
     to some extent. However the healing process is inadequate since no functional hyaline
     cartilage but fibrocartilage is formed (Vachon, Bramlage et al. 1986; Altman, Kates et al.
     1992). Nonetheless, these methods are cheap and easy to perform and are therefore seen
     as the currently best option to relieve the complaints. Other clinical studies have
     suggested that any beneficial effect is related to the arthroscopic procedure itself. A
     nonspecific effect might be related to joint lavage rather than the penetration of the
     subchondral bone (Jackson 1986; Ogilvie-Harris and Fitsialos 1991). In conclusion, these
     techniques may have some benefit with regard to small defects but no effect has been
     proven in relation to large defects, osteoarthritic joints or older patients (Kim, Moran et
     al. 1991).

ii. Implants vary from non-degradable and degradable, cells, periosteum or
     perichondrium, Osteochondral Autograft Transfer System (OATS or Mosaicplasty) and
     Osteochondral Allografts (Elford, Graeber et al. 1992; Freed, Vunjak-Novakovic et al.
     1993; Nixon, Sams et al. 1993; Hendrickson, Nixon et al. 1994; Reddi 1994; Chu, Coutts
     et al. 1995; Grande, Halberstadt et al. 1997). The biomaterials and periosteum can be
     combined with cells or growth factors. Periosteal Arthroplasty is an interesting way of
     treating cartilage defects since many have reported the chondrogenic potential of
     periosteum (O'Driscoll, Keeley et al. 1986; O'Driscoll, Keeley et al. 1988; Zarnett and
     Salter 1989; Nakahara, Bruder et al. 1990; Nakahara, Dennis et al. 1991; Nakahara,
     Goldberg et al. 1991; Nakata, Nakahara et al. 1992; Iwasaki, Nakata et al. 1993; Gallay,
     Miura et al. 1994; Iwasaki, Nakahara et al. 1994; Iwasaki, Nakahara et al. 1995;
     O'Driscoll, Saris et al. 2001; Emans, Surtel et al. 2005). Over 90 percent of collagen type II
     in the hyaline cartilage formed in the cartilage defects treated with periosteal grafts has
     been reported (O'Driscoll, Keeley et al. 1986; O'Driscoll, Keeley et al. 1988).
     Perichondrial Arthroplasty used for human cartilage repair was first described by
     Skoog et al. (Skoog and Johansson 1976). This technique has been reported to give an
     initial cartilage repair (Homminga, Bulstra et al. 1990; Homminga, Bulstra et al. 1991).
     On the long term poor results related to overgrowth of the graft and calcification are
     reported by Bouwmeester *et al.* (Bouwmeester, Beckers et al. 1997). These authors
     concluded that a better fixation of the graft might improve the results. In a study
     comparing periosteum with perichondrium, chondrogenesis was observed significantly
     more using periosteal grafts (Vachon, McIlwraith et al. 1989). This finding and the
     accessibility make periosteum to be preferred over perichondrium.

iii. Osteochondral Grafts can be divided in autologous and allogenic. Mosaicplasty or
     OATS involves harvesting one or more osteochondral plugs from a relatively less
     weight-bearing region of the joint and subsequent implantation of these plugs into an
     articular defect. Possible donor site morbidity is bypassed if osteochondral allografts
     are used (Gross, McKee et al. 1983; Garrett 1986; Czitrom, Keating et al. 1990; Convery,
     Meyers et al. 1991; Garrett 1994; Ghazavi, Pritzker et al. 1997; Garrett 1998; Horas,
     Schnettler et al. 2000; Gross, Aubin et al. 2002).

The role of endochondral ossification in cartilage repair. When using progenitor cells for cartilage repair, ossification of the repaired tissue may impair clinical results. Examples hereof are ossification and formation of interlesional osteophytes when applying techniques such as microfracture and periosteum or perichondrium plasty (Bouwmeester, Beckers et al. 1997; Cole, Farr et al. 2011). These findings illustrate that maintaining differentiated progenitor cells in their chondrogenic state remains challenging in cartilage repair. It appears that in contrast to chondrocytes, progenitor cells have the tendency to follow the different phases of endochondral ossification towards hypertrophy and mineralisation when triggered to differentiate into cartilage. As such, locking cells in their desired differentiation state is of the utmost importance when applying these cells for RM purposes. Findings of Hendriks and co-workers showed that chondrocytes stimulate progenitor cells towards chondrogenesis when both cell types are co-cultured (Hendriks, Riesle et al. 2007). These findings were later bolstered by Fisher and co-workers showing that human articular cartilage-derived soluble factors and direct co-culture are potent means of improving chondrogenesis and suppressing the hypertrophic development of mesenchymal stem cells (Fischer, Dickhut et al. 2010). In this study and other work of the group of Richter the PTHrP is an important candidate soluble factor involved in this effect. PTHrP is primarily known as a key regulator in the process of endochondral ossification. Furthermore, we have recently shown that cyclooxygenase (COX) inhibitors are also able to decrease hypertrophy of chondrocytes (unpublished data). Thus studying the process of endochondral ossification and further unravelling how and why articular chondrocytes maintain their phenotype as well as prevention of hypertrophy may enhance cartilage repair techniques by generating stable cartilage which does not lead to intra-lesional osteophytes. Finally, cartilage defects lead to early OA, also in the process of OA more evidence is found that articular chondrocytes loose their capacity to maintain their phenotype and seem to undergo endochondrogenesis since they become hypertrophic and express collagen type X (Saito, Fukai et al. 2010). As such understanding and controlling the process of endochondrogenesis may be of relevance for future insight and treatment of OA.

3.3 Scaffolds

Scaffold or carrier material refers to a wide variety of artificial 2D or 3D structures that are designed for the purpose of tissue engineering. Scaffolds may be seeded with cells before implantation or are designed to recruit or retain cells at the desired place. (Bentley and Greer 1971; Wakitani, Kimura et al. 1989). For bone and cartilage regeneration, relevant cells are (mesenchymal) stem cells of different origins (bone marrow, adipose tissue, dental pulp, iPS etc.) as well as differentiated cells like chondrocytes. Different variables are important parameters for scaffold design: pore diameter, shape, kind of material, (bio)degradability, implantation site, functionalization, mechanical stability and others. Several materials have been and are being explored for this purpose. Generally scaffold materials can be divided in natural or synthetic. Examples of natural material-based scaffolds for cartilage and bone regeneration are: fibrin, hyaluronan, alginate, agarose, demineralized bone matrix, collagen etc. Synthetic scaffold materials include ceramics and copolymers PolyGlycolic Lactic acid (PGLA) and PolyethyleneGlycol-terephthalate/PolyButylene Terephthalate (PEGT/PBT) (Figure 3) etc. When applying a collagen as carrier material, some authors find enhanced cartilage healing, while others conclude that collagen scaffolds have a limited usefulness for chondrocyte grafting in large defects (Wakitani, Kimura et al. 1989; Nixon, Sams et al. 1993;

Sams, Minor et al. 1995; Sams and Nixon 1995). The use of fibrin as carrier material was reported to give superior cartilage healing compared to controls (empty defect) (Hendrickson, Nixon et al. 1994). Within time an ideal scaffold should degrade or allow the populated cells to take over functionality of the artificial tissue implant. Breakdown products and biomechanical features of the scaffold should not negatively interfere with differentiation towards this tissue. It is therefore challenging to design a scaffold with all the optimal characteristics; proper initial mechanical stability, timed release of required growth factors, timed degradation which allows biomechanical stimuli to remodel the formed tissue, no release of degradation products which interfere with tissue repair, good handling properties, etc. Next generation scaffolds will be so called "smart scaffolds". These scaffolds will be loaded with bioactive factors (e.g. TGF-β1 and members of its superfamily such as BMPs) that can directly influence the differentiation pathways (Sellers, Peluso et al. 1997; Sellers, Zhang et al. 2000; Huang, Goh et al. 2002). Effort is being put in e.g. functionalized scaffolds with specific affinity peptides to retain cells (Dong, Wei et al. 2009). Also, the release of e.g. growth factors may be regulated by "on demand" smart systems that depend on incorporated microspheres or proteolytic degradation of linker-peptides. Unfortunately, an ideal material for artificial scaffolds for cartilage and bone regeneration has not been identified yet, as the biological processes involved are far more complex than anticipated.

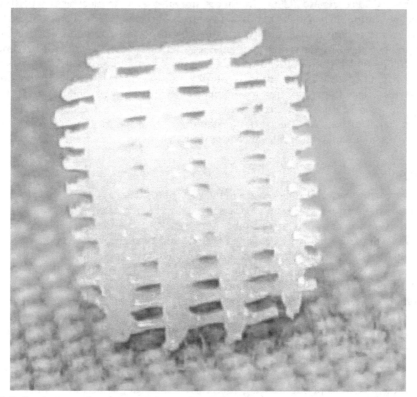

Fig. 3. A PolyethyleneGlycol-terephthalate/PolyButylene Terephthalate (PEGT/PBT) scaffold produced by using a three dimensional rapid prototyping technique.

The endochondral scaffold. During endochondral ossification nature creates its own scaffold. Hypertrophic chondrocytes die and leave a large scaffold. During this process multiple growth factors are released in an orchestrated manner. The scaffold itself is used as a template for invading cells to deposite bone and provide vascularisation. The scaffold itself is resorbed by osteoclasts which in turn respond to biomechanical and biochemical stimuli. As such the scaffold degrades and simultaneously the proper factors are released. The repair tissue remodels to the appropriate architecture as defined by Wolff's law. Studying this process in detail reveals the challenge when "artificial" scaffolds are designed from a material science point of view, and so far no scaffolds have been created with the same properties capable to dictate the same processes of endochondral remodelling.

3.4 Cells

Cells for "orthopaedic" tissues, such as bone and cartilage, originate from the mesenchymal cell lineage and may be derived from different autologous or allogenic sources. Interestingly, cells used for bone regeneration are almost always progenitor cells, whereas for cartilage regeneration also differentiated cells are used, next to progenitor cells. Some authors prefer the use of chondrocytes for transplantation while others prefer the use of undifferentiated multipotent cells (Skoog and Johansson 1976; O'Driscoll, Keeley et al. 1986; Homminga, Bulstra et al. 1991; Brittberg, Lindahl et al. 1994; Lindahl, Brittberg et al. 2003; Nathan, Das De et al. 2003; Emans, Surtel et al. 2005; Park, Sugimoto et al. 2005).Mature chondrocytes can be released from their cartilaginous matrix, selected and expanded *in vitro*. In this way a relatively small amount of autologous tissue can be used as an appropriate cell source. Both chondrocytes and progenitor cells originating from different cell sources have been studied in combination with various biomaterials (Bentley and Greer 1971; Haynesworth, Baber et al. 1992; Freed, Marquis et al. 1993; Freed, Vunjak-Novakovic et al. 1993; Iwasaki, Nakata et al. 1993; Brittberg, Lindahl et al. 1994; Bruder, Fink et al. 1994; Freed, Grande et al. 1994; Gallay, Miura et al. 1994; Wakitani, Goto et al. 1994; Iwasaki, Nakahara et al. 1995). Bone marrow, adipose tissue, synovium, dental pulp, perichondrium and periosteum can serve as a source for multipotent cells (Skoog and Johansson 1976; Homminga, Bulstra et al. 1991; Bouwmeester, Beckers et al. 1997; Chu, Dounchis et al. 1997; O'Driscoll, Saris et al. 2001; Nathan, Das De et al. 2003; Emans, Surtel et al. 2005; Park, Sugimoto et al. 2005). Numerous publications described subpopulations of progenitor cells in these donor tissues that might be more optimal cell sources than e.g. whole cell pool isolates. However, lots of these studies were only performed *in vitro* and one can question whether selection of subtypes based on cell surface markers may bias the outcome of the intervention in a difficult to predict way. The involvement of subchondral bone may play a role in cell source selection as chondrocytes are capable of producing cartilage under the appropriate conditions, but in a situation where simultaneous bone formation is required (involvement of the subchondral bone), multipotent cells might be a better cell source. After selection and expansion, the main challenge is to keep these cells in the damaged area of the joint and this challenge becomes even bigger in larger defects (Bentley and Greer 1971). Grande *et al.* reported that only 8 percent of the total number of cells in the healing tissue originated from transplanted chondrocytes (Grande, Pitman et al. 1989). Chondrocytes can be maintained in the defect by suturing a periosteal flap or a collagen mesh over the defect (Grande, Pitman et al. 1989; Brittberg, Lindahl et al. 1994; Bartlett, Skinner et al. 2005). As discussed above, chondrocytes can also be seeded in a matrix or scaffold. This matrix can be implanted in a cartilage defect. This Matrix Assisted Chondrocyte Transplantation (MACT) is technically less demanding and has shown identical results compared to Autologous Chondrocyte Transplantation on the short term (Bartlett, Skinner et al. 2005) The use or allogenic chondrocytes has been reported to be successful in rabbits but experiments in horses do not support this finding (Wakitani, Kimura et al. 1989; Freed, Grande et al. 1994; Sams, Minor et al. 1995; Sams and Nixon 1995). Immunological rejection or allogenic chondrocytes upon implantation in rabbits has been reported and this remains a major concern when applying allogenic cells. The use of periosteal tissue or cells has been suggested by several authors and is one of the most clear examples of the use of endochondral ossification as a blueprint for cartilage and bone regenerative medicine. The periosteum is populated with mesenchymal progenitor cells that normally contribute to endochondral bone fracture healing. The differentiation capacity of these cells can also be used to create cartilage or bone for regenerative purposes. This principle is further explained below (see paragraph 3.6).

When using differentiated or undifferentiated cells for cartilage, bone or osteochondral repair it is a challenge to differentiate these cells into their desired state and maintain their desired phenotype. As cells from the mesenchymal lineage, once differentiated into chondrocytes, have a natural tendency for terminal differentiation via the endochondral pathway. This is a big concern for regenerative applications. Much effort is being put in technologies that prevent hypertrophic differentiation of transplanted chondrocytes, while on the other hand for bone regeneration hypertrophic differentiation may be a prerequisite for success (Fischer, Dickhut et al. 2010; Scotti, Tonnarelli et al. 2010).

3.5 Biochemical signaling pathways

Growth factors. In growth plate development, homeostasis of articular cartilage as well as bone formation and maintenance, several signaling pathways are interacting or shared between the different tissues. Indian hedgehog (Ihh) and Parathyroid hormone related peptide (PTHrP) coordinate chondrocyte proliferation and differentiation in the so-called PTHrP-Ihh feedback loop (Kronenberg 2003). This coordination influences the length of proliferative chondrocyte columns as well as chondrocyte hypertrophy. Next to the Ihh and PTHrP loop, fibroblast growth factor crucially regulates chondrocyte proliferation and differentiation. Many of the 22 distinct FGF genes and their four receptor genes are expressed at every stage of endochondral bone formation (Ornitz and Marie 2002). Also Bone Morphogenic Proteins (BMPs) have multiple roles during bone and cartilage formation, as well as growth plate development. Interestingly, BMPs were discovered because of their remarkable ability to induce endochondral bone formation when injected subcutaneously in mice. In a cartilage context, BMPs are involved in early chondrogenesis, cartilage maintenance and hypertrophic differentiation. In a bone context they drive differentiation of progenitor cells to osteocytes and induce alkaline phosphatase activity in osteocytes. TGF-β isoforms are also involved in similar processes and interestingly were found to trigger the formation of osteophytes upon intra-articular injection and during OA (Elford, Graeber et al. 1992; van Beuningen, van der Kraan et al. 1993; van Beuningen, van der Kraan et al. 1994; Hunziker 2001). As osteophyte formation itself is an example of endochondral ossification, the role of TGF-β isoforms in endochondral ossification is supported by this finding. Remarkably, some characteristics of OA resemble chondrocyte differentiation processes during skeletal development by endochondral ossification. Resemblances are: chondrocyte proliferation, chondrocyte hypertrophic marker expression (e.g. Collagen type X and MMP-13), vascularisation and focal calcification of joint cartilage. This suggests that during OA the articular cartilage is terminally differentiating via "normal" endochondral pathways. However, how the mature articular cartilage is kept in its cartilaginous state and why it starts a terminal differentiation program in OA is currently poorly understood. In the final stage of endochondral bone formation secretion of pro-angiogenic factors such as VEGF is essential. Sox9 and RunX2 are important transcription factors. Sox9 is the master regulator of chondrogenesis and acts as a negative regulator for chondrocyte hypertrophy, cartilage vascularisation and bone marrow formation (Hattori, Muller et al. 2010). Amongst others it does this via negatively regulating expression of RunX2 via Nkx3.2 (also known as BapX1) (Yamashita, Andoh 2009). RunX2 is a central regulator for the transition from proliferating to hypertrophic chondrocytes, as it drives the transcription of Collagen type X. Interestingly, RunX2 also drives multiple osteogenic developmental programs. Inflammatory pathways are other key players in endochondral ossification (Einhorn, Majeska et al. 1995; Mountziaris and Mikos 2008). Bone fracture healing by endochondral ossification depends on a haematoma-induced inflammatory environment (Grundnes and Reikeras 1993) and several inflammatory molecules (e.g. IL-6, TNFα, COX-2 and iNOS) are involved in bone fracture repair (Einhorn, Majeska et al. 1995; Mountziaris and Mikos 2008) by influencing chondrocyte maturation and osteogenic development. An important chondrogenic growth factor is Insulin Growth Factor 1 (IGF-1). Together with its receptors and several IGF binding proteins it determines chondrocyte proliferation and differentiation. Importantly IGF-1 appears to play a role in preventing chondrocyte apoptosis. Hence, it determines the pace of hypertrophic differentiation and thus growth plate development and fracture callus maturation. It was shown that IGF-1 exerts its action via NF-κB/p65 signaling (Wu, Gong et al. 2008). Furthermore, IGF-1 also directly influences osteocyte biology. It has been reported that IGF-1 stimulates cancellous bone formation and increases the activity of resident osteoblasts (Zhao, Monier-Faugere et al. 2000). RANK is crucially important for bone homeostasis and remodelling. Activation of RANKL on monocytic cells by RANK on osteoblasts induces osteoclastogenesis of committed monocytic cells. Multinucleation is induced, ultimately leading to the generation of mature bone resorbing osteoclasts (Novack and Faccio 2011). This process is counterbalanced by the soluble factor osteoprotegerin (OPG), thereby preventing bone loss due to osteoclast activation. Activation of the RANKL system is potentiated by prostaglandins. PGE$_2$, one of the main cyclooxygenase metabolites is reported to increase bone resorption.

In conclusion, the process of endochondral ossification is dictated by spatiotemporal expression and use of variable interacting growth factors and other molecules. It is clear that mimicking this complex, yet incompletely known, tissue formation in an *in vitro* setting on the same scale as TE was expected to do is quite challenging. Several findings such as endochondral ossification after subcutaneous injection of BMPs show that, *in vivo*, this process may be triggered using stimuli which trigger and enhance the regenerative capacity of the tissue itself. In such an approach the amount of unknown stimuli is expected to be limited and the body's own regenerative capacity is used to generate cartilage or bone, which in turn can be transplanted into the damaged site. As such, this approach applies more to the principles of RM than to the principles of TE. The application of a specific *in vivo* trigger to stimulate endochondral bone formation has many advantages; no expensive culture procedures, no more harvesting of cells, and no introduction of factors which possibly conflict with the natural tissue repair and integration. Table 1 summarises the differences in tissue features, currently applied (TE) techniques for restoration, and remaining challenges.

3.6 Examples of endochondral ossification as blueprint for regenerative medicine

Currently for TE purposes cells are harvested during the first operation and the implantation of the graft/cells is performed during the second procedure. A question that remains is the amount of cells that survives the transplantation. It has been shown that periosteal cells show a much poorer survival compared to chondrocytes after transplantation into the hostile environment of a fresh osteochondral defect (Emans, Pieper et al. 2006). However, the disadvantage of using chondrocytes is the fact that the joint is further damaged. It would be ideal to generate cartilage in an ectopical place which does not further interfere with the joint homeostasis, survives the transplantation and is capable to adapt and repair the defect. In line with this, an interesting variation for cartilage repair is a reported by Takahashi *et al.* who used the early fracture callus, induced at the iliac crest (Takahashi, Oka et al. 1995). The early fracture callus was implanted into osteochondral defects of rabbit knees with excellent results. A paper of our group also reported excellent results after transplantation of periosteum derived cartilage callus into osteochondral defects (Emans, van Rhijn et al. 2010). Stevens *et al.* published an interesting paper on inducing chondrogenesis by subperiosteal injection of a hyaluronan-based gel containing the antiangiogenic factor Suramin. The resulting tissue also resembled cartilage of early fracture callus (Stevens, Marini et al. 2005). The main advantage of this approach is that the body is used as its own "*in situ* incubator"; cells provide their own matrix and complex and costly isolation, selection and culturing procedures are bypassed. After this first report focussing on bone, we aimed to control the local environment by injecting a gel into the space between bone and periosteum which would initiate endochondrogenesis. Both agarose and a gel loaded with TGF-β1 were successful to trigger endochondrogenesis. This tissue was harvested during its first chondrogenic phase and successfully implanted into an osteochondral defect where an excellent lateral integration and no calcification of the cartilage adjacent to the joint was observed (Emans, van Rhijn et al. 2010).

It was recognised by the group of Martin that TE and RM attempts to create bone using the intramembranous pathway (Scotti, Tonnarelli et al. 2010). In contrast, during development most bones are formed by endochondral ossification and the parts that do not ossify forms articular cartilage. In addition, during fracture healing bone gaps and defects are often repaired by endochondral bone formation, during which large amounts of callus can be formed. Depending on the phase in which specific tissue is generated by endochondrogenesis, this tissue can be harvested for different purposes. If tissue in the early chondrogenic phase is harvested this may be ideal to heal both bone and cartilage. If this tissue is harvested at a later stage it resembles trabecular bone which has the potential to be used for bone impaction grafting. Compared to the frequently used TE approach to create bone directly (intra-membranous), it seems more logical that endochondral bone formation which is capable to produce large amounts of cartilage and bone, even in an ectopic site, may fuel further research

Challenges in Tissue Engineering		
Tissue characteristics		
	Bone	Cartilage
Function	Weight bearing	Weight bearing and joint articulation
Cells	Osteoblasts/osteocytes and osteoclasts	Chondrocytes
Origin	Mesenchymal and monocyte lineage	Mesenchymal
ECM	Collagen I and Calcium phosphate	Collagen II, Proteoglycans, GAGs and Hyaluronic acid
Functional ECM water content	No	Yes, important
Cell-cell contact	Yes and important	No, 'communication' via ECM
Vascularisation	Yes	No, hypoxic tissue
Nutrient/oxygen supply	Via vascularisation	Via diffusion
Remodelling	Constant (Wolff's law)	Low grade of remodelling?
Regenerative capacity	High	Low
Access to progenitor cells	Bloodstream, Periosteum, Bone marrow	Superficial layer cartilage? Synovium?
Endochondral ossification	Complete	Has to stop at chondrocyte-phase

Current approaches in TE					
Bone			**Cartilage**		
	Advantages	Disadvantages		Advantages	Disadvantages
Auto- and Allografts	Osteoconductive Osteoinductive? Native bone	Expensive Host-vs-graft reaction Infection Freezing cells? Donor site morbidity	Osteochondral grafts	Native cartilage	Expensive Host-vs-graft reaction (allografts) Infection Donor site morbidity Fixation Cell morbidity during storage
Decellularized bone	Osteoconductive Resembles native bone	Not osteoinductive Host-vs-graft reaction Infection	**Subchondral drilling, abrasion, microfracture**	Activation of bone marrow Very effective Cheap and easy	Fibrocartilage
HA/TCP/ Bonefillers	Osteoconductive Resembles native bone properties Can be loaded with cells/growth factors	Not osteoinductive Mechanical features Handling properties Interference with biomechanical signalling	**ACI/ACT MACT**	Good integration Native cartilage	Infection Time consuming Expansion of cells Fixation Expensive
Growth factors	Osteoinductive	Not osteoconductive Expensive Overload of growth factor Ectopic bone formation	**Implants/ biomaterials**	Can be loaded with cells/growth factors Initial cartilage repair	Calcification of cartilage Fixation Toxic degradation products

Challenges		
Current advantages		**Remaining challenges**

Scaffolds	Conductive
	Can be loaded with cells and/or growth factors to recruit, retain and/ or differentiate the cells
	Immediate initial mechanical stability
		Scaffold design: pore diameter and shape
		(bio)Material: natural or synthetic
		Biodegradability and degradation at right time
		Breakdown products
		Integration / fixation
		Release of growth factors at right time
		Interference with tissue environment
		Cartilage: Nutrient supply in scaffold
		                 Allow ECM formation,
		but prevent mineralisation
		                 Allow articulation, repetitive mechanical
		loading and load damping
		Bone: Nutrient and oxygen supply
		           Stimulate vascularisation
		           Allow bone mineralisation
		           Support high mechanical loading
		Endochondral: progenitors differentiate to hypertrophic chondrocytes which leave a natural 'scaffold' for bone cells to adhere and remodel and provides in essential growth factors and vascularisation at appropriate time points.

Growth factors (BMPs, TGF-βs, PTHrP, VEGF, etc)	Inductive Can regulate differentiation of cells Easy	Does not recapitulate total physiological repair response Keep growth factors at damaged area Effect on tissue *in vivo* incompletely known Still expensive

Progenitor cells	High potential to differentiate into required tissue
	Various origins (bone marrow, dental pulp, adipose tissue, periosteum, blood etc.)
		Have to differentiate and remain differentiated into required tissue
		Infection
		If allografts: host-vs-graft reaction
		Keep cells at damaged area
		Cartilage: Nutrient and oxygen supply
		                 Have to stop differentiating at chondrocyte
		phase
		Bone: Nutrient and oxygen supply
		           Vascularisation
		Cell isolation and culturing is still time consuming and expensive

Adult cells	Inductive of natural tissue Only for cartilage cells?	Donor site morbidity Cells are out of natural environment, can lead to cell death or dedifferentiation If allografts: allogenic reaction Keep cells at damaged area **Cartilage:** Nutrient supply Prevent further differentiation towards hypertrophic chondrocytes

Table 1. Differences in: tissue characteristics, currently applied Tissue Engineering, and remaining challenges for bone and cartilage.

for generating both bone and cartilage. Creating cartilage or bone by triggering endochondrogenesis in an ectopic site bypasses expensive and time consuming culture techniques, logistics, and when triggered by injection of a specific stimulus may even limit the total approach to one operation.

4. Conclusion

From nature it is known that vast amounts of cartilage are formed in the process of endochondrogenesis. Chondrocytes in this cartilage tissue are replaced by a matrix deposited by hypertrophic chondrocytes which die by apoptosis. This matrix is used as an active scaffold for cells that contribute to bone formation. Following embryonic joint formation and post natal growth, the adult skeleton maintains the cellularity and phenotype of articular cartilage, whereas growth plate cartilage completely disappears. This process entitled endochondral ossification can be recapitulated in other places than growth plates. Examples hereof are fracture healing, osteophyte formation and peri-articular ossifications. Even in the process of OA endochondrogenesis plays a role. Next to the formation of osteophytes in OA, evidence has been reported that during the process of OA, articular chondrocytes are triggered to follow the final phase of endochondral ossification (Saito, Fukai et al. 2010).

A scaffold which serves as a template for tissue generation has also been introduced in the field of TE. Thusfar TE has not met initial expectations. Materials used as a scaffold to engineer bone are often engineered to be biocompatible and have good initial biomechanical properties. These properties may interfere with biomechanical stimuli needed for tissue organisation and degradation products from these artificial scaffolds may interfere with the natural healing response. In contrast to a natural endochondral scaffold, artificial scaffolds do not orchestrate ingress of progenitor cells, vascularisation etc.

Periosteum seems to play an important role in postnatal endochondrogenesis. However subcutaneous injection of growth factors leads to generation of bone via the endochondral pathway. The first examples of successful generation of bone and cartilage by triggering the progenitor cells of periosteum are found in literature (Emans, Surtel et al. 2005; Emans, van Rhijn et al. 2010). Also repair of cartilage and bone has been reported to be successful in animal studies using this approach. Using the postnatal endochondrogenic capacity for generation of cartilage and bone has many advantages: expensive culture procedures and logistics are bypassed and sufficient amounts of tissue are likely to be generated. Depending on the stage in which endochondral tissue is harvested, different clinical needs could be treated varying from (osteo)chondral defects to bone defects (Scotti, Tonnarelli et al. 2010). Finally, studying the process of endochondrogenesis may not only be a logical direction for tissue generation, but is also expected to provide useful information how to lock progenitors in the desired phase and will contribute to our understanding of diseases like OA.

5. Acknowledgment

The authors wish to acknowledge the Dutch Arthritis Association and Dutch Stichting Annafonds, as well as Prof. V. Prasad Shastri for the collaboration which has led to further insight into periosteal chondrogenesis.

6. References

Aglietti, P., Buzzi, R., Bassi, P. B. (1994). "Arthroscopic drilling in juvenile osteochondritis dissecans of the medial femoral condyle." *Arthroscopy* 10(3): 286-91.

Altman, R. D., Kates, J., Chun, L. E. (1992). "Preliminary observations of chondral abrasion in a canine model." *Ann Rheum Dis* 51(9): 1056-62.

Anderson, H. (1962). "Histochemical studies of the human hip joint." *Acta Anat* 48: 258-292.

Aydelotte, M.&Kuettner, K. (1992). Heterogeneity of articular chondrocytes and cartilage matrix. New York, Marcel Dekker.

Aydelotte, M. B., Greenhill, R. R.&Kuettner, K. E. (1988). "Differences between sub-populations of cultured bovine articular chondrocytes. II. Proteoglycan metabolism." *Connect Tissue Res* 18(3): 223-34.

Bartlett, W., Skinner, J. A., Gooding, C. R. (2005). "Autologous chondrocyte implantation versus matrix-induced autologous chondrocyte implantation for osteochondral defects of the knee: a prospective, randomised study." *J Bone Joint Surg Br* 87(5): 640-5.

Bentley, G.&Greer, R. B., 3rd (1971). "Homotransplantation of isolated epiphyseal and articular cartilage chondrocytes into joint surfaces of rabbits." *Nature* 230(5293): 385-8.

Blaney Davidson, E. N., Vitters, E. L., van Beuningen, H. M. (2007). "Resemblance of osteophytes in experimental osteoarthritis to transforming growth factor beta-induced osteophytes: limited role of bone morphogenetic protein in early osteoarthritic osteophyte formation." *Arthritis Rheum* 56(12): 4065-73.

Blunk, T., Sieminski, A. L., Gooch, K. J. (2002). "Differential effects of growth factors on tissue-engineered cartilage." *Tissue Eng* 8(1): 73-84.

Bostrom, M. P., Lane, J. M., Berberian, W. S. (1995). "Immunolocalization and expression of bone morphogenetic proteins 2 and 4 in fracture healing." *J Orthop Res* 13(3): 357-67.

Bouwmeester, S. J., Beckers, J. M., Kuijer, R. (1997). "Long-term results of rib perichondrial grafts for repair of cartilage defects in the human knee." *Int Orthop* 21(5): 313-7.

Boyle, W. J., Simonet, W. S.&Lacey, D. L. (2003). "Osteoclast differentiation and activation." *Nature* 423(6937): 337-42.

Bradley, J.&Dandy, D. J. (1989). "Results of drilling osteochondritis dissecans before skeletal maturity." *J Bone Joint Surg Br* 71(4): 642-4.

Brittberg, M., Lindahl, A., Nilsson, A. (1994). "Treatment of deep cartilage defects in the knee with autologous chondrocyte transplantation." *N Engl J Med* 331(14): 889-95.

Buckwalter, J.&Mankin, H. (1998). "Articular cartilage: tissue design and chondrocyte matrix interactions." *AAOS Instr Cours Lect* 47: 487-504.

Chu, C. R., Coutts, R. D., Yoshioka, M. (1995). "Articular cartilage repair using allogeneic perichondrocyte-seeded biodegradable porous polylactic acid (PLA): a tissue-engineering study." *J Biomed Mater Res* 29(9): 1147-54.

Cole, B. J., Farr, J., Winalski, C. S. (2011). "Outcomes After a Single-Stage Procedure for Cell-Based Cartilage Repair: A Prospective Clinical Safety Trial With 2-year Follow-up." *Am J Sports Med* 39(6): 1170-9.

Convery, F. R., Meyers, M. H.&Akeson, W. H. (1991). "Fresh osteochondral allografting of the femoral condyle." *Clin Orthop Relat Res*(273): 139-45.

Czitrom, A. A., Keating, S.&Gross, A. E. (1990). "The viability of articular cartilage in fresh osteochondral allografts after clinical transplantation." *J Bone Joint Surg Am* 72(4): 574-81.

Dong, X., Wei, X., Yi, W. (2009). "RGD-modified acellular bovine pericardium as a bioprosthetic scaffold for tissue engineering." *J Mater Sci Mater Med*.

Donohue, J. M., Buss, D., Oegema, T. R., Jr. (1983). "The effects of indirect blunt trauma on adult canine articular cartilage." *J Bone Joint Surg Am* 65(7): 948-57.

Dowthwaite, G. P., Bishop, J. C., Redman, S. N. (2004). "The surface of articular cartilage contains a progenitor cell population." *J Cell Sci* 117(Pt 6): 889-97.

Einhorn, T. A. (2005). "The science of fracture healing." *J Orthop Trauma* 19(10 Suppl): S4-6.

Elford, P. R., Graeber, M., Ohtsu, H. (1992). "Induction of swelling, synovial hyperplasia and cartilage proteoglycan loss upon intra-articular injection of transforming growth factor beta-2 in the rabbit." *Cytokine* 4(3): 232-8.

Emans, P. J., Pieper, J., Hulsbosch, M. M. (2006). "Differential cell viability of chondrocytes and progenitor cells in tissue-engineered constructs following implantation into osteochondral defects." *Tissue Eng* 12(6): 1699-709.

Emans, P. J., Surtel, D. A., Frings, E. J. (2005). "In vivo generation of cartilage from periosteum." *Tissue Eng* 11(3-4): 369-77.

Emans, P. J., van Rhijn, L. W., Welting, T. J. (2010). "Autologous engineering of cartilage." *Proc Natl Acad Sci U S A* 107(8): 3418-23.

Fischer, J., Dickhut, A., Rickert, M. (2010). "Human articular chondrocytes secrete parathyroid hormone-related protein and inhibit hypertrophy of mesenchymal stem cells in coculture during chondrogenesis." *Arthritis Rheum* 62(9): 2696-706.

Freed, L. E., Grande, D. A., Lingbin, Z. (1994). "Joint resurfacing using allograft chondrocytes and synthetic biodegradable polymer scaffolds." *J Biomed Mater Res* 28(8): 891-9.

Freed, L. E., Vunjak-Novakovic, G.&Langer, R. (1993). "Cultivation of cell-polymer cartilage implants in bioreactors." *J Cell Biochem* 51(3): 257-64.

Furukawa, T., Eyre, D. R., Koide, S. (1980). "Biochemical studies on repair cartilage resurfacing experimental defects in the rabbit knee." *J Bone Joint Surg Am* 62(1): 79-89.

Gallay, S. H., Miura, Y., Commisso, C. N. (1994). "Relationship of donor site to chondrogenic potential of periosteum in vitro." *J Orthop Res* 12(4): 515-25.

Garrett, J. C. (1986). "Treatment of osteochondral defects of the distal femur with fresh osteochondral allografts: a preliminary report." *Arthroscopy* 2(4): 222-6.

Garrett, J. C. (1994). "Fresh osteochondral allografts for treatment of articular defects in osteochondritis dissecans of the lateral femoral condyle in adults." *Clin Orthop Relat Res*(303): 33-7.

Garrett, J. C. (1998). "Osteochondral allografts for reconstruction of articular defects of the knee." *Instr Course Lect* 47: 517-22.

Gerber, H. P., Vu, T. H., Ryan, A. M. (1999). "VEGF couples hypertrophic cartilage remodeling, ossification and angiogenesis during endochondral bone formation." *Nat Med* 5(6): 623-8.

Ghazavi, M. T., Pritzker, K. P., Davis, A. M. (1997). "Fresh osteochondral allografts for post-traumatic osteochondral defects of the knee." *J Bone Joint Surg Br* 79(6): 1008-13.

Gibson, G. (1998). "Active role of chondrocyte apoptosis in endochondral ossification." *Microsc Res Tech* 43(2): 191-204.

Glowacki, J. (1998). "Angiogenesis in fracture repair." *Clin Orthop Relat Res*(355 Suppl): S82-9.

Gold, G. E., Burstein, D., Dardzinski, B. (2006). "MRI of articular cartilage in OA: novel pulse sequences and compositional/functional markers." *Osteoarthritis Cartilage* 14 Suppl 1: 76-86.

Grande, D. A., Halberstadt, C., Naughton, G. (1997). "Evaluation of matrix scaffolds for tissue engineering of articular cartilage grafts." *J Biomed Mater Res* 34(2): 211-20.

Grande, D. A., Pitman, M. I., Peterson, L. (1989). "The repair of experimentally produced defects in rabbit articular cartilage by autologous chondrocyte transplantation." *J Orthop Res* 7(2): 208-18.

Gray, D. J.&Gardner, E. (1950). "Prenatal development of the human knee and superior tibiofibular joints." *Am J Anat* 86(2): 235-87.

Gross, A. E., Aubin, P., Cheah, H. K. (2002). "A fresh osteochondral allograft alternative." *J Arthroplasty* 17(4 Suppl 1): 50-3.

Gross, A. E., McKee, N. H., Pritzker, K. P. (1983). "Reconstruction of skeletal deficits at the knee. A comprehensive osteochondral transplant program." *Clin Orthop Relat Res*(174): 96-106.

Grundnes, O.&Reikeras, O. (1993). "The importance of the hematoma for fracture healing in rats." *Acta Orthop Scand* 64(3): 340-2.

Guyer, R. D., Collier, R., Stith, W. J. (1988). "Discitis after discography." *Spine (Phila Pa 1976)* 13(12): 1352-4.

Hall, B. K.&Jacobson, H. N. (1975). "The repair of fractured membrane bones in the newly hatched chick." *Anat Rec* 181(1): 55-69.

Harada, S.&Rodan, G. A. (2003). "Control of osteoblast function and regulation of bone mass." *Nature* 423(6937): 349-55.

Hasler, E. M., Herzog, W., Wu, J. Z. (1999). "Articular cartilage biomechanics: theoretical models, material properties, and biosynthetic response." *Crit Rev Biomed Eng* 27(6): 415-88.

Hendrickson, D. A., Nixon, A. J., Grande, D. A. (1994). "Chondrocyte-fibrin matrix transplants for resurfacing extensive articular cartilage defects." *J Orthop Res* 12(4): 485-97.

Hendriks, J., Riesle, J.&van Blitterswijk, C. A. (2007). "Co-culture in cartilage tissue engineering." *J Tissue Eng Regen Med* 1(3): 170-8.

Homminga, G. N., Bulstra, S. K., Bouwmeester, P. S. (1990). "Perichondral grafting for cartilage lesions of the knee." *J Bone Joint Surg Br* 72(6): 1003-7.

Homminga, G. N., Bulstra, S. K., Kuijer, R. (1991). "Repair of sheep articular cartilage defects with a rabbit costal perichondrial graft." *Acta Orthop Scand* 62(5): 415-8.

Horas, U., Schnettler, R., Pelinkovic, D. (2000). "[Osteochondral transplantation versus autogenous chondrocyte transplantation. A prospective comparative clinical study]." *Chirurg* 71(9): 1090-7.

Huang, Q., Goh, J. C., Hutmacher, D. W. (2002). "In vivo mesenchymal cell recruitment by a scaffold loaded with transforming growth factor beta1 and the potential for in situ chondrogenesis." *Tissue Eng* 8(3): 469-82.

Huitema, G. C., van Rhijn, L. W.&van Ooij, A. (2006). "Screw position after double-rod anterior spinal fusion in idiopathic scoliosis: an evaluation using computerized tomography." *Spine* 31(15): 1734-9.

Hunter, W. (1995). "Of the structure and disease of articulating cartilages. 1743." *Clin Orthop Relat Res*(317): 3-6.

Hunziker, E. (1992). Articular cartilage structure in humans and experimental animals. New York, Raven Press.

Hunziker, E. B. (1999). "Articular cartilage repair: are the intrinsic biological constraints undermining this process insuperable?" *Osteoarthritis Cartilage* 7(1): 15-28.

Hunziker, E. B. (2001). "Growth-factor-induced healing of partial-thickness defects in adult articular cartilage." *Osteoarthritis Cartilage* 9(1): 22-32.

Hunziker, E. B., Kapfinger, E.&Geiss, J. (2007). "The structural architecture of adult mammalian articular cartilage evolves by a synchronized process of tissue resorption and neoformation during postnatal development." *Osteoarthritis Cartilage* 15(4): 403-13.

Insall, J. (1974). "The Pridie debridement operation for osteoarthritis of the knee." *Clin Orthop Relat Res*(101): 61-7.

Iwasaki, M., Nakahara, H., Nakase, T. (1994). "Bone morphogenetic protein 2 stimulates osteogenesis but does not affect chondrogenesis in osteochondrogenic differentiation of periosteum-derived cells." *J Bone Miner Res* 9(8): 1195-204.

Iwasaki, M., Nakahara, H., Nakata, K. (1995). "Regulation of proliferation and osteochondrogenic differentiation of periosteum-derived cells by transforming growth factor-beta and basic fibroblast growth factor." *J Bone Joint Surg Am* 77(4): 543-54.

Iwasaki, M., Nakata, K., Nakahara, H. (1993). "Transforming growth factor-beta 1 stimulates chondrogenesis and inhibits osteogenesis in high density culture of periosteum-derived cells." *Endocrinology* 132(4): 1603-8.

Jackson, R. W. (1986). "The scope of arthroscopy." *Clin Orthop Relat Res*(208): 69-71.

Kim, H. K., Moran, M. E.&Salter, R. B. (1991). "The potential for regeneration of articular cartilage in defects created by chondral shaving and subchondral abrasion. An experimental investigation in rabbits." *J Bone Joint Surg Am* 73(9): 1301-15.

Kim, S. S., Park, M. S., Gwak, S. J. (2006). "Accelerated bonelike apatite growth on porous polymer/ceramic composite scaffolds in vitro." *Tissue Eng* 12(10): 2997-3006.

Kronenberg, H. M. (2003). "Developmental regulation of the growth plate." *Nature* 423(6937): 332-6.

Kuettner, K.&Pauli, B. (1983). Vascularity of cartilage. New York, Academic Press.

Kuijer, R., Emans, P. J., Jansen, E. (2003). "Isolation and Cultivation of Chondrogenic Precursors from Aged Human Periosteum." *49th Trans ORS* 28: 101.

Kuijer, R., Jansen, E. J., Emans, P. J. (2007). "Assessing infection risk in implanted tissue-engineered devices." *Biomaterials*.

Macchiarini, P., Jungebluth, P., Go, T. (2008). "Clinical transplantation of a tissue-engineered airway." *Lancet* 372(9655): 2023-30.

Mankin, H., Mow, V.&Buckwalter, J. (2000). Articular cartilage repair and osteoarthritis. Rosemont, American Academy of Orthopaedic Surgeons.

Mankin, H., Mow, V.&Buckwalter, J. (2000). Articular cartilage structure, composition, and function. Rosemont, AAOS.

Martin, I., Shastri, V. P., Padera, R. F. (2001). "Selective differentiation of mammalian bone marrow stromal cells cultured on three-dimensional polymer foams." *J Biomed Mater Res* 55(2): 229-35.

Masquelet, A. C.&Begue, T. (2010). "The concept of induced membrane for reconstruction of long bone defects." *Orthop Clin North Am* 41(1): 27-37; table of contents.

McKibbin, B.&Maroudas, A. (1979). "Adult articular cartilage." *Piman Medical* 2E: 461 - 486.

Meachim, G.&Roberts, C. (1971). "Repair of the joint surface from subarticular tissue in the rabbit knee." *J Anat* 109(2): 317-27.

Mitchell, N.&Shepard, N. (1976). "The resurfacing of adult rabbit articular cartilage by multiple perforations through the subchondral bone." *J Bone Joint Surg Am* 58(2): 230-3.

Miyazono, K., Maeda, S.&Imamura, T. (2005). "BMP receptor signaling: transcriptional targets, regulation of signals, and signaling cross-talk." *Cytokine Growth Factor Rev* 16(3): 251-63.

Nakahara, H., Bruder, S. P., Goldberg, V. M. (1990). "In vivo osteochondrogenic potential of cultured cells derived from the periosteum." *Clin Orthop Relat Res*(259): 223-32.

Nakahara, H., Dennis, J. E., Bruder, S. P. (1991). "In vitro differentiation of bone and hypertrophic cartilage from periosteal-derived cells." *Exp Cell Res* 195(2): 492-503.

Nakahara, H., Goldberg, V. M.&Caplan, A. I. (1991). "Culture-expanded human periosteal-derived cells exhibit osteochondral potential in vivo." *J Orthop Res* 9(4): 465-76.

Nakata, K., Nakahara, H., Kimura, T. (1992). "Collagen gene expression during chondrogenesis from chick periosteum-derived cells." *FEBS Lett* 299(3): 278-82.

Nixon, A. J., Sams, A. E., Lust, G. (1993). "Temporal matrix synthesis and histologic features of a chondrocyte-laden porous collagen cartilage analogue." *Am J Vet Res* 54(2): 349-56.

Novack, D. V.&Faccio, R. (2011). "Osteoclast motility: putting the brakes on bone resorption." *Ageing Res Rev* 10(1): 54-61.

O'Driscoll, S. W. (1998). "The healing and regeneration of articular cartilage." *J Bone Joint Surg Am* 80(12): 1795-812.

O'Driscoll, S. W., Keeley, F. W.&Salter, R. B. (1986). "The chondrogenic potential of free autogenous periosteal grafts for biological resurfacing of major full-thickness defects in joint surfaces under the influence of continuous passive motion. An experimental investigation in the rabbit." *J Bone Joint Surg Am* 68(7): 1017-35.

O'Driscoll, S. W., Keeley, F. W.&Salter, R. B. (1988). "Durability of regenerated articular cartilage produced by free autogenous periosteal grafts in major full-thickness defects in joint surfaces under the influence of continuous passive motion. A follow-up report at one year." *J Bone Joint Surg Am* 70(4): 595-606.

O'Driscoll, S. W., Saris, D. B., Ito, Y. (2001). "The chondrogenic potential of periosteum decreases with age." *J Orthop Res* 19(1): 95-103.

Oberpenning, F., Meng, J., Yoo, J. J. (1999). "De novo reconstitution of a functional mammalian urinary bladder by tissue engineering." *Nat Biotechnol* 17(2): 149-55.

Ogilvie-Harris, D. J.&Fitsialos, D. P. (1991). "Arthroscopic management of the degenerative knee." *Arthroscopy* 7(2): 151-7.

Park, Y., Sugimoto, M., Watrin, A. (2005). "BMP-2 induces the expression of chondrocyte-specific genes in bovine synovium-derived progenitor cells cultured in three-dimensional alginate hydrogel." *Osteoarthritis Cartilage* 13(6): 527-36.

Petite, H., Viateau, V., Bensaid, W. (2000). "Tissue-engineered bone regeneration." *Nat Biotechnol* 18(9): 959-63.

Poole, A. R., Kojima, T., Yasuda, T. (2001). "Composition and structure of articular cartilage: a template for tissue repair." *Clin Orthop Relat Res*(391 Suppl): S26-33.

Radin, E. L., Martin, R. B., Burr, D. B. (1984). "Effects of mechanical loading on the tissues of the rabbit knee." *J Orthop Res* 2(3): 221-34.

Rae, P. J.&Noble, J. (1989). "Arthroscopic drilling of osteochondral lesions of the knee." *J Bone Joint Surg Br* 71(3): 534.

Reddi, A. H. (1994). "Symbiosis of biotechnology and biomaterials: applications in tissue engineering of bone and cartilage." *J Cell Biochem* 56(2): 192-5.

Saito, T., Fukai, A., Mabuchi, A. (2010). "Transcriptional regulation of endochondral ossification by HIF-2alpha during skeletal growth and osteoarthritis development." *Nat Med* 16(6): 678-86.

Sams, A. E., Minor, R. R., Wootton, J. A. (1995). "Local and remote matrix responses to chondrocyte-laden collagen scaffold implantation in extensive articular cartilage defects." *Osteoarthritis Cartilage* 3(1): 61-70.

Sams, A. E.&Nixon, A. J. (1995). "Chondrocyte-laden collagen scaffolds for resurfacing extensive articular cartilage defects." *Osteoarthritis Cartilage* 3(1): 47-59.

Schenk, R., Eggli, P.&Hunziker, E. (1986). Articular cartilage morphology. New York, Raven Press.

Sellers, R. S., Peluso, D.&Morris, E. A. (1997). "The effect of recombinant human bone morphogenetic protein-2 (rhBMP-2) on the healing of full-thickness defects of articular cartilage." *J Bone Joint Surg Am* 79(10): 1452-63.

Sellers, R. S., Zhang, R., Glasson, S. S. (2000). "Repair of articular cartilage defects one year after treatment with recombinant human bone morphogenetic protein-2 (rhBMP-2)." *J Bone Joint Surg Am* 82(2): 151-60.

Shastri, V. P. (2006). "Future of regenerative medicine: challenges and hurdles." *Artif Organs* 30(10): 828-34.

Skoog, T.&Johansson, S. H. (1976). "The formation of articular cartilage from free perichondrial grafts." *Plast Reconstr Surg* 57(1): 1-6.

Steinberg, M. S. (1962). "Mechanism of tissue reconstruction by dissociated cells. II. Time-course of events." *Science* 137: 762-3.

Stevens, M. M., Marini, R. P., Schaefer, D. (2005). "In vivo engineering of organs: the bone bioreactor." *Proc Natl Acad Sci U S A* 102(32): 11450-5.

Stevenson, S. (1998). "Enhancement of fracture healing with autogenous and allogeneic bone grafts." *Clin Orthop Relat Res*(355 Suppl): S239-46.

Takahashi, S., Oka, M., Kotoura, Y. (1995). "Autogenous callo-osseous grafts for the repair of osteochondral defects." *J Bone Joint Surg Br* 77(2): 194-204.

Urist, M. (1976). Biogenesis of bone: Calcium and phophorus in the skeleton and blood in vertebrate evolution. Washington DC, Am. Phys. Soc.

Vachon, A., Bramlage, L. R., Gabel, A. A. (1986). "Evaluation of the repair process of cartilage defects of the equine third carpal bone with and without subchondral bone perforation." *Am J Vet Res* 47(12): 2637-45.

Vachon, A., McIlwraith, C. W., Trotter, G. W. (1989). "Neochondrogenesis in free intra-articular, periosteal, and perichondrial autografts in horses." *Am J Vet Res* 50(10): 1787-94.

van Beuningen, H. M., van der Kraan, P. M., Arntz, O. J. (1993). "Does TGF-beta protect articular cartilage in vivo?" *Agents Actions Suppl* 39: 127-31.

van Beuningen, H. M., van der Kraan, P. M., Arntz, O. J. (1994). "Transforming growth factor-beta 1 stimulates articular chondrocyte proteoglycan synthesis and induces osteophyte formation in the murine knee joint." *Lab Invest* 71(2): 279-90.

van der Kraan, P. M.&van den Berg, W. B. (2007). "Osteophytes: relevance and biology." *Osteoarthritis Cartilage* 15(3): 237-44.

Volk, S. W.&Leboy, P. S. (1999). "Regulating the regulators of chondrocyte hypertrophy." *J Bone Miner Res* 14(4): 483-6.

Vortkamp, A., Lee, K., Lanske, B. (1996). "Regulation of rate of cartilage differentiation by Indian hedgehog and PTH-related protein." *Science* 273(5275): 613-22.

Wakitani, S., Kimura, T., Hirooka, A. (1989). "Repair of rabbit articular surfaces with allograft chondrocytes embedded in collagen gel." *J Bone Joint Surg Br* 71(1): 74-80.

Wu, L. N., Ishikawa, Y., Sauer, G. R. (1995). "Morphological and biochemical characterization of mineralizing primary cultures of avian growth plate chondrocytes: evidence for cellular processing of Ca2+ and Pi prior to matrix mineralization." *J Cell Biochem* 57(2): 218-37.

Yoon, B. S.&Lyons, K. M. (2004). "Multiple functions of BMPs in chondrogenesis." *J Cell Biochem* 93(1): 93-103.

Yoon, B. S., Pogue, R., Ovchinnikov, D. A. (2006). "BMPs regulate multiple aspects of growth-plate chondrogenesis through opposing actions on FGF pathways." *Development* 133(23): 4667-78.

Zarnett, R.&Salter, R. B. (1989). "Periosteal neochondrogenesis for biologically resurfacing joints: its cellular origin." *Can J Surg* 32(3): 171-4.

Zhao, F., Grayson, W. L., Ma, T. (2006). "Effects of hydroxyapatite in 3-D chitosan-gelatin polymer network on human mesenchymal stem cell construct development." *Biomaterials* 27(9): 1859-67.

7

Novel Promises of Nanotechnology for Tissue Regeneration

Abir El-Sadik

Anatomy and Embryology, Basic Sciences Department,
King Saud Bin Abdulaziz University for Health Sciences, Riyadh
Kingdom of Saudi Arabia

1. Introduction

The term 'nanotechnology' refers to technology that deals with structures and devices of nanometer (10 $^{-9}$ meter) size. It involves the design, fabrication and utilization of materials of nanoscale dimensions (Gao & Xu, 2009). The resulting nanomaterials exhibit chemical, physical and biological properties that can differ significantly from those of bulk material. These products can be categorized into metals, ceramics, polymers or composite materials that have nanoscale features. The limited size of their particles leads to a high surface area to volume ratio, improved solubility, multifunctionality, high electrical and heat conductivity and improved surface catalytic activity. (El-Sadik et al., 2010). All these phenomena allow give nanoparticles to interact with biological systems at cellular and molecular levels. These interactions enhance the biomedical applications of nanotechnology giving great promise for improving disease prevention, diagnosis, treatment and in particular tissue regeneration (Murthy, 2007).

Since natural human tissues include nano-scale subcellular and extracellular components, artificial nanomaterials mimic the scales of tissue components (Zhang & Webster, 2009). Cells make contact with other cells and with the extracellular matrix with membrnes that have nanoscale features. It has been shown that nanomaterials, with their biomimetic features, can accelerate the rate of cell growth and proliferation and promote tissue acceptance due to reduced immune response (Oh et al., 2009). One of the most useful properties of nanomaterials, which have been extensively investigated, is their ability to interact with proteins that control cell functions. This may make nanomaterials very useful, and perhaps even necessary, tools for regenerating various tissues such as those of the bone, cartilage, blood vessels and nervous system (Liu & Webster, 2007).

Although a series of technological improvements in tissue regeneration have been acheived using conventional methods, a variety of problems still faces current implants. Nanotechnology could provide several solutions to these problems. A wide range of nanomaterials have been made from organic and inorganic composites, just like conventional materials. However, nanotehnology has the ability to control material properties more closely by assembling components at the nanoscale. These nanomaterials (nanoparticles, nanotubes, nanofibers, nanoclusters, nanocrystals, nanowires, nanorods and nanofilms) can be fabricated by multiple and available nanotechnologies. Electrospining, self assembly, phase separation, photolithography, thin film deposition, chemical etching, chemical vapor deposition and electron beam lithography are all techniques currently used to synthesize nanomaterials with ordered or random nanotopographies (Chen & Ma, 2004).

Conventional tissue replacement, using allografts and autografts, cannot satisfy high performance demands and improvements are necessary. Nanotechnology has been used to fabricate cytocompatible biomimetic nanomaterials that provide biological substitutes useful in restoring and improving tissue functions. Moreover, 2-dimensional tissue cell culture systems on flat glass, coated petri dishes or plastic substrates cannot simulate the natural tissue microenvironments. Normal tissue cells are located in a complex network of 3 dimensional extracellular matrix with nanoscale fibers. Nanomaterials could be fabricated that accurately simulate the dimensions and architecture of natural human tissue, allowing significantly improved performance of the cultured cells (Gelain et al., 2006). The composition and topography of a tissue engineered material could even produce cell-environment interactions that determine the implant fate. Nanomaterials need to be designed to be biocompatible and to function without interrupting other physiological processes. In principle, they can promote normal cell growth and differentiation without any adverse tissue reaction. These nanomaterials must be biodegradable either to be removed via degradation or absorption to leave only native tissue. In addition, nanomaterials used in tissue regeneration should possess biomimetic features that allow cells to react normally to internal and external stimuli and to exchange the signals between those cells and the external environment.

This chapter reviews recent progress in the synthesis of nanomaterials for improving stem cell behavior and tissue regeneration. In addition, it highlights potentially valuable applications of nanotechnology in specific tissue regeneration.

2. Effects of nanomaterials on stem cell behaviour and development of tissue regeneration

Nanotechnology is an extremely promising advancement in synthetic methodologies used to functionalize nanomaterials with biomolecules. Nanomolecules could be modified to desired sizes, shapes, compositions and properties producing different types applied in tissue regeneration such as nanoparticles, nanosurfaces and nanoscaffolds.

2.1 Nanoparticles

Several studies have investigated the influences of different types of nanoparticles on the behaviour of stem cells applied in tissue regeneration. The effects of mesoporous silica nanoparticles conjugated with fluorescein isothiocyanate on human bone marrow mesenchymal stem cells has been investigated by several researchers. Internalization of silica nanoparticles into stem cells is mediated by both clathrin and actin-dependent endocytosis. Once inside the cell, the nanoparticles escaped the endolysosomal vesicles and did not affect stem cell viability or proliferation. They enhanced actin polymerization in mesenchymal stem cells. Moreover, regular osteogenic differentiation was successfully induced in the mesenchymal stem cells after the uptake of mesoporous silica nanoparticles in highly chondrogenic synovium (Huang et al., 2008 & Shi et al., 2009). Fibrin polylactide caprolactone nanoparticles have been designed to induce chondrogenic differentiation in mesenchymal stem cells. These complex nanoparticles facilitated the upregulation of chondrogenesis marker genes. In addition, they effectively sustained chondrogenic differentiation and enhanced chondral extracellular matrix deposition by human adipogenic stem cells. Fibrin polylactide caprolactone nanoparticle complexes could be effectively used for in situ cartilage tissue regeneration from human stem cells (Jung et al., 2009).

The application of nanotechnology to stem cell biology might help to maximize therapeutic benefits and minimize possible undesired effects of stem cell therapy, through delivery of sufficient stem cells to the regions of interest with the smallest number of cells to untargeted regions. Tracking the fate, distribution, proliferation, differentiation of engulfed stem cells employed in tissue regeneration is essential to understand the mechanisms of participation of the cells in tissue repair. Nanotechnology can improve several techniques that would enable non-invasive detection of transplanted stem cells within the desired organs. Iron oxide nanoparticles are inorganic nanoparticles that can be synthesized easily in large quantities and different sizes using simple methods. Several studies reported that when iron oxide nanoparticles bind to the external cell membrane, they do not affect cell viability, although they may detach from the cell membrane or interfere with cell surface interactions (Bulte & Kraitchman, 2004). Superparamagnetic iron oxide nanoparticles are successfully internalized via endocytosis in human mesenchymal stem cells. After their uptake, they are located inside cytoplasmic vesicles. Then, they are transferred to lysosomes in which degradation of the nanoparticles occurs, releasing free iron into the cytoplasm (Jing et al., 2008). Coating the surface of iron oxide nanoparticles modifies the surface of the particles for efficient uptake with minimum side effects on the cells. Coating superparamagnetic iron oxide nanoparticles with dextran improves their stability and solubility and prevents their aggregation. Another example of coating the surface of nanoparticles is provided by coating the superparamagnetic iron oxide nanoparticles with gold. The gold provides an inert shell around the nanoparticles and protects them from rapid dissolution within cytoplasmic endosomes and enhances magnetic resonance imaging (MRI) contrast. It has been shown, however, that dissolved iron oxide nanoparticles may produce free hydroxyl radicals which increase the rate of apoptosis and alterations in cellular metabolism (Emerit et al., 2001).

Concerning the effects of iron oxide nanoparticles on stem cell behaviour, magnetite iron oxide cationic liposomes can be applied efficiently to mesenchymal stem cell techniques. Mesenchymal stem cells incubated in osteogenic medium with these nanoparticles changed their shape from fibroblastic to polygonal, formed calcium nodules and increased in number five-fold compared with controls (Ito et al., 2004). In addition, superparamagnetic iron oxide nanoparticles have been shown to enhance the survival rate of stem cells up to 99%, indicating that these nanoparticles improve stem cell viability (Delcroix et al., 2009). Moreover, superparamagnetic iron oxide nanoparticles did not influence the morphology, cell cycle, telomerase activity, proliferation or differentiation ability of labelled neural stem cells (Kea et al., 2009). Superparamagnetic iron oxide nanoparticles have been successfully applied to tracking the fate of several types of stem cells. For example, the migration of embryonic stem cells and bone marrow mesenchymal stem cells labelled with iron oxide nanoparticles towards a lesion site has been tracked using MRI. This labelling technique offers high resolution, speed, easy access and 3-dimensional capabilities and provides information not only for the transplanted cells, but also for the surrounding tissues, reporting edema or inflammation that may affect the fate of the grafted cells and reduce the recovery of damaged tissue (Sykova & Jendelova, 2007). Another example is tracking human mesenchymal stem cells labelled with superparamagnetic iron oxide nanoparticles after transplantation for articular cartilage repair using MRI (Au et al., 2009). These observations have demonstrated the ability of using iron oxide nanoparticles to be useful in monitoring and tracking the fate of transplanted stem cells apparently without affecting their behaviour, although, selection of the type and concentration of nanoparticles is critically important.

In addition to iron oxide nanoparticles, quantum dots have been much used for cell tracking in in tissue regeneration. Quantum dots are fluorescent semiconducting nanocrystals that overcome the limitations of conventional labelling methods. Several researchers have studied the application of quantum dots to monitoring physiological changes inside living cells by labelling the intracellular organelles or specific proteins with quantum dots. They could monitor cellular migration, track cell lineage and investigate stem cell behaviour. Quantum dots can bind to individual molecules on the cell surface and serve in tracking the motion of those molecules. For example, quantum dots have been applied to demonstrate changes in integrin dynamics during osteogenic differentiation of human bone marrow cells (Chen et al., 2007). Numerous studies have demonstrated a variety of techniques of the cellular uptake of quantum dots. These nanoparticles can be delivered into cells by microinjection, endocytosis, liposome-mediated transfection and special peptide delivery (Chang et al., 2008). Delivered quantum dots were found to escaping lysosomal degradation at the beginning of the uptake. Thereafter, lysosome expression was enhanced and all cellular quantum dots were shown in lysosome vesicles. After the uptake of quantum dots, into several types of stem cells, such as mesenchymal stem cells, cytoskeletal reorganization took place. This action revealed the formation of wide and flat leading lamellipodia filled with a dense actin network (Chang et al., 2009). Human mesenchymal stem cells labelled with quantum dots represented the same viability comparing with the unlabelled human mesenchymal stem cells from the same subpopulation (Shah et al., 2007), suggesting that quantum dots could be used safely for long term labelling of stem cells. Moreover, embryonic stem cells could be labelled with quantum dots for cellular tracking in vivo without affecting the viability, proliferation or differentiation of the embryonic stem cells (Lin et al., 2007). These studies demonstrated that quantum dots could enable cellular and molecular imaging and tracking the fate of stem and progenitor cells used in tissue regeneration with high sensitivity and high spatial resolution. These applications are supported by an extensive number of advanced imaging techniques, giving a great impact on tissue regeneration studies.

2.2 Nanosurfaces

Mammalian cells are surrounded by nanostructures formed by biomolecules arranged geometrically in different configurations. These arrangements affect cell behaviour by producing chemical signals such as growth factors or physical signals such as tensile forces caused by interactions with the surrounding nanostructured extracellular matrix. Nanotechnology provides nanotopographical surfaces that can guide cellular adhesion, spreading, morphology, proliferation and differentiation. Cells react differently according to the nanotopography of their environment, which influences their cytoskeletal organization, attachment, and migration. Nanofabrication techniques provide several types of nanosurfaces for tissue regeneration.

Nanosurfaces of different materials with structural modification, such as the presence of large, medium and small nanoscale grooves, pores, pits, ridges and nodules can be recognized by cultured cells. A wide range of cell types, such as fibroblasts (Dalby et al., 2003b), osteoblasts (Lenhert et al., 2005) and mesenchymal stem cells (Biggs et al., 2008), are influenced by nanoscale grooves with dimensions that mimic those in vivo. Cellular morphology depends on cell type and on groove depth and width. Mesenchymal stem cells seeded on nanogrooves respond by aligning their shape and elongation in the direction of the grooves (Dalby et al., 2003b). Human osteoblasts cultured on ordered nanoscale groove/ridge arrays, fabricated by photolithography, were affected significantly (Biggs et al., 2008). The authors seeded human osteoblasts on grooves of 330 nm depth and different widths (10, 25 and 100 μm in width). They concluded that adhesion formation was not affected in 100 μm wide groove/ridge arrays, although upregulation of genes involved in skeletal development was induced. In addition, increased osteospecific functions were observed. 25 μm wide grooves/ ridges were shown to be associated with a reduction in supermature adhesions and an increase in focal complex formation. However, that osteoblast adhesion was significantly reduced in 10 μm wide groove/ridge arrays. Moreover, grooves manufactured on nanosurfaces promoted the elongation and nuclear polarization in the cultured cells (Charest et al., 2004). Cell membranes stopped at the largest grooves but bridged over the narrowest and deepest ones (Matsuzaka et al., 2003). Electron beam lithography has also been used to generate nanoscale patterns for culturing mesenchymal stem cells (Dalby, 2009). The patterns ranged from highly ordered through controlled disorder, to total randomness. The authors concluded that nanoscale change in surface topography altered mesenchymal stem cell differentiation. Successful osteoconversion of the cultured cells using ± 50 nm level of disorder was demonstrated. The cells focal adhesions interacted with the material surface and affected by several signalling pathways, such as G protein and cytoskeletal signalling. These signalling factors modulated cell sensing, morphology, contractility, proliferation and differentiation. Altering the nanotopography of the surface material influenced the cytoskeletal arrangements (Curtis et al., 2006). Mechanical changes were transmitted from the cytoskeleton to the nucleus, affecting the genomic expression patterns and cell phenotype (Dalby et al., 2007).

Among hard carbon coatings, nanocrystalline diamond has been applied successfully to cultured osteogenic and endothelial cells. Nanocrystalline diamond possesses promising electrical and optical properties, high hardness, low friction coefficient and good compatibility (Bacakova et al., 2007). Nanocrystalline diamond has been used in the form of films to improve the mechanical and physical properties of body implants. In addition, it has been shown to attract cell colonization, its surface nanostructure simulating the architecture of extracellular matrix molecules. Nanocrystalline diamond layers deposited on silicon substrates improves the adhesion and growth of osteogenic and endothelial cells (Grausova et al., 2008). The authors concluded that these nanostructured surfaces gave good support for cellular viability and proliferation and could be applied usefully in tissue regeneration. Furthermore, ultrasmooth nanostructured diamond has been used in orthopaedic implants. Several studies were performed on this material, the authors describing their surface modification techniques and cytocompatability (Clem et al., 2008). The studies demonstrated that hydrogen-terminated ultrasmooth nanostructured diamond surfaces supported robust mesenchymal stem cell adhesion and survival. However oxygen and fluorine terminated surfaces resisted cell adhesion. It was concluded that chemical and physical modifications of ultrasmooth nanostructured diamond could promote or prevent cell/biomaterial interactions. Moreover, mesenchymal stem cell adhesion and proliferation were significantly improved on ultrasmooth nanostructured diamond compared with the commonly used and biocompatible cobalt-chrome. There was also osteoblastic differentiation and deposition of mineralized matrix in mesenchymal stem cells. Ultrasmooth nanostructured diamond was found to reduce debris particle release from orthopaedic implants without influencing osseointegration.

Controllable self-assembly of nanonodules has been demonstrated to occur during chemical depositioning of materials on specifically conditioned microtopographical surfaces (Ogawa et al., 2008). The substrate could be a nonmetalic material such a as biodegradable polymer. The biological potential of the nanonodular surfaces affecting the behaviour of cultured cells using titanium dioxide has been investigated (Kubo et al., 2009). Titanium as a substrate material was proven to be non cytotoxic and was applied in therapeutic and implantable devices used in tissue regeneration. Micro-nano-hybrid surfaces, consisting of nanoscale nodules within microscale pits, were created by applying nanonodular self assembly techniques. These surfaces mimicked the biomineralized matrices with greater surface area and roughness. Changing the assembly time controlled the size of the nanonodules. The addition of nanonodules of different sizes (100 – 300 – 500 nm) to micropits selectively promoted osteoblast functions. In addition, these nanonodular topographies enhanced osteoblastic proliferation and differentiation. These advantages were 3 times greater in the nanonodules with a diameter of 300 nm within the micropits, when implanted in a rat femur model. Cell spread was enhanced on the micro- nano-hybrid surfaces. After 3 hours incubation, osteoblasts were shown to be larger and their cell processes and cytoskeletons started to develop on the nanonodular surfaces, while they remained small and circular on the micropit surface alone. Meanwhile, marked cytoplasmic localization of the focal adhesion protein vinculin was shown on the micro-nano-hybrid surfaces, compared with those on the micropit surface which had faint expression.

Another application of titanium in tissue regeneration is the use of nanocrystalline titanium surfaces. This type of nanometer surface roughness promotes osteoblasted adhesion. This nanosurface enhances cell growth and demonstrates extensive wear resistance due to high hardness and strength (Wang & Li, 2003). Cell compatability studies on nanosized titanium particles showed enhanced osteoblast function and largeer deposition of calcium minerals (Webster et al., 2000). One of the most effective nanostructured titanium surfaces for enhancing the attachment, proliferation and spreading of mesenchymal stem cells is layer-by-layer assembled titanium dioxide nanoparticle thin films. This technique depends on electrostatic attraction between oppositely charged species such as titanium dioxide nanoparticles. The advantage of layer-by-layer assembly is that the adsorption of material cn be controlled with nanometer precision. Titanium dioxide thin films have been proved to be an optimal surface for rapid attachment and spreading of cells (Kommireddy et al., 2005). Increasing the number of layers in titanium dioxide thin films has been shown to increase surface roughness. Higher numbers of attached cells were observed on 4-layer titanium dioxide thin film than on a 1-layer thin film, with a faster rate of spreading on the rougher surface (Kommireddy et al., 2006). Moreover, multilayered and functionalized titanium films composed of chitosan and plasmid DNA demonstrated significant high transfection efficiency in mesenchymal stem cells (Hu et al., 2009). The authors reported high production levels of alkaline phosphatase and osteocalcin. They concluded that multilayered titanium films with chitosan and plasmid DNA promoted the differentiation of osteoprogenitor cells into mature osteoblasts over long time.

2.3 Nanoscaffolds

Nanotechnology provides the tissue regeneration field with nanostructures that might accurately simulate the natural 3-dimensional microenvironment of cells. This approach provides a complex network of nanoscale fibers and extracellular ligands, such as many types of collagens, laminin and fibronectin, that are poorly reproduced in the conventional 2-dimensional systems. Growth of cells in 2-dimensional cultures has been shown to reduce the production of particular extracellular matrix proteins, with consequent morphological changes and increase in spreading. The advancement in the technology of nanostructures enhances the scope of fabricating 3-dimensional nanoscaffolds that could potentially mimic the architecture of natural human tissue. These nanostructured scaffolds could control and direct cellular behaviour and interactions with the extracellular matrix. Scaffolds have been designed in the form of nanofibers, nanotubes, nanowires, nanorods, nanocrystals and nanofilms. These nanostructured scaffolds with their biomimetic features and excellent physicochemical properties, stimulated cellular adhesion, growth, morphology, proliferation, altered gene expression and promoted cellular differentiation. The structural features of these nanoscaffolds were engineered according to the nature of cell response which was desired. The scaffolds were designed in a manner that provided a surface to promote cell attachment, spreading and growth while encouraging the formation of a porous network that offered a suitable path for nutrient transmission and tissue ingrowth (Chen & Ma, 2004). These novel nanoscaffolds had excellent mechanical properties that offered structural support until the new tissue would be formed, as they degraded at a rate matching the new tissue formation and provided substrate for cell migration and survival. They were biocompatible and the products of their degradation were also biocompatible (Smith et al., 2010). These nanostructured scaffolds provided the functional role of the native extracellular matrix with growth factors that regulated the cell fate and bioactive peptide sequences that could bind receptors and activate intracellular signalling pathways (Boudreau & Jones, 1999).

Several techniques have been designed for the fabrication of nanofibrous scaffolds to be employed in tissue regeneration. Electrospinning techniques have been the most commonly used. An electric field is applied to draw a polymer solution from an orifice to a collector, producing polymer fibers with diameters ranging in size from 50 nm to several microns. These resulted lengths mimicked that of native collagen fibrils (Baker et al., 2009). Several types of synthetic and natural biomaterials have been used to form nanofibrous scaffolds such as poly (caprolactone) (PCL), poly (lactic-co-glycolic acid) (PLGA) poly (L-lactic acid) (PLLA), collagen, gelatine and fibrinogen; molecules that have been applied extensively in tissue regeneration. Another technique for nanofibrous fabrication is self-assembly. Molecular self-assembly has been applied to produce supramolecular architectures (Silva et al., 2004). This technique produces nanofiber diameters much smaller than those produced using electrospinning. Molecular self-assembly has been less effective in producing macropores for mass transport and cell accommodation. Phase separation techniques have also been also employed to fabricate nanofibers with diameters ranging from 50 – 500 nm and much higher surface –to-volume ratios than produced by other techniques (Chen et al., 2006).

3. Applications of nanotechnology in specific tissue regeneration

Recent studies have been conducted on the promises and applications of nanotechnology in the regeneration of specific tissues, such as bone, cartilage, vascular and neural tissues.

3.1 Bone and cartilage regeneration

Various types of traumatic bone and cartilage damage – bone fractures, osteoarthritis, osteoporosis or bone tumours – represent common and significant clinical problems. However, the treatment of such problems with traditional implant materials only lasts 10 – 15 years on average and implant failures originating from implant loosening, inflammation, infection, osteolysis and wear debris frequently occur. There is a very urgent need to develop a new generation of cytocompatible bone and cartilage substitutes to regenerate bone and cartilage tissues at diseased sites that could last the life time of the patient (Zhang & Webster, 2009).

Bone is effectively a nanocomposite that consists of a protein-based soft hydrogel template formed of collagen, non-collagenous proteins such as laminin, fibronectin and vitronectin, water, and hard inorganic components such as hydroxyapatite, calcium and phosphate. Specifically, 70% of the bone matrix is composed of nanocrystalline hydroxyapatite which is typically 20-80 nm long and 2-5 nm thick. Nanostructured bone extracellular matrix closely surrounds and affects adhesion, proliferation and differentiation of mesenchymal stem cells, osteoblasts, osteoclasts and fibroblasts. Moreover, cartilage is a poorly regenerating tissue composed of a small percentage of chondrocytes but dense nanostructured extracellular matrix rich in collagen fibers, proteoglycans and elastin fibers. The limited regenerative properties of cartilage originate from a lack of chondrocyte mobility in the dense extracellular matrix as well as an absence of progenitor cells and the vascular network necessary for efficient tissue repair (Vasita & Katti, 2006). Development of nanotechnology might provide clinical medicine with new prospects in bone and cartilage reconstruction. Nanotechnology employs engineered materials with the smallest functional organization called nanomaterials that are able to interact with biological systems at a nanoscale (El-Sadik et al., 2010). Nanomaterials could be grown or self-assembled to stimulate the dimensions of natural entities, such as collagen fibers. After decreasing material size into nanoscale, dramatically increased surface area, surface roughness and surface area to volume ratios could be created, leading to superior physiochemical properties such as mechanical, electrical, optical, catalytic, magnetic properties. These biomimetic features with the nanostructured extracellular matrix of bone and cartilage played a key role in stimulating cell growth as well as guided tissue regeneration (Jang et al., 2009). Numerous researchers fabricated cytocompatible biomimetic nanomaterial scaffolds encapsulating cells, such as stem cells, chondrocytes and osteoblasts. In addition, to the dimensional similarity to bone/cartilage tissue, nanomaterials also exhibited unique surface properties, such as surface topography, surface chemistry, surface wettabilty and surface energy, due to their significantly increased surface area and roughness compared to conventional or micron structured materials. As is known, material surface properties mediate specific protein adsorption and bioactivity, such as fibronectin, vitronectin and laminin, before cells adhere on implants, further, they regulate cell behaviour and dictate tissue regeneration. Furthermore, an important criterion for designing orthopaedic implant materials is the formation of sufficient osseointegration between synthetic materials and bone tissue. Studies have demonstrated that nanostructured materials with cell-favourable surface properties could promote greater amounts of specific protein interactions to more efficiently stimulate new bone growth compared to conventional materials (Webster et al., 2001). This is one of the underlying reasons that nanomaterials are superior to conventional materials for bone growth. Therefore, by controlling surface properties, various nanophase ceramic, polymer, metal and composite scaffolds have been designed for bone/cartilage tissue engineering applications (Zhang & Webster, 2009).

There have been significant advances in the development of bone scaffolds with various compositions and 3 dimensional configurations using a variety of techniques such as the electrospining process for the fabrication of nanofibrous matrices. Several studies have reported the performance of nanofibrous materials in guiding cells to initially adhere to, and spread over, the nanostructures, as well as triggering them to secrete appropriate extracellular matrix molecules targeted to the bone and cartilage tissues. The bone-associated cells and the progenitor/stem cells showed initial responses which were anchorage-dependant. The nanofibrous substratum provided favourable conditions for cell anchorage and growth. Further osteoblastic differentiation and mineralization have also been reported to be regulated in a positive manner on nanofibrous surfaces (Woo et al., 2007). One particular requirement of bone tissue regeneration was that the scaffold should be porous, to incorporate large number of cells. The 3-dimensional scaffolds provided the necessary support for bone cells to attach, grow and differentiate and defined the overall shape of a bone tissue cultured transplant (Jang et al., 2009). Nanofibrous and nanotubular scaffolds were fabricated to mimic collagen fibers in bone and cartilage. Natural collagen is a triple helix self assembled into nanofibers of 300 nm in length and 1.5 nm in diameter. A new nanofiber composite was designed with the same self-assembly pattern as collagen and hydroxyapatite crystals in bone by directly nucleating and aligning the hydroxyapatite on the long axis of a nanofiber. Mesenchymal stem cell behaviour on self-assembled peptide amphiphile nanofiber scaffolds was investigated. Significantly enhanced osteogenic differentiation of mesenchymal stem cells was recorded in the 3-dimensional scaffolds compared to 2-dimensional static conventional tissue cultures.

Other types of nanofibers used in bone regeneration include the natural polymers. Natural polymeric nanofibers, such as poly(caprolactone) (PCL), poly(lactic-co-glycolic acid) (PLGA) poly(L-lactic acid) (PLLA), collagen, gelatine and fibrinogen, are excellent candidates for bone and cartilage tissue engineering applications. These biomaterials possess properties that are useful for bone regeneration, such as biodegradability, flexibility, shape availability and ease of fabrication. Nanoporous polymer matrices can be fabricated via electrospinning, phase separation, particulate leaching, chemical etching and 3 dimensional printing techniques (Zhang & Webster, 2009). Poly(caprolactone) (PCL) was first suggested to be a degradable nanofiber matrix for bone regeneration, and it demonstrated good support of the rat bone marrow stromal cells and *in vitro* matrix formation at 4 weeks, including collagen I and calcium phosphate (Yoshimoto et al., 2003). A cell-nanofiber construct was implanted in rat omenta for 4 weeks (Shin et al., 2004). It revealed the formation of collagen I and mineralization similar to bone like extracellular matrix, highlighting its usefulness in bone tissue regeneration. A combination of degradable polymeric nanofibers with bioactive inorganic metals was proved to enhance osteogenic differentiation and calcification of bone matrix. The inorganic phase improved the biological properties of polymers in the bone forming process. Gelatin-hydroxyapatite nanofibers was fabricated (Kim et al., 2005). Hydroxyapatite nanocrystals were distributed in the gelatin matrix and produced an organized hybrid matrix. This composite enhanced osteoblastic differentiation and could be applied usefully in dentistry. In a similar way, collagen-hydroxyapatite (Song et al., 2008) and chitosan-hydroxyapatite (Zhang et al., 2008) nanofibers were generated mimicking the extracellular matrices.

An additional excellent choice of nanomaterials for the reconstruction of bone tissue was the bone-bioactive inorganics such as bioactive glass, ceramics and calcium phosphates. Silica based sol-gel glass mixed with a polymer binder was generated into a nanofibrous mesh by an electrospining technique. Fibers ranging from 84 nm to 640 nm in size were produced (Kim et al., 2006). The large surface area of the nanofibers, and the consequent ionic reaction with the surrounding medium, induced the formation of a bone mineral-like apatite phase on their surfaces. Osteogenic proliferation and differentiation of rat mesenchymal stem cells were found to be enhanced on the bioactive glass nanofiber substrates more than on conventional bioactive glass. Nanophase metals were investigated for orthopaedic tissue regeneration. They are characterized by the presence of more particle boundaries at their surfaces than the conventional micron metals. Linear patterns of nano-features of titanium were created via electron beam evaporation. These patterns induced greater osteoblast adhesion than the micron-rough regions and guided osteoblast morphology and alignment. Highly porous titanium dioxide nanotube layers were fabricated on titanium by anodization. Titanium was anodized electrochemically in dilute hydrofluoric acid electrolyte solutions to produce nanotubes with diameters of 100 nm and lengths of 500 nm into the titanium dioxide layers of titanium. Nanotubular anodized titanium greatly improved osteoblastic function and significantly increased chondrocytic adhesion, promoting bone and cartilage cellular growth (Zhang & Webster, 2009).

3.2 Vascular tissue regeneration

Researchers have come a long way to develop vascular grafts of great efficacy to replace damaged blood vessels, using materials that produce minimal interactions with the inflowing blood and adjacent tissues. Nanomaterials have been found to improve vascular endothelial and smooth muscle functions. Aligned biodegradable poly(L-lactid-co-epsilon-caprolactone) PLLA-CL (75:25) nanofibrous scaffolds have been tested for their ability to fabricate tubular scaffolds for vessels. These nanofibers demonstrated the mechanical strength needed to sustain high pressure of the human circulatory system and the necessary properties that mimic the dimensions of natural extracellular matrix of human coronary artery. They provided an excellent architecture for endothelial and smooth muscle cell adhesion and proliferation. The aligned fibers affected the behaviour of the smooth muscle cells, and the cytoskeleton is organized to follow the direction of the nanofibers (Xu et al., 2004). Electrospun nanofibers fabricated from natural polymers have been established to develop constructs for vascular tissue regeneration. Electrospun collagen and elastin nanofibers were shown to be good scaffolding systems for the engineering of artificial blood vessels (Boland et al., 2004). Another polymer that promoted the endothelial and vascular smooth muscle cell proliferation was the biodegradable poly(lactic-co-glycolic acid) (PLGA), which produced vascular grafts with nanometer surface features. These nanostructures enhanced fibronectin and vitronectin adsorption from serum leading to better vascular cell responses (Miller et al., 2007). Moreover, self-assembled peptides have been fabricated into scaffolds that mimic the vascular basement membrane with excellent cytocompatability. These peptide scaffolds promote endothelialisation and enhance nitric oxide release and laminin and collagen IV deposition by the endothelial cell monolayer (Genove et al., 2005). Titanium nanostructures have been reported to enhance vascular cell adhesion and proliferation greatly. Competitive endothelial cell functions were promoted over that of vascular smooth muscle cells, solving the problem of the overgrowth of smooth muscle cells in vascular stents (Choudhary et al., 2007).

3.3 Neural tissue regeneration

Nanostructure designs have been shown to promote the functional performance of neuronal cells and neural tissue repair. They possess the necessary cytocompatibilty properties for improved neuronal growth, mechanical properties that last long enough to physically support neural tissue regeneration, and electrical properties that stimulate and control neuron behaviour and guide neural tissue repair. Biodegradable and biocompatible novel nanofibers and nanotubes have been fabricated with controlled architecture and components and efficient topography; they promoted neural tissue regeneration. Nanofibrous poly (L-lactic acid) (PLLA) and poly (caprolactone) (PCL) scaffolds designed via electrospining and phase separation demonstrated significant cytocompatibility properties useful for neural tissue regeneration. Incorporation of laminin into the nanofibers created a biomimetic scaffolds for peripheral nerve repair as laminin is an extracellular protein that promotes neurite outgrowth (Koh et al., 2008). Another example for the addition of laminin onto the poly (L-lactic acid) (PLLA) nanofibers was investigated for the culture of the tissues of rat dorsal root ganglia (Patel et al., 2007). Cultures revealed significant longer neurite length more than those cultured on poly (L-lactic acid) (PLLA) nanofibers without laminin. These findings demonstrated the advantages of biosynthetic nanomaterials over the synthetic ones. Moreover, the topography of the electrospun nanofibers scaffolds affected the behaviour of the cultured dorsal root ganglia. Significant extension and elongation of neurites were shown on aligned fibers compared with cultured on randomly oriented nanofibers. The neurites grew in a radial manner on the aligned nanofibers. Those that grew in the direction of the fibers had a faster growth rate than the others indicating that the aligned nanofibrous scaffolds served in guiding neurite orientation and cell alignment (Chow et al., 2007).

Electrospun Chitosan on poly(caprolactone) (PCL) nanofibrous scaffolds provided excellent mechanical properties that enhanced Schwann cell proliferation (Zhang & Webster, 2009).

Chitosan micro and nanofiber mesh tubes have also been investigated for nerve reconstruction (Wang et al., 2008). The authors observed early recovery of sensory functions and elongation of the regenerating axons in 10 mm rat sciatic nerve gap after implantation of the nanofiber mesh tubes. Covalent binding of synthetic and natural materials have been demonstrated in the conjugation of collagen onto a copolymer of methyl methacrylate and acrylic acid electrospun nanofibers (Cao et al., 2009). Increased neurite length of cortical neural stem cells, in proportion to collagen content, was found, indicating that this combination improved the attachment and viability of the cultured neural stem cells. Peptide nanofibrous scaffolds fabricated by self-assembly induced favourable neural cell responses and enhanced neuronal cell functions, outgrowth and functional synapse formation (Zhang & Webster, 2009). Other types of scaffolds are the carbon nanotubes and nanofibers. They were found to guide axon regeneration and improve neural activity as a result of good electrical conductivity, strong mechanical properties and their similar nanoscale dimensions to neurites. Multiwalled carbon nanotubes have been applied for the growth of neurons: a 200 % increase in total neurite length and a 300 % increase in the number of branches and neurites have been demonstrated. In addition, decreased astrocyte proliferation, and consequent decreased glial scar tissue formation, was shown on carbon nanofibers with a polymer composite. Moreover, it was found that astrocytes attached and proliferated less on carbon nanofibers with the smallest nanometer diameter and the highest surface energy (Mckenzie et al., 2004). Carbon nanofibers were shown to limit astrocyte functions, leading to decreased glial scar tissue formation which is essential for increased neuronal implant efficacy.

4. Safety issues involved in the use of nanotechnology

Despite the wide range of applications of nanotechnology in the tissue regeneration studies, still there is a lack of information concerning the influence of nanomaterials on human health. Data available for the safety of nanomaterials, particularly in the field of tissue regeneration, are limited and the mechanisms of their toxicity are still poorly understood. Several studies indicated that a small size, a large surface area and the ability to generate reactive oxygen species increase the potential of nanomaterials to induce cell injury. However, other studies have indicated that, for example, ceramic nanoparticles were safer to osteoblasts than conventional ceramic microparticles. On the other hand, cellular uptake of nanoparticles and their effects on the physiological processes of the cells and their organelles should be deeply investigated before such materials are applied to human tissues. It has been shown, for example, that degradation of nanomaterials used in artificially engineered joints produced toxic responses due to the use of heavy metals such as iron, nickel and cobalt catalysts (Zang & Webster, 2009).

Recent researches in the field of tracking the engrafted stem cells have demonstrated that the safety of quantum dots depends on their physiochemical properties, dose and exposure. Cytotoxicity of quantum dots has been observed owing to the presence of heavy metals such as cadmium and selenium in their cores. Coating the core of quantum dots was recorded to effectively reduce their toxicity to a significant level. Several strategies have been applied to decrease the toxicity of quantum dots. Coating the core with a shell of zinc sulphide reduces the toxicity by blocking the oxidation of the core by air, making them biologically inert. Another technique uses large protein molecules such as bovine serum albumin to could slow the photo-oxidation of the core. Moreover, labelling quantum dots with biomolecules such as arginine-glycine-aspartic acid removed all the toxic effects on cultured stem cells (Solanki et al., 2008). It is recommended to study the appropriate properties and concentrations of different nanoparticles used in cultured and transplanted cells and their safety limits and to deeply understand the physicochemical, molecular and physiological processes of nanomaterials before introducing them into the human bodies.

5. Conclusion

Nanotechnology has shown great potential for numerous tissue regeneration applications. Nanomaterials have achieved one of the major challenges of tissue regeneration which is mimicking the architecture of natural extracellular matrix. Designed nanostructures such as nanoparticles, nanosurfaces and nanoscaffolds have been used to promote stem cell cultures which will speed up understanding, controlling and guiding tissue regeneration studies of different tissues, such as bone, cartilage, vascular and neural tissues. It is suggested that the creation of such nanostructures would advance greatly the field of tissue regeneration. However, nanomaterials require more testing and investigations before full use in human tissue repair. Further understanding of their interactions with biological systems is still needed.

6. References

Au, K.; Liao, S.; Lee, Y. et al. (2009). Effects of Iron Oxide Nanoparticles on Cardiac Differentiation of Embryonic Stem Cells. *Biochem Biophys Res Commun*, Vol.379, (2009), pp. 898-903

Bacakova, L.; Grausova, L.; Vacik, J. et al. (2007). Improved Adhesion and Growth of Human Osteoblast-Like MG 63 Cells on Biomaterials Modified with Carbon Nanoparticles. *Diamond Relat Mater*, Vol.16, No.12 (December 2007), pp. 2133-2140

Baker, B.M.; Handorf, A.M.; Ionescu, L.C.; Li, W. & Mauck, R.L. (2009). New Directions in Nanofibrous Scaffolds for Soft Tissue Engineering and Regeneration. *Expert Rev Med Devices*, Vol.6, No.5, (September 2009), pp. 515-532

Biggs, M.J.P.; Richards, R.G.; McFarlane, S.; Wilkinson, C.D.W.; Oreffo, R.O.C. & Dalby M. J. (2008). Adhesion Formation of Primary Human Osteoblasts and The Functional Response of Mesenchymal Stem Cells to 330? nm Deep Microgrooves. *J R Soc Interface*, Vol.5, (2008), pp. 1231-1242

Boland, E.D.; Matthews, J.A.; Pawlowski, K.J. et al. (2004). Electrospinning Collagen and Elastin: Preliminary Vascular Tissue Engineering. *Front Biosci*, Vol.9, (2004), pp. 1422-1432

Boudreau, N.J. & Jones, P.L. (1999). Extracellular Matrix and Integrin Signalling: The Shape of Things to Come. *Biochem J*, Vol.339, No.3, (1999), pp. 481-488

Bulte, J.W.M. & Kraitchman, D.L. (2004). Monitoring Cell Therapy Using Iron Oxide MR Contrast Agents. *Curr Pharm Biotechnol*, Vol.5, No.6, (2004), pp. 567-584

Cao, H.; Liu, T. & Chew, S.Y. (2009). The Application of Nanofibrous Scaffolds in Neural Tissue Engineering. *Advanced Drug Delivery Reviews*, Vol.61, No.12, (October 2009), pp. 1055-1064

Chang, J.; Su, H. & Hsu, S. (2008). The Use of Peptide- Delivery to Protect Human Adipose- Derived Adult Stem Cells from Damage Caused by The Internalization of Quantum Dots. *Biomaterials*, Vol.29, (2008), pp. 925-936

Chang, J.; Hsu, S. & Su, H. (2009). The Regulation of The Gap Junction of Human Mesenchymal Stem Cells Through The Internalization of Quantum Dots. *Biomaterials*, Vol.30, (2009), pp. 1937-1946

Charest, J.L.; Bryants, L.E.; Garcia, A.J. & King, W.P. (2004). Hot Embossing for Micropatterned Cell Substrates. *Biomaterials*, Vol.25, (2004), pp. 4767-4775

Chen, V.J. & Ma, P.X. (2004). Nano-Fibrous Poly(L-Lactic Acid) Scaffolds with Interconnected Spherical Macropores. *Biomaterials*, Vol.25, No.11, (2004), pp. 2065-2073

Chen, V.J.; Smith, L.A. & Ma, P.X. (2006). Bone Regeneration on Computer-Designed Nano- Fibrous Scaffolds. *Biomaterials*, Vol.27, (2006), pp. 3973-3979

Chen, H.; Titushkin, I.; Stroscio, M. & Cho, M. (2007). Altered Membrane Dynamics of Quantum Dot-Conjugated Integrins During Osteogenic Differentiation of Human Bone Marrow Derived Progenitor Cells. *Biophys J*, Vol.92, (2007), pp. 1399-1408

Choudhary, S.; Haberstroh, K.M. & Webster, T.J. (2007). Enhanced Functions of Vascular Cells on Nanostructured Ti for Improved Stent Applications. *Tissue Engineering*, Vol.13, (2007), pp. 1421-1430

Chow, W.N.; Simpson, D.G.; Bigbee, J.W. & Colello, R.J. (2007). Evaluating Neuronal and Glial Growth on Electrospun Polarized Matrices: Bridging the Gap in Percussive Spinal Cord Injuries. *Neuron Glia Biol*, Vol.3, (2007), pp. 119-126

Clem, W.C.; Chowdhury, S.; Catledge, S.A. et al., (2008). Mesenchymal Stem Cell Interaction with Ultra-Smooth Nanosrtuctured Diamond for Wear-Resistant Orthopaedic Implants. *Biomaterials*, Vol.29, No.24-25, (August-September 2008), pp. 3461-3468

Curtis, A.S.G.; Dalby, M.J. & Gadegaard, N. (2006). Cell Signaling Arising from Nanotopography: Implications for Nanomedical Devices. *Nanomedicine*, Vol.1, (2006), pp. 67-72

Dalby, M.J.; Riehle, M.O.; Yarwood, S.J.; Wilkinson, C.D. & Curtis, A.S. (2003b). Nucleus Alignment and Cell Signaling in Fibroblasts: Response to a Micro-Grooved Topography. *Exp Cell Res*, Vol.284, (2003b), pp. 274-282

Dalby, M.J.; Biggs, M. J.; Gadegaard, N.; Kalna, G.; Wilkinson, C.D. & Curtis, A.S. (2007). Nanotopographical Stimulation of Mechanotransduction and Changes in Interphase Centromere Positioning. *J Cell Biochem*, Vol.100, (2007), pp. 326-338

Dalby, M.J. (2009). Nanostructured Surfaces: Cell Engineering and Cell Biology. *Nanomedicine*, Vol.4, No.3, (April 2009), pp. 247-248

Delcroix, G.J.; Jacquart, M.; Lemaire, L. et al., (2009). Mesenchymal and Neural Stem Cells Labelled with HEDP-coated SPIO Nanoparticles: In Vitro Characterization and Migration Potential in Rat Brain. *Brain Res*, Vol.1255, (2009), pp. 18-31

El-Sadik, A.O.; El-Ansary, A. & Sabry, S.M. (2010). Nanoparticle-Labeled Stem Cells: A Novel Therapeutic Vehicle. *Clinical Pharmacology: Advances and Applications,* Vol.2, (2010), pp. 9-16

Emerit, J.C.; Beaumount; C. & Trivin, F. (2001). Iron Metabolism, Free Radicals, and Oxidative Injury. *Biomed Pharmacother,* Vol.55, No.6, (2001), pp. 333-339

Gao, J. & Xu, B. (2009). Applications of Nanomaterials Inside Cells. *Nanotoday,* Vol.4, (2009), pp. 37-51

Gelain, F.; Bottai, D.; Vescovi, A. & Zhang, S. (2006). Designer Self-Assembling Peptide Nanofiber Scaffolds for Adult Mouse Neural Stem Cell 3-Dimensional Cultures. *PLoS ONE,* Vol.1, No.1, (2006), e119

Genove, E.;Shen, C.; Zhang, S. & Semino, C.E. (2005). The Effect of Functionalized Self-Assembling Peptide Scaffolds on Human Aortic Endothelial Cell Function. *Biomaterials,* Vol.26, No.16, (June 2005), pp. 3341-3351

Grausova, L.; Kromka, A.; Bacakova, L.; Potocky, S.; Vanecek, M. & Lisa, V. (2008). Bone and Vascular Endothelial Cells in Cultures on Nanocrystalline Diamond Films. *Diamond and Related Materials,* Vol.17, No.7-10, (July-October 2008), pp. 1405-1409

Hu, Y.; Cai, K.; Luo, Z. et al. (2009). Surface Mediated in Situ Differentiation of Mesenchymal Stem Cells on Gene-Functionalized Titanium Films Fabricated by Layer-by- Layer Technique. *Biomaterials,* Vol.30, No.21, (July 2009), pp. 3626-3635

Huang, D.; Chung, T.; Hung, Y. et al. (2008). Internalization of Mesoporous Silica Nanoparticles Induces Transient but not Sufficient Osteogenic Signals in Human Mesenchymal Stem Cells. *Toxicol Appl Pharmacol,* Vol.231, (2008), pp. 208-215

Ito, A.; Hibino, E.; Honda, H. et al. (2004). A New Methodology of Mesenchymal Stem Cell Expansion Using Magnetic Nanoparticle. *Biomechemical and Engineering J,* Vol.20, (2004), pp. 119-125

Jang, J.; Castano, O. & Kim, H. (2009). Electrospun Materials as Potential Platforms for Bone Tissue Engineering. *Advanced Delivery Reviews,* Vol.61, (2009), pp. 1065-1083

Jing, X.; Yang, L.; Duan, X. et al. (2008). Invivo MR Imaging Tracking of Magnetic Iron Oxide Nanoparticle Labelled, Engineered, Autologus Bone Marrow Mesenchymal Stem Cells Following Intra-Articular Injection. *Joint Bone Spine,* Vol.75, (2008), pp. 432-438

Jung, Y.; Chung, Y.; Kim, S.H. et al. (2009). In situ Chondrogenic Differentiation of Human Adipose Tissue-Derived Stem Cells in a TGF-b1 Loaded Fibrin-Poly(Lactide-Caprolactone) Nanoparticulate. *Biomaterials,* Vol.30, (2009), pp. 4657-4664

Kea, Y.; Hu, C.; Jianga, X. et al. (2009). In vivo Magnetic Resonance Tracking of Feridex-Labelled Bone MarroDerived Neural Stem Cells after Autologous Transplantation in Rhesus Monkey. *J Neurosci Methods,* Vol.179, (2009), pp. 45-50

Kim, H.W.; Song, J.H. & Kim, H.E. (2005). Nanofiber Generation of Gelatin-Hydroxyapatite Biomimetics for Guided Tissue Regeneration. *Adv Funct Matr,* Vol.15, (2005), pp. 1988-1994

Kim, H.W.; Kim, H.E. & Knowles, J.C. (2006). Production and Potential of Bioactive Glass Nanofibers as a Next-Generation Biomaterial. *Adv Funct Mater,* Vol.16, (2006), pp. 1529-1535

Koh, H.S.; Yong, T.; Chan, C.K. & Ramakrishna, S. (2008). Enhancement of Neurite Outgrowth Using Nanostructured Scaffolds Coupled with Laminin. *Biomaterials,* Vol.29, No.26, (September 2008), pp. 3574-3582

Kommireddy, D.S.; Ichinose, I.; Lvov, Y.M. & Mills, D.K. (2005). Nanoparticle Thin Films: Surface Modification for Cell Attachment and Growth. *J Biomed Nanotechnol,* Vol.3, (2005), pp. 286-290

Kommireddy, D.S.; Sriram, S.M.; Lvov, Y.M. & Mills, D.K. (2006). Stem Cell Attachment to Layer-by-Layer Assembled TiO2 Nanoparticle Thin Films. *Biomaterials,* Vol.27, No.24, (August 2006), pp. 4296-4303

Kubo, K.; Tsukimura, N.; Iwasa, F. et al.   (2009). Cellular Behavior on TiO2 Nanonodular Structures in a Micro-to-Nanoscale Hierarchy Model. *Biomaterials,* Vol.30, No.29, (October 2009), pp. 5319-5329

Lenhert, S.; Meier, M.B.; Meyer, U.; Chi, L. & Wiesmann, H.P. (2005). Osteoblast Alignment, Elongation and Migration on Grooved Polystrene Surfaces Patterned by Langmuir-Blodgett Lithography. *Biomaterials,* Vol.26, (2004), pp. 563-570

Lin, S.; Xie, X. & Patel, M.R. (2007). Quantum Dot Imaging for Embryonic Stem Cells. *BMC Biotechnol,* Vol.7, (2007), pp. 67

Liu, H. & Webster, T.J. (2007). Nanomedicine for Implants: A Review of Studies and Necessary Experimental Tools. *Biomaterials,* Vol.28, No.2, (January 2007), pp. 354-369

Mckenzie, J.L.; Waid, M.C.; Shi, R. & Webster, T.J. (2004). Decreased Functions of Astrocytes on Carbon Nanofiber Materials. *Biomaterials,* Vol.25, No.7-8, (March-April 2004), pp. 1309-1317

Matsuzaka, K.; Walboomers, X.F.; Yoshinari, M.; Inoue, T. & Jansen, J.A. (2003). The Attachment and Growth Behavior of Osteoblast-like Cells on Microtextured Surfaces. *Biomaterials,* Vol.24, (2003), pp. 2711-2719

Miller, D.C.; Haberstroh, K.M. & Webster, T.J. (2007). PLGA Nanometer Surface Features Manipulate Fibronectin Interactions for Improved Vascular Cell Adhesion. *J Biomed Mater Res A,* Vol.81, No.3, (June 2007), pp. 678-684

Murthy, S.K. (2007). Nanoparticles in Modern Medicine: State of the Art and Future Challenges. *International Journal of Nanomedicine,* Vol.2, (2007), pp. 129-141

Ogawa, T.; Saruwatari, L.; Takeuchi, K.; Aita, H. & Ohno, N. (2008). Ti Nano-Nodular Structuring for Bone Integration and Regeneration. *J Dent Res,* Vol.87, (2008), pp. 751-756

Oh, S.; Brammer, K.S.; Julie Li, Y.S.; et al.   (2009). Stem Cell Fate Dictated Solely by Altered Nanotube Dimension. *Proc Natl Acad Sci USA,* Vol.106, No.7, (February 2009), pp. 2130-2135, ISSN 1729-8806

Patel, S.; Kurpinski, K.; Quigley, R. et al., (2007). Bioactive Nanofibers: Synergistic Effects of Nanotopography and Chemical Signaling on Cell Guidance. *Nano Lett,* Vol.7, (2007), pp. 2122-2128

Shah, B.S.; Clark, P.A.; Moioli, E.K.; Stroscio, M.A. & Mao, J.J. (2007). Labelling of Mesenchymal Stem Cells by Bioconjugated Quantum Dots. *Nano Lett,* Vol.7, (2007), pp. 3071-3079

Shi, X.; Wang, Y.; Varshney, R.R. et al., (2009). In-vitro Osteogenesis of Synovium Stem Cells Induced by Controlled Release of Bisphosphate Additives from Microspherical Mesoporous Silica Composite. *Biomaterials*, Vol.30, (2009), pp. 3996-4005

Shin, M.; Yoshimoto, H. & Vacanti, J.P. (2004). In Vivo Bone Tissue Engineering Using Mesenchymal Stem Cells on a Novel Electrospun Nanofibrous Scaffold. *Tissue Eng*, Vol.10, (2004), pp. 33-41

Silva, G.A.; Czeisler, C.; Niece, K.L. et al. (2004). Selective Differentiation of Neural Progenitor Cells by High-Epitope Density Nanofibers. *Science*, Vol.303, (2004), pp. 1352-1355

Smith, I.O.; Liu, X.H.; Smith, L.A. & Ma, P.X. (2010). Nano-Structured Polymer Scaffolds for Tissue Engineering and Regenerative Medicine. *Wiley Interdiscip Rev Nanomed Nanobiotechnol*, Vol.1, No.2, (March 2010), pp. 226-236

Song, J.H.; Kim, H.E. & Kim, H.W. (2008). Electrospun Fibrous Web of Collagen-Apatite Precipitated Nanocomposite for Bone Regeneration. *J Mater Sci Mater Med*, Vol.19, (2008), pp. 2925-2932

Sykova, E. & Jendelova, P. (2007). Migration, Fate and In vivo Imaging of Adult Stem Cells in the CNS. *Cell Death Differ*, Vol.14, (2007), pp. 1336-1342

Vasita, R. & Katti, D.S. (2006). Nanofibers and Their Applications in Tissue Engineering. *International Journal of Nanomedicine*, Vol.1, No.1, (2006), pp. 15-30, ISSN 11769114

Wang, L. & Li, D. Y. (2003). Mechanical, Electrochemical and Tribological Properties of Nanocrystalline Surface of Brass Produced by Sandblasting and Annealing. *Surface and Coatings Technology*, Vol.167, No.2-3, (April 2003), pp. 188-196

Wang, W.; Itoh, S.; Matsuda, A. et al. (2008). Influences of Mechanical Properties and Permeability on Chitosan Nano/Microfiber Mesh Tubes as a Scaffold for Nerve Regeneration. *J Biomed Mater Res A*, Vol.84, No.A, (2008), pp. 557-566

Webster, T.J.; Ergun, C.; Doremus, R.H.; Siegel, R.W. & Bizios, R. (2000). Enhanced Functions of Osteoblasts on Nanophase Ceramics. *Biomaterials*, Vol.21, No.17, (September 2000), pp. 1803-1810

Webster, T.J.; Schadler, L.S.; Siegel, R.W. & Bizios, R. (2001). Mechanisms of Enhanced Osteoblast Adhesion on Nanophase Alumina Involve Vitronectin. *Tissue Engineering*, Vol.7, No.3, (2001), pp. 291-301, ISSN 10763279

Woo, K.M.; Jun, J.H.; Chen, J.H.; et al. (2007). Nano-Fibrous Scaffolding Promotes Osteoblast Differentiation and Biomineralization. *Biomaterials*, Vol.28, (2007), pp. 335-343

Xu, C.Y.; Inai, R.; Kotaki, M. & Ramakrishna, S. (2004). Aligned Biodegradable Nanofibrous Structure: A Potential Scaffold for Blood Vessel Engineering. *Biomaterials*, Vol.25, No.5, (February 2004), pp. 877-886

Yoshimoto, H.; Shin, H.; Terai, H. & Vacanti, A. (2003). Biodegradable Nanofiber Scaffolds by Electrospinning and its Potential for Bone Tissue Engineering. *Biomaterials*, Vol.24, (2003), pp. 2077-2082

Zhang, Y.; Venugopal, J.R.; El-Turki, A.; Ramakrishna, S.; Su, B. & Lim, C.T. (2008). Electrospun Biomimetic Nanocomposite Nanofibers of Hydroxyapatite/Chitosan for Bone Tissue Engineering. *Biomaterials*, Vol.29, (2008), pp. 4314-4322

Zhang, L. & Webster, T.J. (2009). Nanotechnology and Nanomaterials: Promises for Improved Tissue Regeneration. *Nanotoday*, Vol.4, No.1, (February 2009), pp. 66-80

Part 3

Modeling and Assessment of Regeneration

8

A Mathematical Model for Wound Contraction and Angiogenesis

Fred Vermolen and Olmer van Rijn
Delft Institute of Applied Mathematics, Delft University of Technology
The Netherlands

1. Introduction

Cutaneous wounds, ulcers or burns, as a result of external damage, such as intensive solar exposure or accidents, occur in high numbers and may cause ever lasting traumas. In some cases, the wounds are very painful and impair an individual's daily life in terms of health, and social interaction with his or her surroundings, but also in terms of mobility and ability to work or to perform leisure activities. Furthermore, the aesthetic feeling of patients is highly improved by the treatment of burns and other wounds since otherwise the wounds can make a detrimental impact on the appearance of the patient's skin. Besides aesthetic appearance, also the functioning of the damaged skin is different since infections are possibly more likely to occur near the (scar tissue of the) burn. Furthermore, the conception of temperature and pain by a patient is also altered by the burn, ulcer or cutaneous wound. Therefore, the treatment of these defects, which occurs in very high numbers, is important and hence it is crucial to improve treatments and to make treatments more efficient.

Nowadays many different treatments, such as, in more serious cases, skin transplantation, injection of cell cultures and the implant of artificial skin, are commonly carried out by plastical surgeons in order to relieve the patient and to minimize the aesthetic effects of scar tissue as much as possible. In order to be able to improve medical treatment of scars, it is important to understand the biological mechanism behind scar formation in terms of plastic deformation and a regenerated excess of collageneous matrix. More information about the treatment of scars and the biology behind the scar formation can, among others, be found in Bloemen (2011); van der Veer (2009). The deformations are caused by the contractile mechanism due to the pulling behavior of the (myo-)fibroblasts. Dallon (2008) experimentally found that the nature of contraction is predominantly determined by the following two mechanisms:

- The degree and orientation of motility of fibroblasts. This motility mechanism of the fibroblasts is caused by the attachment and movement of the lamellipodia of the fibroblasts onto the collageneous fibres;
- The attachment of the philapods of the less motile myofibroblasts onto the extra cellular matrix.

These mechanisms were simulated by Dallon (2010) by the use of a spring model. Since Dallon's two-dimensional model tracks the forces exerted by each individual philapod or lamellipodium of the individual (myo)fibroblast, the formalism becomes very expensive from a computational point of view when applied to burns of realistic dimensions with millions of fibroblasts and collageneous fibres. However, his observations and calculations are very useful for a thorough understanding of the implications of the fundamental processes and for the calibration of continuum models that are based on partial differential equations.

The severity of a wound is determined by the thickness of the damaged skin layer of the patient. A minor injury concerns the damage on the corneum, which is replaced with the patient's tissues relatively quickly. This type of injury is referred to as a first degree skin burn or wound. A more severe damage concerns the impairment of the epidermis. In this case reepithialialization has to repair the epidermis by migration and proliferation of keratinocytes. This damage is classified as a second degree burn or wound, but this type of wound will heal without many problems for healthy patients. Contraction does not take place and hence the burn or wound will recover entirely without any plastic deformations or significant scars. Third degree burns or wounds pose a more serious damage in the sense that also (part of) the dermis, and even the subcutis could be disrupted. Here the fibroblast rich dermis, consisting of the collageneous fibrous tissue has to be repaired. This takes place by a sequence of signaling processes to initiate proliferation and movement of fibroblasts and the restoration of the vascular network. As the fibroblasts produce an excess of collageneous fibres, on which they, and the myofibroblasts to a larger extent, exert contractile forces, wound contraction takes place. The process of wound contraction is a useful mechanism for a rapid minimization of exposure of the underlying tissues to hazardous external environments, when the wound is caused by mechanical damage. In particular, in skins of rabbits, percentages of up to 80 percent of the initial wound area have been reported in various experimental studies. In humans, experimental studies evidence that wound contraction is much less significant, being in the order of 5–10 percent. However, in the case of healing of burns, this contraction phenomenon is undesirable, as it gives rise to significant deformations, which can be plastic and furthermore, the patient is left with an excess of collageneous fibres and unpleasantly looking scars. Remodeling is a very slow process which cannot remove all wrinkles as a result of the plastic deformations due to wound contraction.

In order to be able to improve surgical treatments, in terms of effectiveness and minimization of invasion into the patient, it is crucial to know which behavior of the (myo-)fibroblasts cause the plastic deformation of the skin. In the case of a third degree burn or wound, fibroblasts enter the wound area during the proliferative stages of the healing process of the dermis. Subsequently, the fibroblasts start to proliferate and to produce extracellular matrix, referred to as fibrous tissue. Furthermore, as a result of exposure to high strains, fibroblasts differentiate into myofibroblasts, which are considered as weak muscle cells. Myofibroblasts increase the measure of contraction of the wound area of the dermis. This differentiation process also takes place under the influence of a growth factor TF-β, which is produced by the fibroblasts and myofibroblasts depending on the amount of extracellular matrix present. The growth factor also stimulates the production of fibroblasts and its regeneration of collagen. Next to the enhancement of the production of several biological entities, the growth factor increases the chemotactic transport of the fibroblasts towards the wound area. To get more quantitative insight into the influences of the growth factors and other agents on the amount of wound contraction caused by the pulling forces of the (myo)fibroblasts, detailed mathematical models with parameter sensitivity analysis are indispensable. This sensitivity analysis can give insight into the quantification of the influence of all biological parameters involved

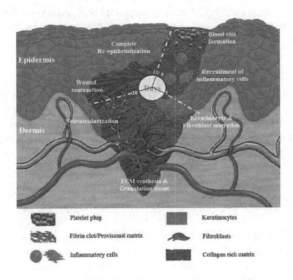

Platelet plug		Keratinocytes	
Fibrin clot/Provisional matrix		Fibroblasts	
Inflammatory cells		Collagen rich matrix	

Fig. 1. A schematic of the events during wound healing. The dermis and epidermis are illustrated. The picture was taken with permission from http://www.bioscience.org/2006/v11/af/1843/figures.htm

in this process on contraction and healing, as well as values such that healing of burns is optimized with respect to a minimal level of wound contraction and maximum healing speed. These results are helpful to surgeons to design innovative minimal invasive treatments that are applicable to patients. Furthermore, the mathematical analysis is helpful to make the treatment patient specific.

In this manuscript, we address two partial processes during the proliferative phase: wound contraction and angiogenesis. When the tissue is provided with enough oxygen and nutrients the process of wound closure starts. Cells in the epidermis, which mainly consist of keratinocytes, start regenerating the upperlayer of the wound. Usually the skin can not be replaced fully and some scars are left where the wound was located, due to excess of regenerated collagen. The second and third stage of wound healing do not take place at the same location in the wound. The former is located in the dermis, the latter is limited to the epidermis. The epidermis and the dermis consist of different type of cells and are separated by a so-called basal membrane, see also Figure 1.

In this manuscript, we first present a selection of the currently available mathematical models that seek to describe the biological processes of wound healing as well as possible. The healing process is very complex and many factors contribute to it, therefore simplifications have to be made. The main topics in this thesis are combining two models for angiogenesis and coupling models for the different stages of wound healing. Currently models exist for angiogenesis and dermal regeneration (fibroblasts and collagen) separately, however, only scarcely have there been attempts to couple the models. This is vital as the various stages of wound healing overlap and hence influence each other. The models that we consider in this study are all formulated in terms of partial differential equations (PDEs) that are based on conservation principles. Such coupled models could give more insights into how the process of wound healing evolves. These insights might lead to treatments that reduce healing time, e.g. the use of certain hormones to speed up the healing process. Also scars and other deformations due to incomplete healing might be prevented or reduced. This issue is especially crucial for the treatment of burns, where hypotrophic scars may result after injury.

A lot of simulations have been done in literature to give more insight on how these models behave. Also the dependence of the models on certain parameters is investigated in the present paper. Finally recommendations are made for future research in the topic of mathematically describing wound healing. Many studies are based on PDEs, for instance the work by Murray (2004); Olsen (1995); Maggelakis (2003); Gaffney (2002); Sherratt (1991); Adam (1999); Javierre (2009); Vermolen (2009; 2010; 2011); Schugart (2008); Xue (2009). Many other modeling studies are based on cell-based or Monte-Carlo methods, such as the cellular Potts models used by Glazier (1992); Merks (2009); Plank (2004) to mention a few. This class of model is lattice-based and minimizes a virtual energy functional. Recently, a semi-stochastic continuous cell-based model was formulated by Vermolen-Gefen (2011).

The present manuscript falls within the class of papers, in which one attempts to combine existing mathematical models for various subprocesses occuring during wound healing. Some recent work by this team are Vermolen (2010), and Vermolen (2011), in which the most simplified models for wound contraction, closure and angiogenesis are coupled. The present model is based on a combination of some more advanced models for wound contraction and angiogenesis and gives a more sophisticated formalism for dermal regeneration. The paper is organized as follows. In Section 2, we present several models for processes of angiogenesis and wound contraction. Here, we also present some results of simulations. This is an innovation with respect to other studies. In Section 3, we consider the coupling of the models, including simulations. In Section 4, we describe the numerical methods. Finally, some conclusions are drawn in Section 5.

The character of the current manuscript is rather informal and descriptive about the mathematical concepts used in the present study. The level of abstract mathematics has been reduced tremendously. Further, we note that the simulations shown in this manuscript are still in a preliminary state.

2. Current models

The mathematical model for the proliferative stage of wound healing is usually separated in three distinct parts representing three stages of wound healing. These three stages are wound contraction, angiogenesis and wound closure. Note that the inflammation stage mentioned in Section 1 is not taken into account. This is due to the fact that inflammation only contains the damage and only after the inflammation stage is finished the real healing process starts.

In this chapter we present some of the currently available models on the above mentioned wound healing stages. In Section 2.1, we first present the model on wound contraction. Next in Section 2.2, a model for angiogenesis is presented. This model is a combination of two accepted models that describe a specific feature in the angiogenesis process. The two models take a very different approach on how to model the growth of new blood vessels in the wound. In Section 2.3, a study that attempts to combine models of dermal regeneration and angiogenesis is briefly discussed. In all the models that we deal with, we consider a bounded simply connected domain $\Omega \subset \mathbb{R}^2$. The boundary is denoted by $\partial\Omega$.

2.1 The wound contraction models

During the wound contraction stage fibroblasts (connective tissue cells) invade the wound site and contract the extracellular matrix (ECM). The contraction decreases the area of contact between the wound and its surroundings, thereby reducing the chance of contamination and infection. Furthermore this process is vital in assuring that new blood vessels can be formed in the wound during angiogenesis, since the fibroblasts invading the wound form the tissue in which the new capillaries can grow. The wound contraction stage is limited to the dermis, however, the contraction of the ECM also effects the tissue in the epidermis.

We use the model for contraction due to Javierre (2009), which deals with the presence of myofibroblasts. Myofibroblasts are a kind of weak muscle cells. They are nonmotile cells that differentiate from fibroblasts and transmit and amplify the traction forces generated by the fibroblasts, Vermolen (2009). Secondly, the model incorporates the effects of a growth factor that triggers wound contraction.

The equation concerning the fibroblast concentration u_{fib} becomes

$$\frac{\partial u_{\text{fib}}}{\partial t} + \nabla \cdot \left(\frac{\partial \mathbf{u}}{\partial t} u_{\text{fib}} - D_{\text{fib}} \nabla u_{\text{fib}} + \frac{a_{\text{fib}}}{(b_{\text{fib}} + c_{\text{ecm}})^2} u_{\text{fib}} \nabla c_{\text{ecm}} \right) =$$

$$\left(\lambda_{\text{fib}} + \frac{\lambda_{\text{fib}}^0 c_{\text{ecm}}}{C_{1/2} + c_{\text{ecm}}} \right) u_{\text{fib}} \left(1 - \frac{u_{\text{fib}}}{K} \right) - \frac{k_1 c_{\text{ecm}}}{C_k + c_{\text{ecm}}} u_{\text{fib}} + k_2 u_{\text{myo}} - d_{\text{fib}} u_{\text{fib}}, \tag{1}$$

where c_{ecm} and u_{myo} respectively denote the growth factor and myofibroblast concentration. The first term in the left-hand side corresponds to the total accumulation, the second term follows from passive convection due to deformation of the tissue. The third and fourth terms of the left-hand side account for random walk and chemotaxis (movement towards the gradient of the growth factor). In the right-hand side of the above equation, we respectively have the logistic proliferation term up to an equilibrium, in which proliferation is enhanced by the presence of the growth factor, the differentiation term to myofibroblasts under presence of the growth factor, back differiation from myofibroblasts and finally a term dealing with cell death. The cell death rate is denoted by d_{fib}, the myofibroblast to fibroblast differentiation rate by k_2 and the fibroblast to myofibroblast differentiation rate by k_1. Furthermore λ_{fib}^0, $C_{1/2}$ and C_k are known constants that monitor the growth factor's influence on the contraction process and K is a parameter that regulates the equilibrium concentration.

The production term, first on the right hand side, now also incorporates growth factor stimulated proliferation. The other three terms on the right hand side respectively account for differentiation to and from myofibroblasts and cell death.

The PDE for the myofibroblast concentration u_{myo} is similar to equation (1). However, since myofibroblast are nonmotile cells, they will only move due to passive convection. The myofibroblast concentration thus obeys

$$\frac{\partial u_{\text{myo}}}{\partial t} + \nabla \cdot \left(\frac{\partial \mathbf{u}}{\partial t} u_{\text{myo}} \right) = \varepsilon_{\text{myo}} \left(\lambda_{\text{fib}} + \frac{\lambda_{\text{fib}}^0 c_{\text{ecm}}}{C_{1/2} + c_{\text{ecm}}} \right) u_{\text{myo}} \left(1 - \frac{u_{\text{myo}}}{K} \right)$$

$$+ \frac{k_1 c_{\text{ecm}}}{C_k + c_{\text{ecm}}} u_{\text{fib}} - k_2 u_{\text{myo}} - d_{\text{myo}} u_{\text{myo}}, \tag{2}$$

where ε_{ecm} is a proportionality constant, further d_{myo} and u_{myo}^0 denote the myofibroblasts death rate and the myofibroblast equilibrium concentration respectively. The terms on the left-hand side account for accumulation and passive convection due to deformation of the tissue. The right-hand side contains proliferation of myofibroblasts under presence of the growth factor, differentiation of fibroblasts to myofibroblasts, back differentiation to fibroblasts, and (programmed) cell death (apoptosis).

Both fibroblasts and myofibroblasts contribute to the production of the ECM, furthermore the production is chemically enhanced by the growth factor, Vermolen (2009). The PDE for the ECM density ρ then is given by

$$\frac{\partial \rho}{\partial t} + \nabla \cdot \left(\frac{\partial \mathbf{u}}{\partial t} \rho \right) = \left(\lambda_\rho + \frac{\lambda_\rho^0 c_{ecm}}{C_\rho + c_{ecm}} \right) \frac{u_{fib} + \eta_b u_{myo}}{R_\rho^2 + \rho^2} - d_\rho (u_{fib} + \eta_d u_{myo}) \rho, \qquad (3)$$

where λ_ρ and d_ρ are the ECM production and death rate respectively. The terms on the left-hand side describe accumulation and passive convection, and the right-hand side describes growth factor enhanced production of collagen, as well as decay of collagen. Furthermore λ_ρ^0 and C_ρ are known constants that monitor the growth factor's influence on the contraction process. Further, R_ρ is a parameter that quantifies how the ECM production rate depends on the ECM density itself and η_b and η_d are proportionality constants.

The dynamics of the growth factor concentration c_{ecm} are mainly determined by the fibroblasts and myofibroblasts as they produce the growth factor. Also the growth factor is motile, so it is subject to active convection. This leads to the following PDE for the growth factor concentration

$$\frac{\partial c_{ecm}}{\partial t} + \nabla \cdot \left(\frac{\partial \mathbf{u}}{\partial t} c_{ecm} - D_c \nabla c_{ecm} \right) = \frac{k_c (u_{fib} + \zeta u_{myo}) c_{ecm}}{\Gamma + c_{ecm}} - d_c c_{ecm}. \qquad (4)$$

Here the second and third term on the left hand side account for passive convection and ordinary diffusion. The terms on the right hand side account for growth factor production and growth factor decay respectively. Furthermore D_c is the growth factor diffusion coefficient, k_c denotes the growth factor production rate and d_c the natural decay rate. Also Γ is a parameter that quantifies how the growth factor production rate depends on the growth factor concentration itself and ζ is a proportionality constant.

The initial and boundary conditions for the fibroblast concentration and the ECM density remain the same as in the model due to Tranquillo. For the myofibroblast and growth factor concentration the following initial conditions are imposed

$$u_{myo}(\mathbf{x}, 0) = 0, c_{ecm}(\mathbf{x}, 0) = c_{ecm}^0$$

for $\mathbf{x} \in \Omega_w$ and

$$u_{myo}(\mathbf{x}, 0) = 0, c_{ecm}(\mathbf{x}, 0) = 0$$

for $\mathbf{x} \in \Omega_u$. Here c_{ecm}^0 denotes the growth factor equilibrium concentration. Furthermore the growth factor concentration satisfy a no flux boundary condition on all boundaries. For the myofibroblast concentration we can apply the same reasoning as for the ECM density ρ and hence no boundary conditions have to be imposed.

The mechanical part of the wound contraction model is based on the linear viscoelastic equations, i.e.

$$- \nabla \cdot \sigma = \mathbf{f}_{\text{ext}}. \tag{5}$$

Here $\sigma = \sigma_{\text{ecm}} + \sigma_{\text{cell}}$, the stresstensor, accounts for the ECM related stress, σ_{ecm}, and the cell stress, σ_{cell}. Furthermore $\mathbf{f}_{\text{ext}}$ represents the external forces acting on the tissue.

In all the below discussed models the ECM related stress tensor σ_{ecm} is given as

$$\sigma_{\text{ecm}} = \mu_1 \frac{\partial \epsilon}{\partial t} + \mu_2 \frac{\partial \theta}{\partial t} \mathbf{I} + \frac{E}{1+\nu} \left(\epsilon + \frac{\nu}{1-2\nu} \theta \mathbf{I} \right). \tag{6}$$

Here the first two terms on the right hand side respresent the viscous effects and the last term the elastic effects. If we let $\mathbf{u} = \mathbf{u}(\mathbf{x}, t)$ denote the displacement of the ECM, then the strain tensor ϵ and the dilation θ in equation (6) are respectively given by

$$\epsilon = \frac{1}{2} \left(\nabla \mathbf{u} + (\nabla \mathbf{u})^T \right) \tag{7}$$

and

$$\theta = \nabla \cdot \mathbf{u}. \tag{8}$$

Furthermore, in relation (6), $\mathbf{I}$ denotes the identity tensor and μ_1, μ_2, E and ν respectively represent the dynamic and kinematic viscosity, Young's modulus and Poisson's ratio.

The external forces acting on the tissue, $\mathbf{f}_{\text{ext}}$, are modelled similarly in all three models, i.e.

$$\mathbf{f}_{\text{ext}} = -s\rho \mathbf{u}. \tag{9}$$

Here $\rho = \rho(\mathbf{x}, t)$ denotes the ECM density and s is the tethering elasticity coefficient.

At time $t = 0$ it is assumed that there is no displacement of the ECM, i.e. $\mathbf{u}(\mathbf{x}, 0) = \mathbf{0}$. Also we assume that $\mathbf{u}$ vanishes at the boundary far away from the wound, i.e. $\mathbf{u}(\mathbf{x}, t) = \mathbf{0}$ for $\mathbf{x} \in \partial \Omega$. This can be justified by taking the computational domain Ω sufficiently large, so that the boundary effects can be ignored.

Since the myofibroblasts transmit and amplify the traction forces generated by the fibroblasts this is also visible in the cell traction term σ_{cell}. For the model due to Olsen et al. this term is given by

$$\sigma_{\text{cell}} = \frac{\tau u_{\text{fib}} \left(1 + \xi u_{\text{myo}} \right) \rho}{R_\tau^2 + \rho^2} \mathbf{I}, \tag{10}$$

where ξ is a constant of proportionality and R_τ quantifies how the cell traction depends on the ECM density.

In Javierre (2009) an extension of the model due to Olsen et al. is presented. Javierre et al. propose the mechanical stress to act as a factor that effects the differentiation from fibroblasts to myofibroblasts. They introduce an estimation of the mechanical stimulus that depends on the dilation $\theta = \nabla \cdot \mathbf{u}$ as

$$p_{\text{cell}}(\theta) = \frac{K_{\text{act}} p_{\text{max}}}{K_{\text{act}} \theta_1 - p_{\text{max}}} (\theta_1 - \theta) \chi_{[\theta_1, \theta^*]}(\theta) + \frac{K_{\text{act}} p_{\text{max}}}{K_{\text{act}} \theta_2 - p_{\text{max}}} (\theta_2 - \theta) \chi_{[\theta_2, \theta^*]}(\theta) + K_{\text{pas}} \theta. \tag{11}$$

Here χ denotes the indicator function, i.e.

$$\chi_I(\theta) = \begin{cases} 1, \text{ if } \theta \in I, \\ 0, \text{ else.} \end{cases}$$

and the first two terms on the right hand side account for the contractile stress generated internally by the myosin machinery and transmitted through the actin bundles, Javierre (2009). The third term on the right hand side establishes the contractile stress supported by the passive resistance of the cell. See also Figure 2 for a plot of $p_{\text{cell}}(\theta)$.

Furthermore, in equation (11), the compression and traction strain limits are respectively denoted by θ_1 and θ_2, p_{max} respresents the maximal contractile force exerted by the actomyosin machinery and K_{max} and K_{pas} the volumetric stiffness moduli of the active and passive components of the cell. Also the parameter θ^* can be computed from K_{act} and p_{max} as $\theta^* = \frac{p_{\text{max}}}{K_{\text{act}}}$, Javierre (2009).

To incorporate the effects of the mechanical stimulus on the fibroblast to myofibroblast differentiation an extra factor is found before the differentiation term (the second term on the right hand side) in equation (1). The fibroblast to myofibroblast differentiation term changes to

$$\frac{p_{\text{cell}}(\theta)}{\tau_d + p_{\text{cell}}(\theta)} \frac{k_1 c_{\text{ecm}}}{C_k + c_{\text{ecm}}} u_{\text{fib}}, \tag{12}$$

where τ_d is a parameter that quantifies how the differentiation rate depends on the mechanical stimulus. Note that this term is also present in the PDE for the myofibroblast concentration and that thus the second term on the right hand side of equation (2) also changes to the above.

The mechanical stimulus also effects the the cell stresses and thus the cell traction term $\boldsymbol{\sigma}_{\text{cell}}$. In Javierre (2009) it is assumed that $\boldsymbol{\sigma}_{\text{cell}}$ depends linearly on $p_{\text{cell}}(\theta)$ and thus that

$$\sigma_{\text{cell}} = p_{\text{cell}}(\theta) \frac{u_{\text{fib}} (1 + \xi u_{\text{myo}}) \rho}{R_\tau^2 + \rho^2} \mathbf{I}. \tag{13}$$

In order to give more insight in the process of wound contraction we did some simulations with the model due to Javierre (2009). We will describe the numerical techniques in Section 4. Further, the input data can be found in the appendix. As a computational domain we use the unit square, i.e. $\Omega = \{\mathbf{x} = (x, y) | \, 0 \le x, y \le 1\}$, and the initial wound is given by $\Omega_w = \{\mathbf{x} | \, |\mathbf{x}| \le \frac{1}{2}\}$. The results are given in Figures 3 to 5, where we show the solution two days after injury. The computations have been done using parameter values taken from Javierre (2009), see also the appendix.

In Figure 3 we show the fibroblast and myofibroblast concentration two days after injury. The myofibroblast concentration is highly concentrated around the wound edge, whereas the fibroblast have invaded the wound. Figure 4 shows the ECM density and the growth factor concentration two days after injury. We see that the ECM density is slightly elevated at the wound edge, which is to be expected since the wound is healing there. Furthermore the growth factor concentration has spread throughout the computational domain, but is still concentrated inside the wound. In Figure 5, the displacement pattern due to contractile forces exerted by fibroblasts and myofibroblasts is plotted. If we compare Figure 5 with Figure 3 we see that the ECM displacement is largest at places of high myofibroblast concentration. Here

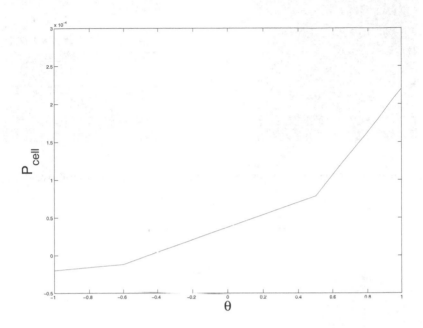

Fig. 2. The mechanical stimulus p_{cell} as a function of the dilation θ, computed with values from Javierre (2009).

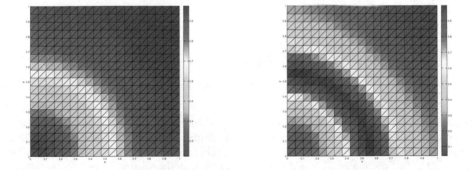

Fig. 3. Normalized fibroblast (left) and myofibroblast (right) densities two days after injury. All input data have been given in the appendix.

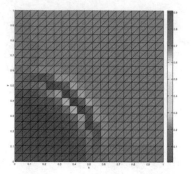 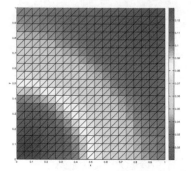

Fig. 4. Normalized ECM density (left) and growth factor concentration (right) two days after injury.

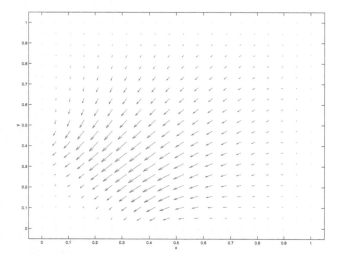

Fig. 5. Displacement of the ECM two days after injury.

the effect of the myofibroblasts, as they transmit and amplify the traction forces generated by the fibroblasts, can clearly be seen.

The normalized solutions in time at $x = 0$, furthest in the wound, are shown in Figure 6. This gives an indication of the development of the solutions in time. We see that the fibroblast concentration increases towards it equilibrium, whereas the myofibroblast concentration first rises and then falls again. This is due to the fact that, as the wound heals, the myofibroblasts either differentiate back to fibroblasts again or undergo apoptosis and hence eventually will disappear completely. Also the growth factor concentration eventually goes to zero as the wound is healed. The ECM density slowly rises in time and will eventually reach its equilibrium, allthough it can take some time before the ECM is completely restored. We finally

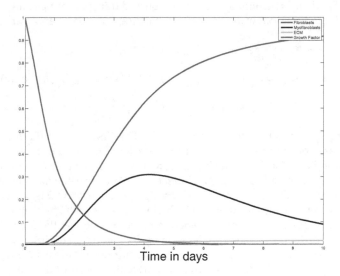

Fig. 6. Normalized solutions furthest in the wound, at $x = 0$, in time.

remark that all the simulations in this subsection were obtained without any coupling with the model for angiogenesis.

2.2 Angiogenesis

In this section, we present the model for angiogenesis. These two models each take a very different approach on how to model this process. Where the model due to Maggelakis (2003) focusses on the relation between a lack of oxygen and capillary growth, the model due to Gaffney (2002), attempts to model the migration of endothelial cells into the wound. Both models adress an important aspect of angiogenesis, but on the other hand both also miss an important aspect.

In this section we present a novel angiogenesis model based on the models of Maggelakis and Gaffney et al. In this model we attempt to unite the two approaches and thus create a model that is suitable for dealing with both aspects of angiogenesis. This gives a new model for angiogenesis. By combining these two aspects in one model we hope to create a more accurate model of the process of angiogenesis. As a basis we take the model of Gaffney et al. and extend it with a negative feedback mechanism for oxygen. This assures that both the endothelial cell migration and the oxygen shortage aspects are covered in this novel angiogenesis model.

The model due to Gaffney et al. is given by

$$\frac{\partial u_{\text{tip}}}{\partial t} - \nabla \cdot (D_1 \nabla u_{\text{tip}} + D_2 \nabla u_{\text{end}}) = f(u_{\text{tip}}, u_{\text{end}}),$$

$$\frac{\partial u_{\text{end}}}{\partial t} - \nabla \cdot \lambda_5 (D_1 \nabla u_{\text{tip}} + D_2 \nabla u_{\text{end}}) = g(u_{\text{tip}}, u_{\text{end}})$$

(14)

where the left-hand sides account for accumulation and transport of tips and endothelial cells by means of a biased random walk process. Further, the functions f and g are given by

$$f(u_{tip}, u_{end}) = \lambda_2 u_{tip} - \lambda_3 u_{tip}^2 - \lambda_4 u_{tip} u_{end},$$

$$g(u_{tip}, u_{end}) = \lambda_6 a u_{end}(u_{end}^0 - u_{end}) + \lambda_6 \chi u_{tip} u_{end}(u_{end}^1 - u_{end})$$

$$+ \lambda_5(\lambda_3 u_{tip}^2 + \lambda_4 u_{tip} u_{end}).$$

These functions were taken from Gaffney (2002). The first term of the function f models tip-branching, as each tip has a likelihood to bifurcate. The second term of the function f accounts for tip-tip anastomosis, which is the process that two tips have a probability to join and hence form a loop, by which a tip is no longer a tip, and hence the number of tips decreases then. The third term of the function f stands for tip-sprout anastomosis, which is the process that a tip may converge into a branch, which closes the network as well and thereby also decreasing the number of tips. For the function g, we distinguish the following terms: The first one contains ordinary logistic proliferation under standard conditions, the second term accounts for an increased logistic growth due to the presence of tips. Finally, the third term accounts for the extent of anastomosis. To incorporate the effects of the macrophage derived growth factor (MDGF) concentration c_{md} on the growth of capillary tips and the proliferation of endothelial cells we assume that λ_2 and λ_6 are functions of the macrophage derived growth factor c_{md}, which is released as a result of a shortage of oxygen. These functions must be zero if there is no MDGF present and rise as the MDGF concentration rises. Furthermore the effects of additional MDGF must be lower if there is already a lot of MDGF present. Therefore we let

$$\lambda_2(c_{md}) = \lambda_2^0 \frac{c_{md}}{c_{md} + \tau_{tip}},$$

$$\lambda_6(c_{md}) = \lambda_6^0 \frac{c_{md}}{c_{md} + \tau_{end}},$$

where τ_{tip} and τ_{end} qualify how respectively λ_2 and λ_6, accounting for tip regeneration and logistic proliferation of endothelial cells respectively, depend on the MDGF concentration. The functions $\lambda_2(c_{md})$ and $\lambda_6(c_{md})$ are given in Figure 7 for $0 \leq c_{md} \leq 1$.

This settles the trigger mechanism that the MDGF concentration fullfills in the growth of new capillaries. To get a good overview of what the model looks like we give the PDEs that drive the model, i.e.

$$\frac{\partial u_{oxy}}{\partial t} = D_{oxy}\Delta u_{oxy} - \lambda_{oxy} u_{oxy} + \lambda_{13}\left(u_{tip} + \frac{\lambda_{oxy} u_\theta u_{end}}{\lambda_{13} u_{end}^0}\right), \tag{15}$$

$$\frac{\partial c_{md}}{\partial t} = D_{md}\Delta c_{md} - \lambda_{md} c_{md} + \lambda_{21} Q(u_{oxy}), \tag{16}$$

$$\frac{\partial u_{tip}}{\partial t} = \nabla \cdot \{D_1 \nabla u_{tip} + D_2 u_{tip} \nabla u_{end}\} + f(u_{tip}, u_{end}), \tag{17}$$

$$\frac{\partial u_{end}}{\partial t} = \lambda_1 \nabla \cdot \{D_1 \nabla u_{tip} + D_2 u_{tip} \nabla u_{end}\} + g(u_{tip}, u_{end}), \tag{18}$$

where we explain the terms occuring in the above PDEs.

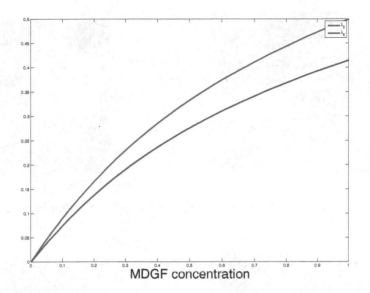

Fig. 7. λ_2 and λ_6 as functions of c_{md}. Here we used $\tau_{tip} = \tau_{end} = 1$, $\lambda_2^0 = 0.83$ and $\lambda_6^0 = 1$.

- the first equation: the first, second and third term in the right-hand side, respectively, stand for diffusion of oxygen (u_{oxy}), consumption of oxygen, and supply of oxygen due to the blood flow in the tips and capillaries (via diffusion through the capillary walls);

- the second equation: the first, second and third term in the right-hand side, respectively, model diffusion of macrophage derived growth factor (VEGF), natural decay of VEGF, and secretion by the macrophages as a result of a shortage of oxygen;

The last two equations were described earlier.

Further, the functions f and g are given by

$$f(u_{tip}, u_{end}) = \lambda_2^0 \frac{c_{md}}{c_{md} + \tau_{tip}} u_{tip} - \lambda_3 u_{tip}^2 - \lambda_4 u_{tip} u_{end},$$

$$g(u_{tip}, u_{end}) = \lambda_6^0 \frac{c_{md}}{c_{md} + \tau_{end}} \left(a u_{end}(u_{end}^0 - u_{end}) + \chi u_{tip} u_{end}(u_{end}^1 - u_{end}) \right)$$

$$+ \lambda_5 (\lambda_3 u_{tip}^2 + \lambda_4 u_{tip} u_{end}).$$

To illustrate how this new model behaves we show some results in Figures 8 to 10. The input-data can be found in the appendix. As a computational domain we use the unit square, i.e. $\Omega = \{\mathbf{x} = (x, y) \mid 0 \le x, y \le 1\}$, and the initial wound is given by $\Omega_w = \left\{ \mathbf{x} \mid |\mathbf{x}| \le \frac{1}{2} \right\}$.

In Figure 8 we see the oxygen and MDGF concentration seven days after injury. The oxygen tension decreases as one moves into the center of the wound. The relation between a lack of oxygen and the production of the macrophage derived growth factor can clearly be seen. In

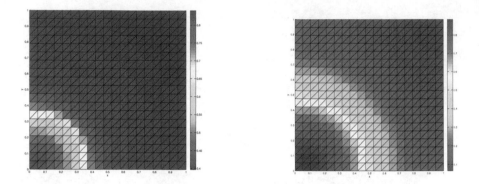

Fig. 8. Normalized oxygen (left) and macrophage derived growth factor (right) concentration seven days after injury.

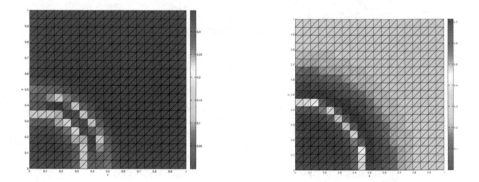

Fig. 9. Normalized capillary tip concentration (left) and endothelial cell density (right) seven days after injury.

areas where the oxygen concentration is low, i.e. inside the wound, the MDGF concentration is at its peak and vice versa. Hence, the MDGF concentration is maximal at the center of the wound. The time for ingress of macrophages has been assumed to be negligible. Also in Figure 10 we see that as the oxygen concentration rises the MDGF concentration drops at approximately the same rate.

Furthermore in Figure 9 we see a front of capillary tips, which slowly moves towards the center of the wound. Also the endothelial cell density is slighty elevated at the wound edge, since this is where the new capillaries are formed. This can also be seen in Figure 10, where the endothelial cell density first peaks and then drops again towards an equilibrium. The capillary tip concentration also peaks, but then drops to zero again. This is to be expected since eventually all capillary tips join together in the newly formed capillary network. The local maximum of the oxygen concentration at $t \approx 18$ days, follows from the peak in capillary tips. As the shortage of oxygen decreases, the concentration of macrophage derived growth factors decreases down to zero.

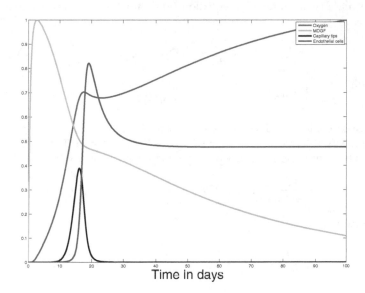

Fig. 10. Normalized solutions furthest in the wound, at $x = 0$, in time.

3. The coupled model

For all the stages during the proliferative phase of wound healing mathematical models have been presented that attempt to describe the processes involved in these stages. These models only focus on one wound healing stage particularly and do not take into account the interactions between these stages. One example of interaction is the need of oxygen for the growth of cells and thus the dependency of the profileration terms on the oxygen concentration. But there are several more interactions that we can think of, including some that will not be taken into account here either.

In Vermolen (2010) and Vermolen (2011) an attempt is made to combine models of the three wound healing stages into one mathematical model. In this chapter we take the novel model on angiogenesis, presented the previous subsection, and make an attempt to couple it with the wound contraction model due to Javierre (2009), given in Section 2.1. We will investigate both the influence of the oxygen concentration on the wound contraction mechanism and the influence of the fibroblast concentration on capillary growth. Furthermore the displacement of the extracellular matrix (ECM) will also effect the angiogenesis process, this will also be taken into account. For now we will not consider wound closure.

In the wound contraction stage several processes require energy to work. The growth of new tissue consumes energy as cells divide and form new cells, i.e. mitosis. Also the active movement of the fibroblasts requires energy since the cells crawl over each other. This energy needed for wound contraction comes primarily from the food that an individual consumes, however, oxygen is needed to put the energy to use, i.e. the cells require oxygen to get the most out of the energy. This means that the oxygen concentration is good indicator for the amount of energy that is available.

If we look at the partial differential equation (PDE) for the fibroblast concentration in the Javierre model,

$$\frac{\partial u_{fib}}{\partial t} + \nabla \cdot \left(\frac{\partial \mathbf{u}}{\partial t} u_{fib} - D_{fib} \nabla u_{fib} + \frac{a_{fib}}{(b_{fib} + c_{ecm})^2} u_{fib} \nabla c_{ecm} \right) =$$

$$\left(\lambda_{fib} + \frac{\lambda^0_{fib} c_{ecm}}{C_{1/2} + c_{ecm}} \right) u_{fib} \left(1 - \frac{u_{fib}}{K} \right) - \frac{p_{cell}(\theta)}{\tau_d + p_{cell}(\theta)} \frac{k_1 c_{ecm}}{C_k + c_{ecm}} u_{fib} + k_2 u_{myo} - d_{fib} u_{fib}, \quad (19)$$

the third term on the left hand side denotes the active mobility due to random walk and the first term on the right hand side represents fibroblast proliferation. To incorporate the effects of the oxygen level on these two processes we replace these terms with the following,

$$\frac{u_{oxy}}{\tau_{oxy} + u_{oxy}} \left(-D_{fib} \nabla u_{fib} + \frac{a_{fib}}{(b_{fib} + c_{ecm})^2} u_{fib} \nabla c_{ecm} \right)$$

for the mobility and

$$\frac{u_{oxy}}{\tau_{oxy} + u_{oxy}} \left(\lambda_{fib} + \frac{\lambda^0_{fib} c_{ecm}}{C_{1/2} + c_{ecm}} \right) u_{fib} \left(1 - \frac{u_{fib}}{K} \right)$$

for the proliferation of fibroblasts. The extra term in front, $\frac{u_{oxy}}{\tau_{oxy} + u_{oxy}}$, assures that if there is no oxygen present, i.e. no energy can be consumed, the two processes are stopped. When the tissue is saturated with oxygen the processes continue at their normal rate (the term then approaches one). Note that due to the PDE for the oxygen concentration the oxygen level will never rise to dangerous levels (the concentration moves towards an equilibrium), i.e. oxygen poisoning will never take place.

The proliferation of myofibroblasts also consumes energy and thus the same dependency on the oxygen concentration can be found in the PDE for the myofibroblasts. This concludes the influence of the oxygen level on wound contraction covered in this model.

The other way around wound contraction also effects the growth of new capillaries. First the displacement of the ECM causes passive convection of the variables of the angiogenesis model. This means that in each of the four equations an extra term is found that describes this passive convection, i.e.

$$\nabla \cdot \left(\frac{\partial \mathbf{u}}{\partial t} u_i \right),$$

where u_i denote the four variables of the novel angiogenesis model.

Furthermore the new capillaries need tissue to grow in. At first all tissue in the wound has been destroyed by the injury and so the capillaries can not grow. Gradually fibroblasts invade the wound and new tissue is formed. Only then can the recovery of the capillary network start. This is why it is reasonable to let the growth of capillaries depend on the fibroblast concentration.

The growth terms in (17) and (18) are given by

$$\lambda^0_2 \frac{c_{md}}{c_{md} + \tau_{tip}} u_{tip}$$

and
$$\lambda_6^0 \frac{c_{md}}{c_{md} + \tau_{end}} \left(a u_{end}(u_{end}^0 - u_{end}) + \chi u_{tip} u_{end}(u_{end}^1 - u_{end}) \right)$$
respectively. Similarly to how the oxygen concentration is coupled with the fibroblast PDE we couple the fibroblasts to the capillary tip and endothelial cell density PDEs. Therefor we introduce the factor
$$\frac{u_{fib}/u_{fib}^0}{\tau_{fib} + u_{fib}/u_{fib}^0}$$
in front of both production terms. This results in no capillary growth if there are no fibroblasts present, i.e. there is no appropriate dermal tissue for them to grow in. As the fibroblast concentration rises the rate of capillary growth also rises towards its normal rate, since the term approaches one.

This concludes the coupling between the wound contraction model due to Javierre and the novel angiogenesis model covered in this thesis. Of course there are several other interaction between them. One can for instance think about the differentation from fibroblasts to myofibroblasts and back, which surely also consumes energy. Alternatively, we could think of also linking the chemotaxis term to the oxygen content. This could be a subject for further study.

Next we present some results of the computation done on the coupled model. The values of the parameters used can be found in appendix. We vary the diffusion speeds of the fibroblasts and the oxygen, since we consider these to be of great importance (the problem seems to be diffusion dominated) and we would like to study the effect of these parameters on the solution.

In Figures 11 to 13 the results of the simulations can be found. The figures show the normalized solutions in time furthest in the wound, i.e. at $x = 0$. The difference in diffusion speeds can clearly be seen in the graphs.

We see that with slow fibroblast diffusion the growth of capillaries start off at a later point in time. This is to be expected since the fibroblasts provide the tissue in which the capillaries can grow. The growth of the capillaries does follow a similar course. First the capillary tips find their way to the center of the wound and after that the capillary network is restored, which decreases the number of tips. As the number of tips decreases down to zero, the oxygen content decreases for a short while due to the lack of this tip-source. Later, the oxygen tension increases to its undamaged equilibrium.

Further, having slower oxygen diffusion, the oxygen concentration depends more on the growth of new capillaries. In Figure 13 we see that the oxygen concentration rises far slower than 11 and 12. The oxygen concentration grows due to capillaries transporting oxygen to the wound side and not primarily due to diffusion.

We see that the varying the diffusion speeds has a major effect on the solutions. This confirms our idea that the problem is diffusion dominated. Although the solutions follow similar patterns in all cases, the differences can also be seen clearly.

Furthermore the coupling between the two models can also be seen. Especially with low diffusion speeds we see that the fibroblast concentration clearly depends on the oxygen concentration. Also the growth of new capillaries starts off later than in the uncoupled model, see Section 2.2. This can also be explained by the coupling, since the growth of capillaries now

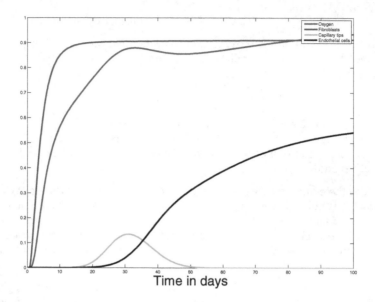

Fig. 11. Normalized solutions furthest in the wound, at $x = 0$, in time for $D_{fib} = 0.02$ cm^2/days and $D_{oxy} = 0.01$ cm^2/days.

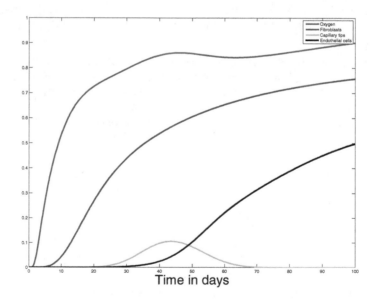

Fig. 12. Normalized solutions furthest in the wound, at $x = 0$, in time for $D_{fib} = 0.002$ cm^2/days and $D_{oxy} = 0.01$ cm^2/days.

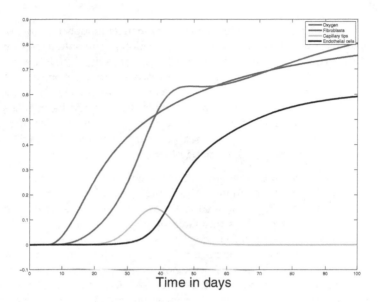

Time in days

Fig. 13. Normalized solutions furthest in the wound, at $x = 0$, in time for $D_{fib} = 0.002$ cm^2/days and $D_{oxy} = 0.001$ cm^2/days.

depends on the fibroblast concentration. So the growth can not begin untill there is enough tissue available, i.e. the fibroblast concentration is non-zero.

4. Numerical methods

We use a Galerkin finite-element method with linear triangular elements to solve the resulting system of PDEs. The reaction-transport equations are solved using a second-order Trapezoidal Time Numerical Integration Method. The nonlinear problem at each time step is solved using a Newton's method, which gives quadratic convergence. For the numerical integration of the spatial integrals in the weak formulation, we use the second order accurate Newton-Cotes integration rule. The numerical solution will thereby have a quadratic accuracy in both element size and time step. For an efficient implementation, the reactive-transport equations are solved as a fully coupled problem in which the degrees of freedom are numbered in a nodewise fashion. The mechanical parameters were taken at the current time step, since at each time-step the mechanical problem is solved before the biological reactive-transport equations are solved numerically.

The visco-elastic equations are solved using a Galerkin finite-element method with linear triangular elements. The system is solved as a fully coupled problem with a nodewise arrangement of the degrees of freedom, being the vertical and horizontal displacement. The concentrations and cellular densities from the previous time step are used in the mechanical balance equations from visco-elasticity. For the time-integration, a Trapezoidal Numerical Integration Method is used as well to have second order accuracy in time as well. The linear elements give a second-order accuracy for the element size.

5. Discussion

In this paper, we described and coupled some mathematical models for wound contraction and angiogenesis as subprocesses for dermal regeneration post-wounding. It can be seen in Figure 10 that in the course of healing, the endothelial cell density, which is the most important measure for the vascular network density, first increases up to value above the equilibrium value, which corresponds to the fully healed state. This increase coincides with the temporary high capillary tip density at these times. After this intermediate stage, the capillary tip density decreases down to zero, and the endothelial cell density decreases to the equilibrium as time proceeds. This qualitatively agrees with the rabbit ear chamber images from the experiments that were carried out by Komori (2005), among others.

Furthermore, the numerical solutions converge to the undamaged state at the longest scales. This is consistent with clinical situations if the initial wound is very small. However, scar formation due to an excessive regeneration of collagen is not taken into account in the present model. Hence, the present model is incapable of predicting the occurrance of ulcers or hypertrophic scars that can result for large wounds or burns. This issue will be dealt with in future, as well as the extension of the present model by the incorporation of the epidermal layer which starts healing as a result of triggering of keratinocytes by the signaling agents that are secreted by the fibroblasts in the dermis. We are also interested in the development of the basal membrane, which separates the dermis from epidermis, in the course of time.

We also note that the model is entirely based on the continuum hypothesis, and that all densities and concentrations should be considered as averaged quantities over a *representative volume element*. At the smaller scale, one has to use a more cellular approach, such as the cellular automata (cellular Potts) models or (semi-) stochastic approaches. A translation between these classes of models is highly desirable and hardly found in literature.

Finally, we note that modeling of wound healing is very complicated, due to the enormous complexity of the healing process. The present model can already help in obtaining insight into the relation between several parameters, such as the influence of various parameters on the speed and quality of wound healing. In future studies, we intend to include the effects of several treatment of wounds, such as pressure or drug treatments, on the kinetics of wound healing. The models can then be used as a tool for medical doctors to evaluate the influence of certain treatments on wound healing, as well as to determine the circumstances for optimal healing with respect to minimization of hypertrophic scars in the case of burns. Here, we also remark that all data are patient-dependent and hence all parameters in the model are exposed to a stochastic nature. In order to deal with the issues of uncertainties, we intend to employ stochastic finite element methods in near future.

6. Conclusions

We presented an advanced model for the coupling of angiogenesis and wound contraction. The model gives a more complete picture than most of the presently existing formalisms in literature. However, still some room for improvement remains. The current model could also be extended with the healing of the epidermis located on top of the dermis. This will be done in a future study.

The first important innovations in the present study are the formulation of a new angiogenesis model, which consists of a driving force due to lack of oxygen (Maggelakis) and a balance of both the capillary tips and capillaries by tracking these quantities as individual parameters. The second important innovation concerns the combination of the wound contraction model due to Javierre (2009) with the newly developed angiogenesis model. As an important factor of communication between both processes, we use the oxygen tension (on fibroblast mobility and proliferation), the presence of macrophage derived growth factor influencing the logistic proliferation rate of endothelial cells and the fibroblast density on the production of endothelial cells. Of course, these coupling terms have been assumed from educated guesses. An experimental validation could be decisive on the validity of the assumptions used in the present model. The calculations in the present manuscript are preliminary and a parameter sensitivity analysis is to be carried out.

We also note that there is a large uncertainty for the values of all the parameters used. We intend to use stochastic methods to better deal with the occurrance of patient dependencies and other uncertainties in the data. This will be tackled in future studies. The present paper was more descriptive, rather than mathematical.

7. Appendix: Parameter values

In this Appendix, we show the data that we used for the calculations. The first two tables show the parameter values for the skin regeneration models ((myo)fibroblasts and collagen). The third table gives the data of the visco-elastic model for wound contraction. The fourth table gives the input for the angiogenesis model. Further, the values of the coupling parameters are scattered throughout the tables as well.

Parameter	Description	Value	Dimension
u_{fib}^0	Fibroblast density in healthy tissue	10^4	cells/cm^3
D_{fib}^0	Fibroblast diffusion rate	$2 \times 10^{-2}/2 \times 10^{-3}$	cm^2/day
a_{fib}	Determines, with b_{fib}, the maximal chemotaxis rate per unit GF conc.	4×10^{-10}	g/cm day
b_{fib}	GF conc. that produces 25% of the maximal chemotactic response	2×10^{-9}	g/cm^3
λ_{fib}	Fibroblast proliferation rate	0.832	day^{-1}
λ_{fib}^0	Maximal GF induced proliferation rate	0.3	day^{-1}
K	Determines the fibroblast equilibrium density	1×10^7	cells/cm^3
$C_{1/2}$	Half-maximal GF enhancement of fibroblasts proliferation	1×10^{-8}	g/cm^3
k_1	Maximal fibroblast to myofibroblast differentation rate	0.8	day^{-1}
k_2	Myofibroblast to fibroblast differentation rate	0.693	day^{-1}
C_k	Half-maximal GF enhancement of fibroblast to myofibroblast differentiation	10^{-8}	g/cm^3
d_{fib}	Fibroblast death rate	0.831	day^{-1}
ε_{myo}	Myofibroblast to fibroblast logistic growth rate proportionality factor	0.5	-
d_{myo}	Myofibroblasts death rate	2.1×10^{-2}	day^{-1}
τ_{oxy}	Determines oxygen enhancement of (myo)fibroblasts proliferation	2×10^{-4}	

Table 1. Parameters related to the fibroblast and myofibroblast equations.

Parameter	Description	Value	Dimension
ρ^0	Collagen concentration in healthy tissue	0.1	g/cm^3
ρ_{ini}	Initial collagen concentration in the wound	10^{-3}	g/cm^3
λ_ρ	Collagen production rate	7.59×10^{-10}	g^3/cm^6 cell day
λ_ρ^0	Maximal rate of GF induced collagen production	7.59×10^{-9}	g^3/cm^6 cell day
C_ρ	Half-maximal GF enhancement of collagen production	10^{-8}	g/cm^3
R_ρ	Half-maximal collagen enhancement of ECM deposition	0.3	g/cm^3
η_b	Myofibroblast to fibroblast collagen production rate proportionality factor	2	-
d_ρ	Collagen degradation rate per unit of cell density	7.59×10^{-8}	cm^3/cell day
η_d	Myofibroblast to fibroblast collagen degradation rate proportionality factor	2	-
c_{ecm}^0	Initial GF concentration in the wound	10^{-8}	g/cm^3
D_c	GF diffusion rate	5×10^{-2}	cm^2/day
k_c	GF production rate per unit of cell density	7.5×10^{-6}	cm^3/cell day
ζ	Myofibroblast to fibroblast chemical production rate proportionality factor	1	-
Γ	Half-maximal enhancement of net GF production	$\times 10^{-8}$	g/cm^3
d_c	GF decay rate	0.693	day^{-1}

Table 2. Parameters related to the collagen and growth factor equations.

Parameter	Description	Value	Dimension
p_{max}	Maximal cellular active stress per unit of ECM	10^{-4}	N g/cm2 cell
K_{pas}	Volumetric stiffness moduli of the passive components of the cell	2×10^{-5}	N g/cm2 cell
K_{act}	Volumetric stiffness moduli of the active filaments of the cell	1.852×10^{-5}	N g/cm2 cell
θ_1	Shortening strain of the contractile element	-0.6	-
θ_2	Lengthening strain of the contractile element	0.5	-
τ_d	Half-maximal mechanical enhancement fo fibroblast to myofibroblast differentation	10^{-5}	N g/cm2 cell
μ_1	Undamaged skin shear viscosity	200	N day/cm2
μ_2	Undamaged skin bluk viscosity	200	N day/cm2
E	Undamaged skin Young's modulus	33.4	N/cm2
ν	Undamaged skin Poisson's ratio	0.3	-
ξ	Myofibroblasts enhancement of traction per unit of fibroblasts density	10^{-3}	cm^3/cell
R_τ	Traction inhibition collagen density	5×10^{-4}	g/cm^3
s	Dermis tethering factor	5×10^2	N/cm g

Table 3. Parameters related to the mechanical behaviour of cells and the ECM.

Parameter	Description	Value	Dimension
u_{oxy}^0	Oxygen concentration in healthy tissue	5	mg/cm^3
D_{oxy}	Oxygen diffusion rate	$10^{-2}/10^{-3}$	day^{-1}
λ_{oxy}	Oxygen decay rate	2×10^{-2}	day^{-1}
λ_{13}	Oxygen transport rate	1	day^{-1}
u_θ	Threshold value for macrophage derived GF	5	mg/cm^3
D_{md}	Macrophage derived GF diffusion rate	0.1	day^{-1}
λ_{md}	Macrophage derived GF decay rate	1	day^{-1}
λ_{21}	Macrophage derived GF production rate	10	day^{-1}
u_{tip}^0	Normalized initial capillary tip concentration in the small strip facing the wound	1	-
D_1	Capillary tip diffusion rate	3.5×10^{-4}	cm^2/day
u_{end}^0	Normalized endothelial cell density in healthy tissue	1	-
D_2	Endothelial cell diffusion rate	3.5×10^{-4}	cm^2/day
λ_2^0	Capillary tip growth rate	0.83	day^{-1}
τ_{tip}	Half-maximal macropahge derived GF enhancement of capillary tip growth	1	-
λ_3	Rate at which two capillary tips meet	0.83	day^{-1}
λ_4	Rate at which a capillary tip meets another capillary	0.85	day^{-1}
λ_6^0	Endothelial cell proliferation rate	1	day^{-1}
τ_{end}	Half-maximal macropahge derived GF enhancement of endothelial cell proliferation	1	-
a	Determines, with χ and u_{end}^1, the equilibrium endothelial cell density	0.25	-
χ	Determines, with a and u_{end}^1, the equilibrium endothelial cell density	0.3	-
u_{end}^1	Determines, with a and χ, the equilibrium endothelial cell density	10	-
λ_5	Capillary tip to capillary proportionality factor	0.25	-
τ_{fib}	Half-maximal fibroblast enhancement of capillary growth and endothelial cell proliferation	1	-

Table 4. Parameters related to angiogenesis.

8. References

Bloemen, M.C.T., van der Veer, W.M. Ulrich, M.M.W., van Zuijlen, F.B., Niessen, F.B., Middelkoop, E.: *Prevention and curative management of hypertrophic scar formation*, to appear in Burns, 2011.

van der Veer, W.M., Bloemen, M.C.T., Ulrich, M.M.W., Molema, G., van Zuijlen, P.P.M., Middelkoop, E., Niessen, F.B.: *Potential cellular and molecular causes of hypertrophic scar formation*, Burns, 35, 15–29, 2009.

Dallon, J.C., Ehrlich, H.P.: *A review of fibroblast populated collagen lattices* Wound repair and regeneration, 16, 472–479, 2008.

Dallon, J.C.: *Multiscale modeling of cellular systems in biology*, Current opinion in colloid and interface science, 15, 24–31, 2010.

urray, J.D.: *Mathematical Biology II: Spatial Models and Biomedical Applications*, New York: Springer-Verlag; 2004.

Olsen, L., Sherratt, J.A. and Maini, P.K.: *A mechanochemical model for adult dermal wound closure and the permanence of contracted tissue displacement*, Journal of Theoretical Biology 1995; 177:113-128.

Maggelakis, A.: *A mathematical model for tissue replacement during epidermal wound healing*, Applied Mathematical Modelling 2003; 27:189-196.

Gaffney, E.A., Pugh, K. and Maini, P.K.: *Investigating a simple model for cutaneous wound healing angiogenesis*, Journal of Theoretical Biology 2002; 45:337-374.

Sherratt, J.A. and Murray, J.D.: *Mathematical analysis of a basic model for epidermal wound healing*, Journal of Theoretical Biology 1991; 29:389-404.

Adam, J.A.: *A simplified model of wound healing (with particular reference to the critical size defect)*, Mathematical and Computer Modelling 1999; 30:23-32.

Javierre, E., Moreo, P., Doblaré, M. and García-Aznar, J.M.: *Numerical modeling of a mechano-chemical theory for wound contraction analysis*, International Journal of Solids and Structures 2009; 46:3597-3606.

Vermolen, F.J. and Javierre, E.: *A suite of continuum models for different aspects in wound healing*, In: Bioengineering research of chronic wounds, studies in mechanobiology, tissue engineering and biomaterials, New York: Springer-Verlag; 2009.

Vermolen, F.J. and Javierre, E.: *Computer simulations from a finite-element model for wound contraction and closure*, Journal of Tissue Viability 2010; 19:43-53.

Vermolen, F.J. and Javierre, E.: *A finite-element model for healing of cutaneous wounds combining contraction, angiogenesis and closure*, submitted, 2011.

Schugart, R.C., riedman, A., Zhao, R., Sen, C.K.: *Wound angiogenesis as a function of tissue oxygen tension: a mathematical model*, Proceedings of the National Academy of Sciences USA, 105(7), 2628–2633, 2008.

Xue, C., Friedman, A., Sen, C.K.: *A mathematical model of ischemic cutaneous wounds*, Proceedings of the National Academy of Sciences USA, 106(39), 16783–16787, 2009.

Graner, F., Glazier, J.: *Simulation of biological cell sorting using a two-dimensional extended Potts model*, Phys. Review Letters, 69, 2013–2016, 1992.

Merks, M.H., Koolwijk, P.: *Modeling morphogenesis in silico and in vitro: towards quantitative, predictive, cell-based modeling*, Mathematical modeling of natural phenomena, 4(4), 149–171, 2009.

Plank, M.J. and Sleeman, B.D.: *Lattice and non-lattice models of tumour angiogenesis*, Bull. Mathem. Biol., 66 (2004), 1785–1819.

Vermolen, F.J. and Gefen, A.: *A semi-stochastic cell-based formalism to model the dynamics of migration of cells in colonies*, to appear, 2011.

Kumar, V., Abbas A. and Fausto, N.: *Robbins and Cotran Pathologic Basis of Disease*, Philadelphia: Elsevier Saunders; 2005.

Komori, M., Tomizawa, Y., Takada, K. and Ozaki, M.: *A single local application of recombinant human basic fibroblast growth factor accelerates initial angiogenesis during wound healing in rabbit ear chamber*, Anesth Analg, 100 (2005), 830–834.

9

Non-Invasive Evaluation Method for Cartilage Tissue Regeneration Using Quantitative-MRI

Shogo Miyata
KEIO University
Japan

1. Introduction

Articular cartilage is an avascular tissue covering articulating surfaces of bones and it functions to bear loads and reduce friction in diarthrodial joints. The cartilage can be regarded as a porous gel, mainly composed of large proteoglycan (PG) aggregates having a negative fixed-charge density (nFCD), a water-swollen network of collagen fibrils, and interstitial water, all of which play important roles in load-bearing properties (Lee et al., 1981; Mow et al., 1980).

Although articular cartilage may function well over a lifetime, traumatic injury or the degenerative changes associated with osteoarthritis (OA) can significantly erode the articular layer, leading to joint pain and instability. Because of its avascular nature, articular cartilage has a very limited capacity to regenerate and repair. It is well-known that the natural response of articular cartilage to damage is variable and, at best, unsatisfactory.

Therefore, numerous studies have reported tissue-engineering approaches to restore degenerated cartilage and to repair defects; these approaches involve culturing autologous chondrocytes *in vitro* to create three-dimensional tissue that is subsequently implanted. In these tissue engineering approaches, it is important to assess the biomechanical and biochemical properties of the engineered cartilage. These material properties of the engineered constructs are detectable only via direct measurements that are invasive and require destructive treatments such as histological analysis, biochemical quantification, and mechanical testing. The application and utilization of these tissue-engineering approaches in a clinical setting requires a non-invasive method of evaluating biomechanical and biochemical properties of the actual regenerated cartilage for transplantation. Moreover, the method should be applicable to various aspects of cartilage regenerative medicine, including the characterization of the regenerated tissue during *in vitro* culture and *in vivo* evaluation after transplantation.

Magnetic resonance imaging (MRI) of articular cartilage is well accepted and has become common in recent years. Quantitative MRI techniques have been successfully developed to measure the macromolecular state within cartilage tissue. For example, the relationship between the water content of the degenerated cartilage and water self-diffusion has been reported (Shapiro et al., 2001), while the transverse relaxation time T2 has been related to collagen concentration (Fragonas et al., 1998) and the spatial distribution of collagen, including both fibril orientation and organization (Nieminen et al., 2001; Xia et al., 2002).

The gadolinium-diethylene triamine pentaacetic acid (Gd-DTPA^{2-})-enhanced T1 imaging technique has been used to predict PG content (Bashir et al., 1996) and spatial distribution (Bashir et al., 1999). Furthermore, nFCD can be estimated from consecutive T1 relaxation time measurements using Gd-DTPA^{2-}-enhanced MRI and related to PG concentration. This MRI technique is already well-known as the "delayed Gadolinium Enhanced Magnetic Resonance Imaging of Cartilage" (dGEMRIC) technique. This technique is based on the utilization of the two-negative charge of the MRI contrast agent (i.e., Gd-DTPA^{2-}). Sulfated glycosaminoglycans (sGAG) in the PGs are negatively charged in the cartilage, giving rise to nFCD; the electric exclusion force between this nFCD and the negatively charged contrast agent result in the inverse distribution of the contrast agent to the PG distribution in the cartilage. Consequently, relaxation time (T1) and nFCD—as determined by dGEMRIC technique — correlate with PG concentration.

Previous studies have reported that, in tissue-engineered cartilage, MR measurements of regenerated cartilage showed correlations with biochemical properties (Potter et al., 2000) and biomechanical properties (Chen et al., 2003). Additionally, the sGAG content and the compressive modulus—the latter of which was determined by unconfined compression tests—showed a trend toward correlation with the nFCD, as determined by the Gd-DTPA^{2-}-enhanced MRI technique (Chen et al., 2003; Ramaswamy et al., 2008). In our earlier study, we reported that the nFCD of tissue-engineered cartilage determined by GD-DTPA^{2-}-enhanced MRI has been found to correlate with sGAG content (Miyata et al., 2006).

Although the non-invasive assessment of tissue integration and the non-destructive evaluation of molecular structure of the engineered cartilage are important, we believe no previous study has fully evaluated the relationships between the biomechanical properties and MRI measurements of regenerated cartilage consisting of articular chondrocytes. Previous study has indicated that MR images of autologous chondrocyte transplants may show clinically significant variations; neither biochemical properties nor the FCD of regenerated articular cartilage has been evaluated.

In this chapter, we introduce our evaluation technique for tissue-engineered cartilage using quantitative-MRI. We tested the hypothesis that MRI measurements of tissue-engineered cartilage correlate with biomechanical and biochemical properties and that these novel approaches can be used to evaluate cartilaginous matrix material properties during tissue regeneration.

2. Quantitative Magnetic Resonance Imaging (MRI) of tissue engineered cartilage

2.1 Isolation of chondrocytes and preparation of chondrocyte-seeded agarose constructs

We used agarose gel culture for tissue-engineered cartilage model, because agarose is a biocompatible, thermosensitive hydrogel that offers superior homogeneity and stability for assessing both biomechanical and biochemical properties during *in vitro* culture, and has been used widely in cartilage mechanobiology. Chondrocyte-seeded agarose gels were prepared as described previously (Miyata et al., 2006; Miyata et al., 2004).

Articular chondrocytes were obtained from the glenohumeral joints of freshly slaughtered 4- to 6-week-old calves, from a local abattoir. Articular cartilage was excised from the humeral head, diced into ~1 mm³ pieces, then shaken gently in Dulbecco's Modified Eagle's Medium/Ham's F12 (DMEM/F12) supplemented with 5% fetal bovine serum (FBS), 0.2% collagenase type II, and antibiotics-antimycotics, for 8–10 h at 37°C. Cells were then isolated from the digest by centrifugation and rinsed twice with phosphate buffered saline (PBS). Finally, after the isolated cells were resuspended with feed medium (DMEM/F12 supplemented with 20% FBS, 50 µg/mL L-ascorbic acid, and antibiotics-antimycotics), and the total number of cells was counted with a hemocytometer.

The isolated chondrocytes in the feed medium were mixed with an equal volume of PBS containing agarose with a low melting temperature (Agarose type VII, Sigma, MO) at 37°C, to prepare 1.5×10^7 cells/mL in 2% (wt/vol) agarose gel; it was then cast in a custom-made mold to make a large gel plate. After gelling at 4°C for 25 minutes, approximately 50 disks of 8-mm diameter, 1.5-mm thickness were cored out from the large gel plate with a biopsy punch. The chondrocyte-seeded agarose disks were fed 2.5 mL feed medium/disk, every other day and maintained in a 5% CO_2 atmosphere at 37°C.

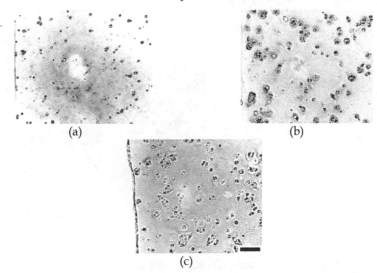

(a)   (b)

(c)

Fig. 1. Histological appearance of tissue-engineered cartilage at day 3 (a), day 10 (b), and day 28 (c), stained with alcian blue (Miyata et al., 2010). Scale bar = 100 µm.

Alcian blue-stained sections of the cultured specimens are shown in Fig. 1. Over the culture period, the chondrocytes in the agarose gel appeared rounded in shape, similar to those in the "native" articular cartilage. As shown in Fig. 1, the chondrocytes synthesized a thin shell of pericellular matrix (~day 10) and expanded the volume of the cartilaginous matrix (~day 28).

2.2 Magnetic Resonance Imaging (MRI) of cultured chondrocyte-seeded agarose gel

Quantitative MRI evaluations were performed on a 2.0-T Biospec 20/30 System with a B-GA20 Gradient System (Bruker, Karlsruhe, Germany) with a maximum gradient strength of 100 mT/m. The MRI data acquisition and reconstruction were performed using the ParaVision (Bruker) software system. In all MRI experiments, three or four sheets of the disks were stacked in layers and placed into glass tubes containing phosphate buffered saline (PBS) (Fig. 2). The measured parameters included longitudinal (T1) and transverse (T2) relaxation time and water self-diffusion coefficient (Diff). A longitudinal relaxation time map (T1-map) was obtained with a short echo time (TE: 15 ms) spin-echo sequence with different repetition time values (TR: 100 ms to 15 s, 16 steps). A transverse relaxation time map (T2-map) was obtained with a long repetition time value (TR: 15 s) spin-echo sequence with different echo time values (TE: 30 ms to 450 ms, 29 steps). A diffusion coefficient map (Diff-map) was calculated from the images obtained using a conventional diffusion weighted spin-echo (SE-DWI, TR: 15 s, TE: 35 ms) sequence with different b values (0, 74, 275, 603, 1059 s/mm^2). All sequences were performed with a field of view (FOV) of 50 × 50 mm^2, matrix size 64 × 64, and slice thickness 3 mm. The values of the relaxation time (T1 and T2) and the relative diffusion coefficient (Diff*) were calculated as the average of the specimen from the obtained T1-, T2-, and Diff-maps. The value of Diff* (= $Diff_S/Diff_P$) was calculated by normalizing the diffusion coefficient of the sample ($Diff_S$) by the diffusion coefficient of PBS ($Diff_P$) around the sample. All MRI measurements were carried out with no contrast agent at room temperature (23°C).

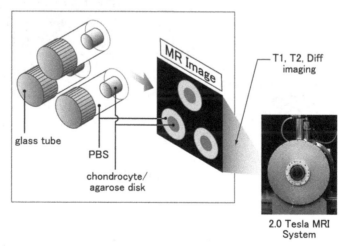

Fig. 2. Schematic diagram of MR Imaging (Miyata et al., 2007).

Figure 3–5 shows the MRI maps of the engineered cartilage. At the first stage of the culture (day 1), T1 and Diff of the engineered cartilage showed values similar to those of the PBS around the cartilage; hence, it was difficult to distinguish the boundaries between the engineered cartilage and the bath solution (PBS) in the MRI maps (Fig. 3a and 5a). By the end of the culture (day 28), the boundaries were distinguished in both T1- and Diff-maps (Fig. 3a–3c and 5a–5c). In contrast, the boundary between the specimen and the PBS remained clear in the T2-map during the culture time (Fig. 4a–4c). The T1, T2, and Diff values of the engineered cartilage were averaged, and the results are summarized in Figure 6. T1 and Diff* of the tissue-engineered cartilage had decreased with an increase in the culture time (Fig. 6a and 6c). On the other hand, T2 of the engineered cartilage showed considerably lower values than those of the PBS in the glass tube throughout the culture time, and these values tended to increase slightly with the culture time (Fig. 6b).

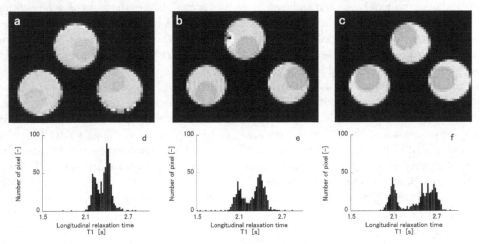

Fig. 3. T1-maps of day 1 (a), day 7 (b), and day 28 (c) post-inoculation specimens, and histograms of the T1 values derived from the MR images on day 1 (d), day 7 (e), and day 28 (f) (Miyata et al., 2007).

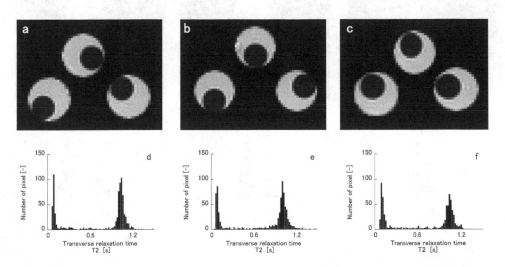

Fig. 4. T2-maps of day 1 (a), day 7 (b), and day 28 (c) post-inoculation specimens, and histograms of the T2 values derived from the MR images on day 1 (d), day 7 (e), and day 28 (f) (Miyata et al., 2007).

Consistent with the results of previous studies (Chen et al., 2003; Potter et al., 1998), our results showed that both T1 and Diff* decreased with an increase in the culture time. On the other hand, T2 tended to increase slightly by the end of the culture time. To understand the MRI properties of the tissue water protons, we have to understand the behavior of water molecules in the tissue at different stages of tissue maturity. With tissue growth and development, proteoglycan and collagen molecules accumulate in the agarose gel, resulting in a large fraction of macromolecule-associated water, which is known as "bound" water. Generally, the water molecules in the "bound" condition show short T1 and T2 relaxation times due to a reduced mobility as compared to "free" water. Thus, water proton relaxation curves, which were described by a single exponential, are derived from the weighted sum of the relaxation behavior of the "free" and "bound" water molecules in the engineered cartilage. This is consistent with our results that the T1 relaxation time and Diff* decreased with an increase in the content of cartilaginous matrix in the agarose gel. In the case of transverse relaxation, the T2 relaxation time of the engineered cartilage showed a value similar to that of the "native" articular cartilage (75–90 ms measured by our MRI system) from the early phase of the culture; further, T2 tended to increase slightly with tissue maturation. Based on this result, we speculate that the transverse relaxation of the water molecules in the engineered construct might be mainly affected by its association with the agarose molecules.

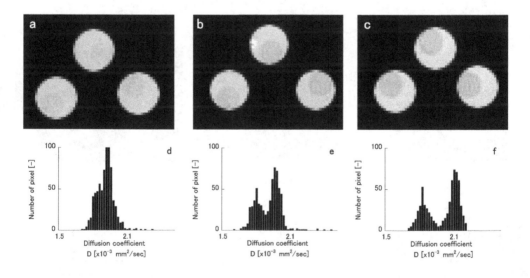

Fig. 5. Diff-maps of day 1 (a), day 7 (b), and day 28 (c) post-inoculation specimens, and histograms of the Diff values derived from the MR images on day 1 (d), day 7 (e), and day 28 (f) (Miyata et al., 2007).

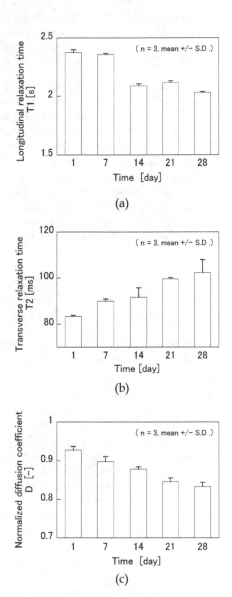

Fig. 6. Longitudinal relaxation time (a), transverse relaxation time (b), and relative diffusion coefficient (c) of the tissue-engineered cartilage during the culture time (Miyata et al., 2007). The values represent mean +/- S.D. (n = 3).

2.3 Evaluation of fixed charge density of tissue-engineered cartilage

For 'native' articular cartilage, the gadolinium-diethylene triamine pentaacetic acid (Gd-DTPA^{2-}) -enhanced T1 imaging technique has been used to predict the PG content (Bashir et al., 1996) and spatial distribution (Bashir et al., 1999). Furthermore, the negative fixed charge density (nFCD) can be estimated from consecutive T1 relaxation time measurement using Gd-DTPA^{2-}-enhanced MRI and be related to the PG concentration. In this study, we used this dGEMRIC technique to monitor and evaluate tissue integration of the engineered cartilage.

The MRI measurements were performed with a 2.0-Tesla Bruker Biospec 20/30 system using Gd-DTPA^{2-} contrast agent. In all MRI measurements, the specimens were put into glass tubes filled with PBS (Fig. 7). The longitudinal relaxation time map, T1-map, was obtained with a short-echo time (TE: 15 ms), spin-echo sequence with different repetition time values (TR: 100 ms to 15 s, 16 steps). Subsequently, the specimens were balanced in PBS containing 1 mM Gd-DTPA^{2-} (Magnevist®, Nihon Schering, Osaka, Japan) for 10–12 hours; the longitudinal relaxation time map in the contrast agent, T1$_{Gd}$-map, was obtained again with a short-echo time (TE: 15 ms), spin-echo sequence with different repetition time values (TR: 30 ms to 5 s, 13 steps). Finally, using the relaxivity (R) value of Gd-DTPA^{2-} in saline (5.24 in our MRI system), the concentration of the contrast agent was estimated using the formula [Gd-DTPA^{2-}] = $1/R(1/T1_{Gd} - 1/T1)$. The negative fixed charge density (FCD) was calculated as follows

$$nFCD = \frac{[Na^+]_b\sqrt{[Gd-DTPA^{2-}]_t}}{\sqrt{[Gd-DTPA^{2-}]_b}} - \frac{[Na^+]_b\sqrt{[Gd-DTPA^{2-}]_b}}{\sqrt{[Gd-DTPA^{2-}]_t}} \qquad (1)$$

where subscript b stands for bath solution and subscript t stands for cartilaginous tissue(Bashir et al., 1996). All MRI measurements were performed at room temperature 23°C.

In the gadolinium-enhanced MR imaging measurements, longitudinal relaxation time of the bulk PBS containing Gd-DTPA reagent showed 0.179 ± 0.06 seconds in our MRI system. The T1$_{Gd}$ of the cultured specimen increased as a function of tissue maturation (0.197 ± 0.001 to 0.222 ± 0.003 seconds). At the first stage of the culture (day 3), T1$_{Gd}$ of the tissue-engineered cartilage showed values proximate to those of the PBS containing the Gd-DTPA^{2-} agent around the engineered cartilage; hence, it was difficult to distinguish the boundaries between the engineered cartilage and the bath solution in the T1$_{Gd}$-maps (Fig. 8a). By the end of the culture (day 28), the boundaries had become distinct in the T1Gd-maps (Fig. 8). The [Gd-DTPA^{2-}] in the engineered cartilage decreased with increases in culture time. The nFCD, as determined from the [Gd-DTPA^{2-}] in the specimen and bath solution, increased with culture time (Fig. 9).

As time in culture lengthened, the gross appearance of the cultured disk became increasingly opaque. The DMMB assay (Farndale et al., 1986) revealed that the sGAG content of the chondrocyte/agarose disks increased as a function of tissue maturation (0.19 ± 0.27 to 13.2 ± 1.9 mg/mL-disk-vol). Finally, the sGAG content of the reconstructed cartilaginous disk reached approximately 20% of the "native" articular cartilage (data not shown).

To correlate gadolinium-enhanced MRI and biochemical properties, the sGAG content of the tissue was plotted as a function of the FCD. From the linear regression analysis, the FCD correlated significantly with the sGAG content (r = 0.95, n = 30, P < 0.001) (Fig. 10), and the tissue [Gd-DTPA^{2-}] correlated with the sGAG content by r = 0.83, n = 30, P < 0.001.

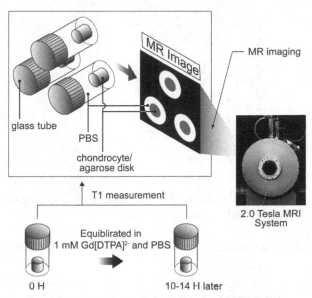

Fig. 7. Schematic diagram of gadolinium-enhanced MRI. In all MRI measurements, the cultured specimens were put into glass tubes filled with phosphate buffered saline (PBS) or 1 mM Gd DTPA^{2-} (Miyata et al., 2010).

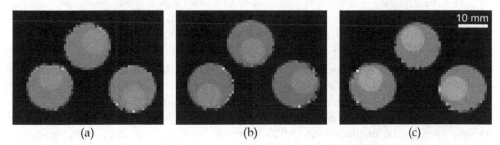

Fig. 8. Quantitative water proton T1 maps in the presence of Gd-DTPA2– at day 3 (a), day 7 (b), and day 28 (c) (Miyata et al., 2010).

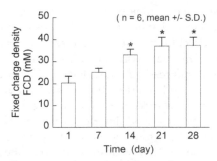

Fig. 9. Tissue fixed-charge density, with time in culture, for tissue-engineered cartilage (Miyata et al., 2010). * indicates significant difference from day 0 ($P < 0.05$).

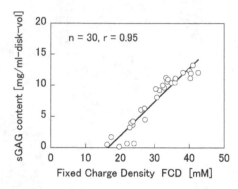

Fig. 10. Scatter plots relating the tissue fixed charge density (FCD) to the sulfated glycosaminoglycan (sGAG) content (Miyata et al., 2006).

2.4 Static and dynamic biomechanical testing of cultured agarose/chondrocyte constructs

Mechanical testing of the disk-shaped specimens was performed with unconfined compression, using impermeable stainless platens in PBS at room temperature. Static compressive properties were measured in a custom-made chamber attached to a material testing device (Autograph 5kNG, Shimadzu, Kyoto, Japan). Stress relaxation tests were performed by applying a ramp displacement at 0.05 mm/min to a 20% static compressive strain, followed by relaxation to equilibrium (2,400 s). The equilibrium compressive modulus (E_{eq}) was calculated from the imposed compressive strain and the equilibrium load, divided by the cross-sectional area of the specimen.

Dynamic compression tests were carried out using a viscoelastic spectrometer (DDV-MF, A&D, Tokyo, Japan) (Miyata et al., 2005). For preconditioning, a 20% static compressive strain was loaded and a sinusoidal displacement of 0.5% compressive strain was then superimposed at a frequency of 1 Hz. After equilibrium had been reached (approximately 20 min), a sinusoidal displacement of 0.5% compressive strain was applied at frequencies ranging from 0.01 to 5.0 Hz. The dynamic compressive modulus (E_{dyn}) was calculated from the ratio of the measured stress amplitude and the applied strain amplitude.

Figure 11 shows the means and standard deviations of the equilibrium compressive modulus E_{eq} and dynamic compressive modulus E_{dyn} versus time in culture, for the tissue-engineered cartilage. With respect to the static compressive property, significant differences were observed in the equilibrium compressive modulus. With increases in culture time, the E_{eq} of the specimens increased and reached approximately 10% of that of "native" cartilage from which the chondrocytes were harvested (0.45 ± 0.12 MPa, n =3). With respect to the dynamic compressive property, significant differences were also observed for testing conditions. The dynamic compressive modulus E_{dyn} of the engineered cartilage depended on both testing frequency and culture time. For each time point, E_{dyn} increased nonlinearly with increases in frequency. The engineered cartilage also exhibited marked stiffening with time in culture. The value of E_{dyn} increased with culture time at each testing frequency (0.01–2.0 Hz).

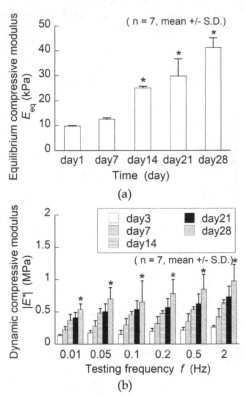

Fig. 11. Equilibrium compressive modulus E_{eq} (a) and dynamic compressive modulus E_{dyn} (b), with time in culture, for the cultured chondrocyte/agarose disks (Miyata et al., 2010). * indicates significant difference from day 0 (P < 0.05).

2.5 Relationships between MRI measurements and biomechanical properties of cultured chondrocyte-seeded constructs

To determine the correlations between the quantitative MRI measurements and the biomechanical and biochemical properties of the tissue-engineered cartilage, we performed linear regression analyses among the MRI-derived parameters (T1, T2, Diff, and FCD), the biochemical composition (sGAG content), and the biomechanical properties (E_{eq}, E_{dyn}) of the engineered cartilage.

To confirm the correlation, the E_{eq} of the engineered cartilage were plotted as functions of the T1, T2, and Diff, respectively. The E_{eq} of the engineered cartilage (Fig. 12a) showed a strong correlation with T1 and Diff but a weak correlation with T2 (Fig. 12b and 12c). Similarly, the tissue sGAG concentration (Fig. 13a and 13c) and were found to be strongly correlated with T1 and Diff. Consistent with the results of the previous investigation (Potter et al., 2000), our results showed that T1 relaxation time and Diff showed a significant correlation with the biomechanical properties and the sGAG content of the tissue-engineered cartilage. The results of recent studies have shown that the articular cartilage degeneration induced by collagenase treatment resulted in changes in T2 relaxation time and the equilibrium modulus (Nieminen et al., 2000). In the present study, slight increase in T2 values was observed during the culture.

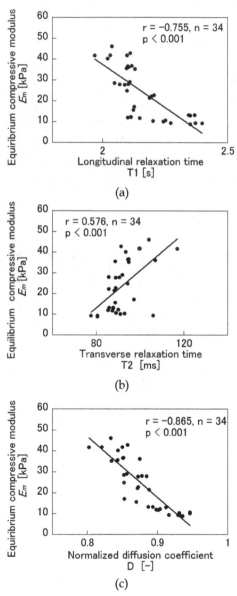

(a)

(b)

(c)

Fig. 12. Scatter plots for the relationship between the equilibrium compressive modulus E_{eq} and longitudinal relaxation time (a), transverse relaxation time (b), and relative diffusion coefficient (c) (Miyata et al., 2007). Solid line represents the linear regression line.

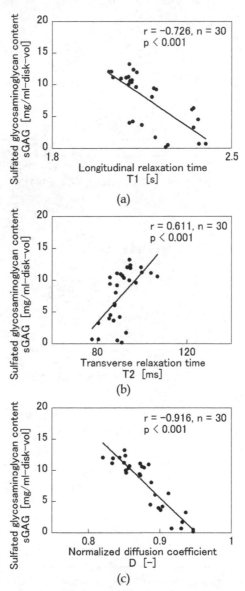

Fig. 13. Scatter plots for the relationship between the equilibrium compressive modulus E_{eq} and longitudinal relaxation time (a), transverse relaxation time (b), and relative diffusion coefficient (c) (Miyata et al., 2007). Solid line represents the linear regression line.

One possible explanation is that the changes in the biophysical properties might be mainly due to the altered sGAG content, and the synthesis of collagen and the reorganization of collagen network might be insufficient in the agarose gel culture.

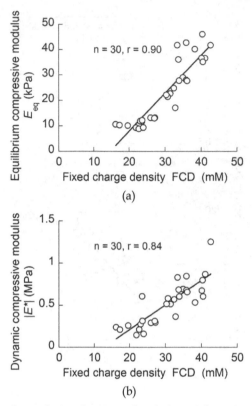

Fig. 14. Typical scatter plots relating the tissue fixed-charge density to equilibrium compressive modulus E_{eq} (a) and dynamic compressive modulus E_{dyn} at 0.5 Hz (b) (Miyata et al., 2010).

	R^2	P
FCD vs. E_{eq}	0.81	< 0.001
FCD vs. E_{dyn}, 0.01 Hz	0.79	< 0.001
FCD vs. E_{dyn}, 0.02 Hz	0.73	< 0.001
FCD vs. E_{dyn}, 0.05 Hz	0.73	< 0.001
FCD vs. E_{dyn}, 0.5 Hz	0.70	< 0.001
FCD vs. E_{dyn}, 2.0 Hz	0.71	< 0.001

Table 1. Linear Pearson correlations between biomechanical and Gd-DTPA^{2-}-enhanced MRI parameters in tissue-engineered cartilage (Miyata et al., 2010).

To evaluate the relationship between Gd-DTPA^{2-}-enhanced MRI parameters and biomechanical properties, the E_{eq} and E_{dyn} of the engineered cartilage were plotted as functions of the nFCD, respectively. From the linear Pearson correlation analysis, it was found that nFCD correlated significantly with E_{eq} and E_{dyn} (Table 1, Fig. 14). The equilibrium compressive modulus showed a higher correlation than the dynamic compressive modulus of all testing frequencies, and the dynamic compressive modulus tended to show a slightly higher correlation at low frequencies (0.01–0.05 Hz). The sGAG of articular cartilage plays a crucial role in static compressive behavior, while collagen bears a dynamic compressive load (Korhonen et al., 2003). Therefore, the nFCD—which is to say, the sGAG content—might show a higher correlation with the equilibrium modulus than with the dynamic modulus. Moreover, the dynamic modulus showed a trend toward correlation with the nFCD at lower frequencies than that of higher frequencies. That might reflect the collagen network levels regenerated in the agarose gel. Nonetheless, the results of recent studies have shown that variations in collagen architecture among varieties of articular cartilage decreased the significance of correlations between Gd-DTPA^{2-}-enhanced MRI and mechanical properties, because the architecture of the collagen network, as well as PGs, plays an important role in the mechanicalproperties of articular cartilage (Nissi et al., 2007). In the present study, the chondrocytes in agarose gel reconstructed the immature collagen network, prompting a low-level effect on the compressive property compared to "native" articular cartilage; therefore, significant correlations might be found between Gd-DTPA^{2-}-enhanced MRI and compressive properties. From these facts, our evaluation methods using Gd-DTPA^{2-}-enhanced MRI could be applicable at the earlier stage of tissue regeneration.

3. Conclusion

In conclusion, we evaluated the changes in the quantitative MRI parameters and matrix FCD of tissue-engineered cartilage that consisted of articular chondrocytes and hydrogels. We found significant linear correlations between the quantitative MRI measurements and the biomechanical and biochemical properties of the engineered cartilage. Finally, we suggest that the quantitative MRI technique can be a useful, non-invasive approach to evaluate the biomechanical properties of regenerated cartilage during *in vitro* culturing process.

4. Acknowledgment

This research was supported in part by a Grant-in-Aid for Young Scientists (B) (No. 18700414) from the Ministry of Education, Science, Sports and Culture of Japan.

5. References

Bashir, A.; Gray, M. L. & Burstein, D. (1996). Gd-DTPA^{2-} as a Measure of Cartilage Degradation. *Magnetic Resonance Medicine*, Vol.36, pp.665-673

Bashir, A.; Gray, M.L.; Hartke, J. & Burstein, D. (1999). Nondestructive Imaging of Human Cartilage Glycosaminoglycan Concentration by MRI. *Magnetic Resonance in Medicine*, Vol.41, pp.857–865

Chen, C. T.; Fishbein, K.W.; Torzilli, P. A.; Hilger, A.; Spencer, R. G. & Horton, W. E., Jr. (2003). Matrix Fixed-Charge Density as Determined by Magnetic Resonance Microscopy of Bioreactor-Derived Hyaline Cartilage Correlates with Biochemical and Biomechanical Properties. *Arthritis and Rheumatism*, Vol.48, pp.1047-1056

Farndale, R. W.; Buttle, D. J. & Barrett, A. J. (1986). Improved Quantitation and Discrimination of Sulphated Glycosaminoglycans by Use of Dimethylmethylene Blue. *Biochimica et Biophysica Acta*, Vol.883, pp.173-177

Fragonas, E.; Mlynárik, V.; Jellús, V.; Micali, F.; Piras, A.; Toffanin, R.; Rizzo, R. & Vittur, F. (1998). Correlation between Biochemical Composition and Magnetic Resonance Appearance of Articular Cartilage. *Osteoarthritis and Cartilage*, Vol.6, pp.24–32

Korhonen, R.K.; Laasanen, M.S.; Töyräs, J.; Lappalainen, R.; Helminen, H.J. & Jurvelin, J.S. (2003). Fibril Reinforced Poroelastic Model Predicts Specifically Mechanical

Behavior of Normal, Proteoglycan Depleted and Collagen Degraded Articular Cartilage. *Journal of Biomechanics*, Vol.36, pp.1373–1379

Lee, R. C.; Frank, E. H.; Grodzinsky, A. J. & Roylance, D. K. (1981). Oscillatory Compressional Behavior of Articular Cartilage and Its Associated Electromechanical Properties. *Journal of Biomechanical Engineering*, Vol.103, pp. 280-292

Miyata, S.; Tateishi, T.; Furukawa, K. & Ushida, T. (2005). Influence of Structure and Composition on Dynamic Visco-Elastic Property of Cartilaginous Tissue: Criteria for Classification between Hyaline Cartilage and Fibrocartilage Based on Mechanical Function. *JSME International Journal: C*, Vol.48, pp.547–554

Miyata, S.; Homma, H.; Numano, T.; Furukawa, K; Tateishi, T. & Ushida, T. (2006). Assessment of Fixed Charge Density in Regenerated Cartilage by Gd-DTPA - Enhanced MR Imaging. *Magnetic Resonance and Medical Science*, Vol.5, No.2, pp. 73-78

Miyata, S.; Numano, T.; Homma, H.; Tateishi, T. & Ushida, T. (2007). Feasibility of Noninvasive Evaluation of Biophysical Properties of Tissue-Engineered Cartilage by Using Quantitative MRI. *Journal of Biomechnaics*, Vol.40, pp. 2990-2998

Miyata, S.; Homma, H.; Numano, T.; Tateishi, T. & Ushida, T. (2010). Evaluation of Negative Fixed-charge Density in Tissue-Engineered Cartilage by Quantitative MRI and Relationship with Biomechanical Properties. *Jounal of Biomechanical Engineering*, Vol.132, No.7, pp.071014

Mow, V.C.; Kuei, S. C.; Lai, W.M. & Armstrong, C.G. (1980). Biphasic Creep and Stress Relaxation of Articular Cartilage in Compression? Theory and Experiments. *Journal of Biomechanical Engineering*, Vol.102, pp.73-84

Nieminen, M.T.; Rieppo, J.; Toyras, J.; Hakumaki, J.M.; Silvennoinen, J.; Hyttinen, M.M.; Helminen, H.J. & Jurvelin, J.S. (2001). T2 Relaxation Reveals Spatial Collagen Architecture in Articular Cartilage: a Comparative Quantitative MRI and Polarized Light Microscopic Study. *Magnetic Resonance in Medicine*, Vol.46, pp.487-493

Nieminen, M.T.; Toyras, J.; Rieppo, J.; Hakumaki, J.M.; Silvennoinen, J.; Helminen, H.J. & Jurvelin, J.S. (2000). Quantitative MR Microscopy of Enzymatically Degraded Articular Cartilage. *Magnetic Resonance in Medicine*, Vol.43, pp.676-681.

Nissi, M.J.; Rieppo, J.; Töyräs, J.; Laasanen, M.S.; Kiviranta, I.; Nieminen, M.T. & Jurvelin, J.S. (2007). Estimation of Mechanical Properties of Articular Cartilage with MRI – dGEMRIC, T2 and T1 Imaging in Different Species with Variable Stages of Maturation. *Osteoarthritis and Cartilage*, Vol.15, pp.24–32

Potter, K.; Butler, J.J.; Adams, C.; Fishbein, K.W.; McFarland, E.W.; Horton, W.E. & Spencer, R.G. (1998). Cartilage Formation in a Hollow Fiber Bioreactor Studied by Proton Magnetic Resonance Microscopy. *Matrix Biology*, Vol.17, pp.513-523

Potter, K.; Butler, J.J.; Horton, W.E. & Spencer, R.G. (2000). Response of Engineered Cartilage Tissue to Biochemical Agents as Studied by Proton Magnetic Resonance Microscopy. *Arthritis and Rheumatism*, Vol.43, pp.1580-1590

Ramaswamy, S.; Uluer, M.C.; Leen, S.; Bajaj, P.; Fishbein, K.W. & Spencer, R.G. (2008). Noninvasive Assessment of Glycosaminoglycan Production in Injectable Tissue-Engineered Cartilage Constructs Using Magnetic Resonance Imaging. *Tissue Engineering Part C: Methods*, Vol.14, pp.243–249

Shapiro, E.M.; Borthakur, A.; Kaufman, J.H.; Leigh, J.S. & Reddy, R. (2001). Water Distribution Patterns Inside Bovine Articular Cartilage as Visualized by 1H Magnetic Resonance Imaging. *Osteoarthritis Cartilage*, Vol.9, pp.533-538

Xia, Y.; Moody, J.B. & Alhadlaq, H. (2002). Orientational Dependence of T2 Relaxation in Articular Cartilage: A Microscopic MRI (microMRI) Study. *Magnetic Resonance in Medicine*, Vol.48, pp.460-469

Permissions

The contributors of this book come from diverse backgrounds, making this book a truly international effort. This book will bring forth new frontiers with its revolutionizing research information and detailed analysis of the nascent developments around the world.

We would like to thank Prof. Jamie Davies, for lending his expertise to make the book truly unique. He has played a crucial role in the development of this book. Without his invaluable contribution this book wouldn't have been possible. He has made vital efforts to compile up to date information on the varied aspects of this subject to make this book a valuable addition to the collection of many professionals and students.

This book was conceptualized with the vision of imparting up-to-date information and advanced data in this field. To ensure the same, a matchless editorial board was set up. Every individual on the board went through rigorous rounds of assessment to prove their worth. After which they invested a large part of their time researching and compiling the most relevant data for our readers. Conferences and sessions were held from time to time between the editorial board and the contributing authors to present the data in the most comprehensible form. The editorial team has worked tirelessly to provide valuable and valid information to help people across the globe.

Every chapter published in this book has been scrutinized by our experts. Their significance has been extensively debated. The topics covered herein carry significant findings which will fuel the growth of the discipline. They may even be implemented as practical applications or may be referred to as a beginning point for another development. Chapters in this book were first published by InTech; hereby published with permission under the Creative Commons Attribution License or equivalent.

The editorial board has been involved in producing this book since its inception. They have spent rigorous hours researching and exploring the diverse topics which have resulted in the successful publishing of this book. They have passed on their knowledge of decades through this book. To expedite this challenging task, the publisher supported the team at every step. A small team of assistant editors was also appointed to further simplify the editing procedure and attain best results for the readers.

Our editorial team has been hand-picked from every corner of the world. Their multi-ethnicity adds dynamic inputs to the discussions which result in innovative outcomes. These outcomes are then further discussed with the researchers and contributors who give their valuable feedback and opinion regarding the same. The feedback is then collaborated with the researches and they are edited in a comprehensive manner to aid the understanding of the subject.

Apart from the editorial board, the designing team has also invested a significant amount of their time in understanding the subject and creating the most relevant covers. They scrutinized every image to scout for the most suitable representation of the subject and create an appropriate cover for the book.

The publishing team has been involved in this book since its early stages. They were actively engaged in every process, be it collecting the data, connecting with the contributors or procuring relevant information. The team has been an ardent support to the editorial, designing and production team. Their endless efforts to recruit the best for this project, has resulted in the accomplishment of this book. They are a veteran in the field of academics and their pool of knowledge is as vast as their experience in printing. Their expertise and guidance has proved useful at every step. Their uncompromising quality standards have made this book an exceptional effort. Their encouragement from time to time has been an inspiration for everyone.

The publisher and the editorial board hope that this book will prove to be a valuable piece of knowledge for researchers, students, practitioners and scholars across the globe.

List of Contributors

Marianna Karagianni, Torsten J. Schulze and Karen Bieback
Institute of Transfusion Medicine and Immunology; Medical Faculty Mannheim, Heidelberg University;
German Red Cross Blood Donor Service Baden-Württemberg – Hessen, Germany

Arnaldo Rodrigues Santos Jr.
Centro de Ciências Naturais e Humanas (CCNH), Universidade Federal do ABC, Santo André, SP, Brazil

Christiane Bertachini Lombello
Centro de Engenharia e Ciências Sociais Aplicadas (CECS), Universidade Federal do ABC, Santo André, SP, Brazil

Selma Candelária Genari
Centro Estadual de Educação Tecnológica Paula Souza, Faculdade de Tecnologia de Bauru (FATEC), Bauru, SP, Brazil

Dilaware Khan, Claudia Kleinfeld and Edda Tobiasch
University of Applied Sciences Bonn-Rhine-Sieg, Rheinbach

Martin Winter
Oralchirurgische Praxis, Rheinbach, Germany

Magdalena Cieslik
Faculty and Institute of Stomatological Materials Science, Medical University of Silesia, Katowice, Bytom, Poland

Jacek Nocoń
Private Dentistry Practice, Oberhausen, Germany

Jan Rauch
NZOZ – Specialist Dentistry Clinic, Wadowice, Poland

Tadeusz Cieslik
Faculty and Clinic of Oral and Maxillofacial Surgery, Medical University of Silesia, Katowice, Poland

Anna Ślósarczyk
Faculty of Glass Technology and Amorphous Coatings, AGH - Krakow University of Science and Technology, Kraków, Poland

Maria Borczuch-Łączka
Faculty of Ceramic Technology, AGH - Krakow University of Science and Technology, Kraków, Poland

Aleksander Owczarek
Division of Statistics, Medical University of Silesia, Katowice, Sosnowiec, Poland

Chao Feng and Yue-min Xu
Department of Urology, Shanghai Jiaotong University-Affiliated 6th People's Hospital, Shanghai, China

Peter J. Emans, Marjolein M.J. Caron, Lodewijk W. van Rhijn and Tim J.M. Welting
Department of Orthopaedic Surgery, Maastricht University Medical Center, The Netherlands

Abir El-Sadik
Anatomy and Embryology, Basic Sciences Department, King Saud Bin Abdulaziz University for Health Sciences, Riyadh, Kingdom of Saudi Arabia

Fred Vermolen and Olmer van Rijn
Delft Institute of Applied Mathematics, Delft University of Technology, The Netherlands

Shogo Miyata
KEIO University, Japan